READER'S DIGEST

THE BODY MAINTENANCE MANUAL

READER'S DIGEST

THE BODY MAINTENANCE MANUAL

A GUIDE TO FLEXIBILITY, FITNESS AND REPAIR

Dr Jenny Sutcliffe MCSP

Consultant: Rupert Eckersley FRCS

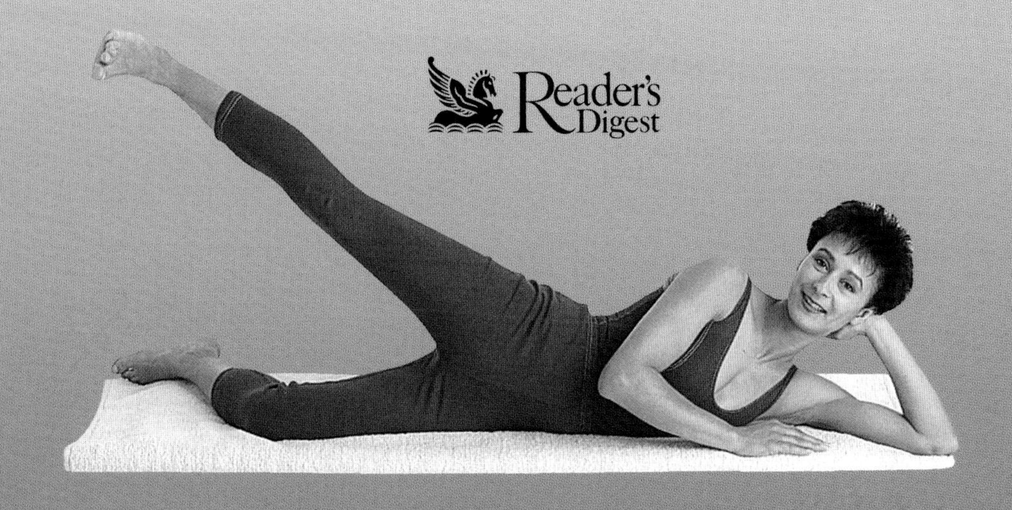

Reader's Digest

To Claire, my oldest friend, without whom my life would be poorer – and who may find this book useful sooner than she would wish.

PLEASE NOTE
This book is not intended as guidance for the diagnosis or treatment of serious health problems; please refer to a medical professional if you are in any doubt about any aspect of your condition. The author, packager and publisher cannot be held responsible for any injuries which may result from the use of information in this book.

A READER'S DIGEST BOOK

Published by The Reader's Digest Association Limited
11 Westferry Circus
Canary Wharf
London E14 4HE

ISBN 0 276 42428 X

A CIP data record for this book is available from the British Library

Edited, designed and produced by
Eddison Sadd Editions Limited
St Chad's House, 148 King's Cross Road
London WC1X 9DH

Phototypeset in Minion and Frutiger using QuarkXPress on Apple Macintosh
Origination by Pixel Graphics, Singapore
Printed by C & C Offset Printing Co. Ltd, Hong Kong

Contents

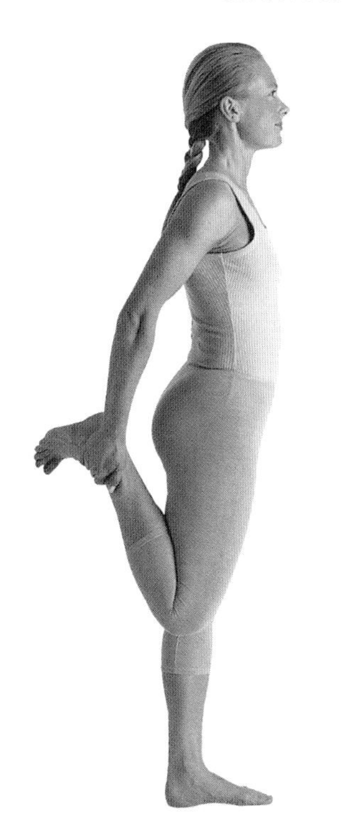

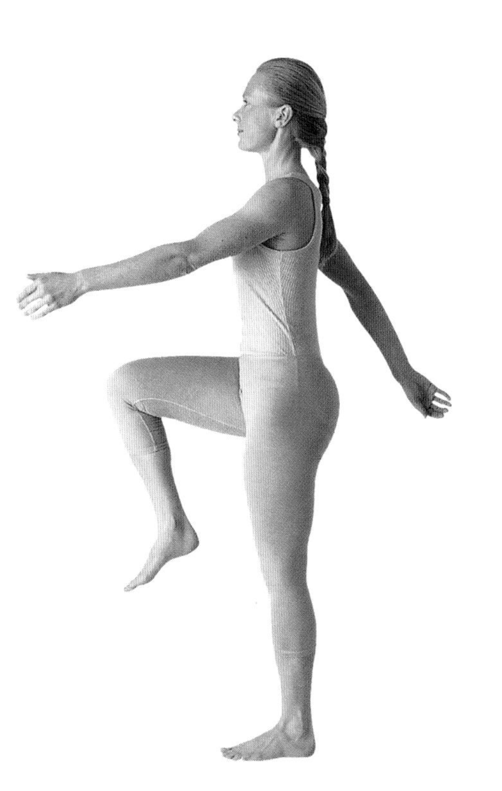

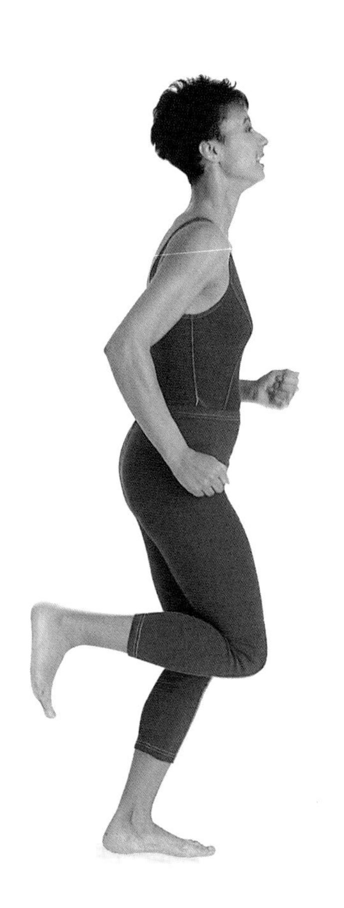

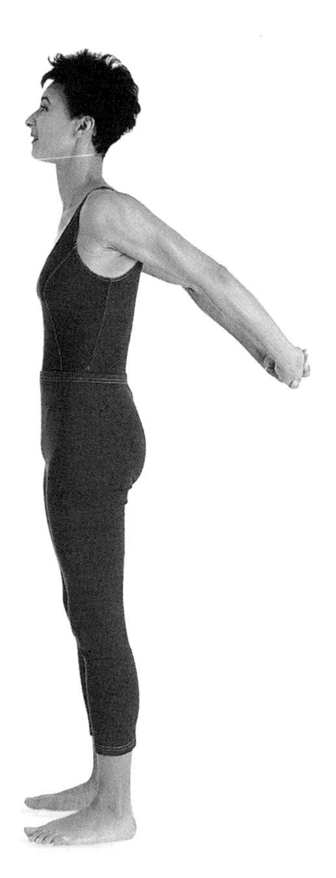

Foreword

There is no doubt that we should all be more active in looking after our bodies and keeping fit. This book is a huge step in that direction, with regard to maintaining a healthy musculo-skeletal system. In my own clinics, I see many patients who would benefit from this book and who could have avoided the need to see me by reading it – and I won't hesitate to recommend it to them.

As our lives get busier and busier – both at work and at play – the physical stresses and strains on our muscles and joints increase accordingly. To prevent us ending up as physical wrecks, we need to know how our bodies work, how to prevent damage and how to treat it when things go wrong.

Jenny Sutcliffe is to be congratulated on putting the complex anatomy and physiology of the musculo-skeletal system into words and diagrams that make it so simple to understand. This book will educate you on how the bones, joints and muscles function normally in your body and how to avoid aches and pains by taking preventative measures. Should you be unlucky enough to injure yourself, there is pertinent information about common musculo-skeletal problems, with advice on how to treat them and when to seek further attention. The book should be seen as a starting point in building up a knowledge of how to deal with common musculo-skeletal problems. The methods described here are not the only ones available and I would encourage readers to write in their own notes and comments about other therapies that they may have tried or heard about to build on Jenny Sutcliffe's simple, straightforward advice.

The aches and pains of everyday life can seem relatively minor in the context of major medical diseases, but they do cause significant difficulties to those who are suffering. And it is precisely these symptoms that cause more working days to be lost than any other medical problem. The modern healthcare system is under tremendous pressure to treat an ever-increasing number of patients with more expensive drugs, technology and surgery. This means that all health professionals are forever balancing this with the opposing need to contain costs. The treatment of musculo-skeletal problems is no exception, with the result that, too often, the simple everyday problems are overlooked. Here is a book to fill this need, and more besides – keep it to hand at all times!

Rupert Eckersley FRCS

Introduction

Once upon a time, I was quite a good tennis player and I loved playing the game. Unfortunately, that was longer ago than I would care to remember – and five children in the past! Nowadays I play just once a year, at my friend Claire's tennis tournament. I enjoy seeing my friends, but I don't enjoy the actual tennis very much these days, because it seems harder and harder to reach the ball each year, and it takes more and more time for me to recover afterwards.

The irritating thing is that I know exactly what I'm doing wrong – and it's almost everything. I shouldn't just charge on to the court without warming up, especially after 365 days of relative inactivity. And I certainly shouldn't expect my muscles and joints to put up with a lot of strain on one day in the year, when they have barely been put through their paces for the whole of the previous 12 months.

Nobody, of course, is sympathetic when I moan about my aches and pains, because I'm meant to know about these things – and I do. 'Physio heal thyself' is a polite version of what I hear around the house. I mutter excuses about work, children and housework, but excuses are all they are. It really is very easy to keep fit and flexible with a routine of exercises that are not even particularly demanding. And instead of relying on a hot bath and a glass of wine to soothe muscle strains and joint problems, it's really not too difficult to sort them out with remedial exercises.

After writing this book, however, everything is going to be different. I'd like to thank Sheila Watson, Nigel Perryman, Sophie Bevan and Elaine Partington, and everybody who has helped with it, and promise them that from now on I'm going to practise what I preach. And I've promised myself that next year I'm going to win the tennis tournament!

Jenny Sutcliffe

How to use this book

Modern life confronts the human body with challenges it has never faced before in its millions of years of evolution. We have more leisure time today than at any period in history, and much of it is spent in sporting or other types of physical activity – whether playing squash, jogging, gardening or simply taking a walk in the park. Yet the pressures of modern living make us uniquely unprepared to enjoy – or to endure – such activities without the risk of pain or even serious injury. This is because so much of our lives is spent in a sedentary position, staring at a computer screen, for example, or driving a car. And sedentary activities bring their own dangers, too, such as bad posture, cramped muscles and tension headaches.

This book is designed to show how you can respond to these challenges, prolong good health and enjoy physical activity to the full. It is divided into four sections. The first, 'Understanding your body', looks at the basic anatomy of the body: how muscle groups and joints work; and how posture, exercise, relaxation and diet combine to keep the body in good working order. Next comes 'What's the problem?', a section that examines different types of muscle and joint pain, looking at their causes and the anatomy behind them, and showing you how to avoid a range of common problems, from housemaid's knee to a frozen shoulder.

The third section, 'Self-help for aches and pains', shows you how to use a whole range of home physiotherapy aids, from ultrasound and massage devices to ice packs and wobble boards. Then, using flow charts, you can diagnose and treat aches and pains in muscles and joints throughout the body. Once a preliminary diagnosis has been made, you are either advised to seek professional help or prescribed short-term treatment and long-term remedial exercises. But prevention, as the saying goes, is better than cure, so 'Keeping up the good work', the fourth section, sets you a practical course in body maintenance, prescribing exercises for each major muscle group and joint – not forgetting the all-important warming-up and warming-down routines. And you will find out how to tailor a ten-minute daily maintenance programme to your own lifestyle, age and special requirements.

The aim of this book is to help you live life to the full, and it's not possible to do that if you have injured or strained yourself as a result of overdoing things. So look out for the safety watchpoints to ensure that exercises are the right ones for you, taking into account your age and level of fitness and suppleness. Keep an eye out, too, for medical alerts. These point out any potential hazards or conditions that may require medical help. It is always sensible to consult your doctor before embarking on any new exercise regime.

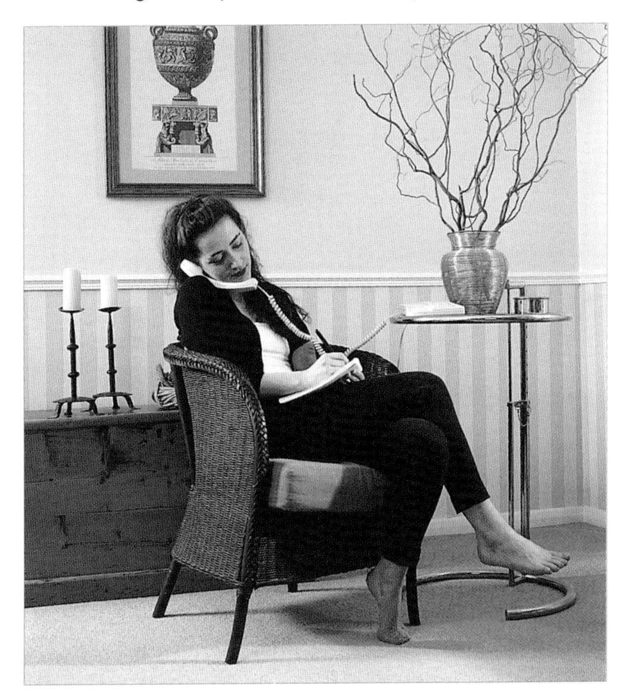

Unnecessary strain
Children have naturally good posture (top), but we all develop bad habits (above) that strain our muscles and joints.

SECTION ONE

UNDERSTANDING YOUR BODY

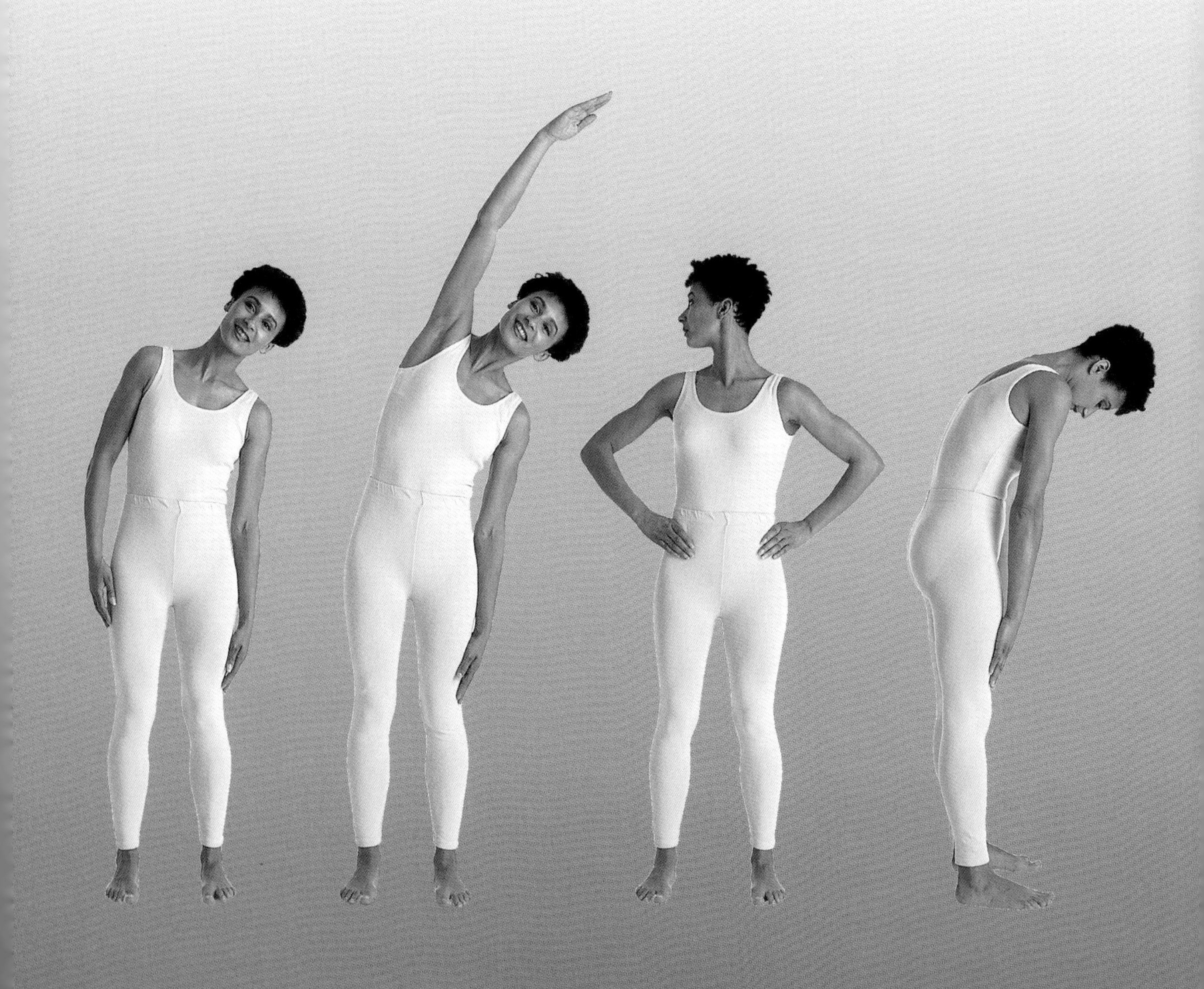

The human body is made up of 11 systems – skeletal, muscular, nervous, cardiovascular, lymphatic, respiratory, digestive, urinary, reproductive, endocrine and the skin – and all these must interact harmoniously if the body is to work with maximum efficiency in good health. So while this book is primarily concerned with the muscles and the skeleton, it is vital to remember that the rest of the body plays its part in ensuring that the musculo-skeletal system works correctly. And this means that exercise, diet and stress management also play a part in the smooth running of the system.

It is easy to think of the skeleton as something rigid and dead: a mass of bone and sinew that has no life, but is just moved around by the muscles. In fact, the ends of the bones are made up of living cells which constantly renew themselves, and the skeleton has a number of functions quite apart from giving the body a framework: it protects the internal organs and the brain, and is a storehouse of minerals, such as calcium and phosphorus, and of the marrow that manufactures red blood cells. Nevertheless, the skeleton forms a marionette-like complex of bones, joints and ligaments that are moved by strings (the muscles and tendons) and precisely controlled by a guiding hand (the nervous system).

This section of the book tells you how the muscles and joints work to move the body. It explains joint design, describes the range of movements possible at each joint, and reveals how joints, muscles and other body systems interact to control posture and movement. Finally, it shows how exercise – or the lack of it – diet and stress impact on the efficient working of the system as a whole.

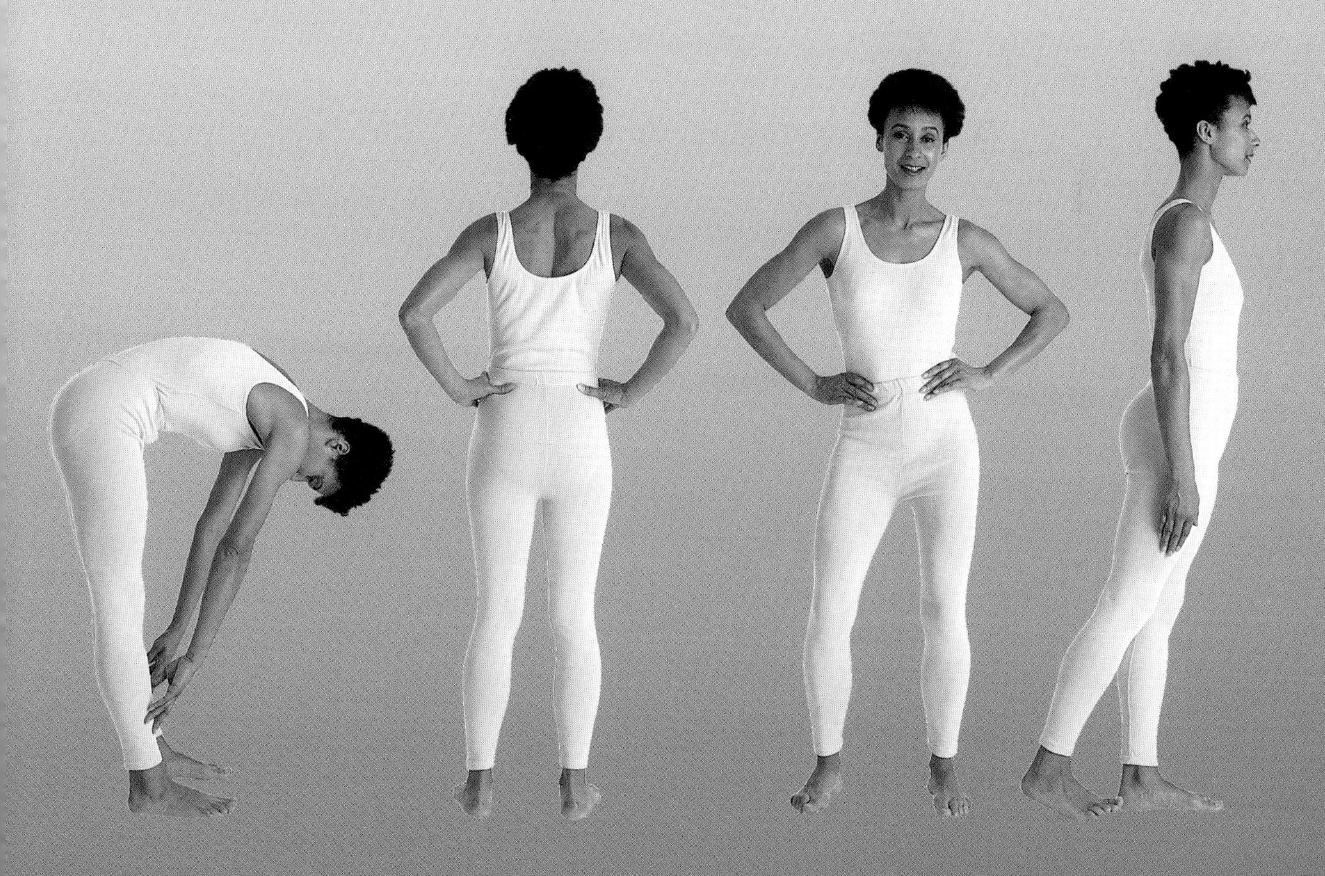

BODY BASICS The musculo-skeletal system

Many millions of years have passed since the ancestors of humankind first became distinguishable from the apes. And during this time, the structure of the body has changed, infinitesimally slowly, but surely, into the one that we now occupy. Today the musculo-skeletal system – the body's building block – is, in overall terms, a triumph of design. Form is fitted to function to create a robust, yet complex, series of checks, balances and opposing, yet complementary, forces.

Despite this, the evolutionary process has not been without its compromises. There are a number of weak points or 'design faults' in the body – such as the shoulder joint and the lower back – that will be discussed in detail later in the book. It is worth remembering, too, that for almost the entire period of human evolution people have not sat for much of the day in front of computer screens or steering wheels. And until recently few people lived sufficiently long to have to cope with the effects of wear and tear on the body.

The next few pages provide a brief outline of the movements the musculo-skeletal system is designed to make possible, and the movements that are not possible without causing damage. For when too much strain is put on one part of the body – if, for example, a movement is attempted that a joint does not allow, or an unnatural strain on one part of the body causes a damaging counter-action in another part – the tissues are likely to be damaged. Repairing them is possible, but it takes time and effort, so prevention is always better than cure.

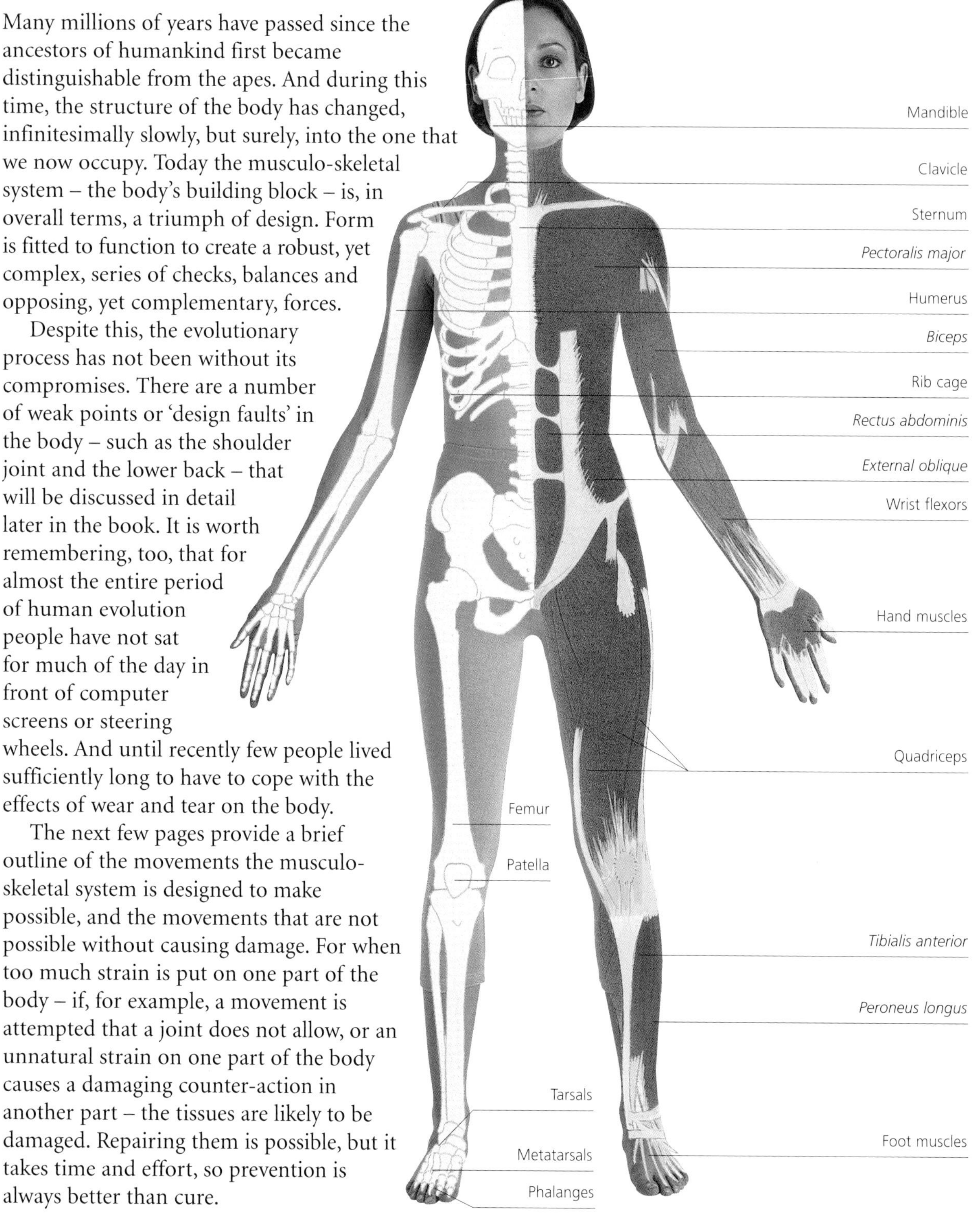

Fitting the pieces together

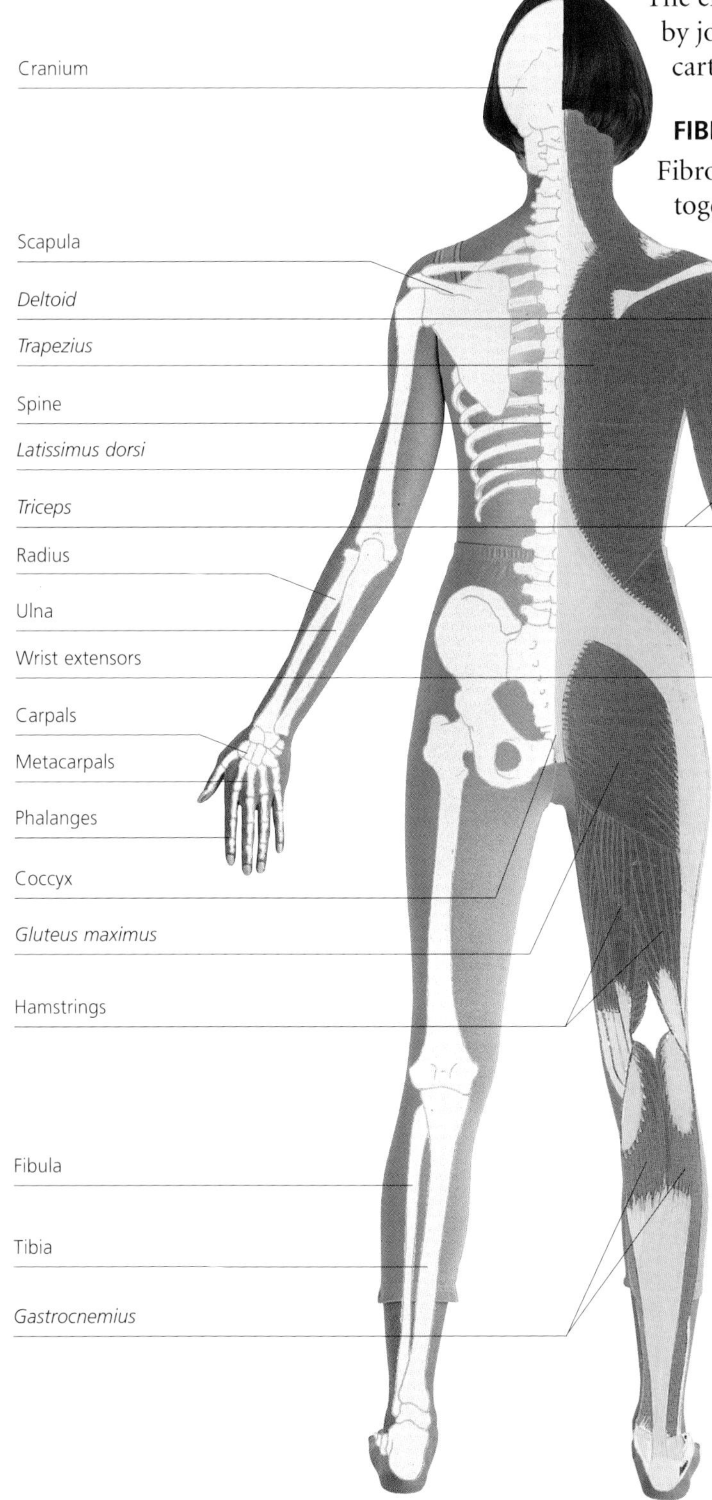

The elements of the skeleton are linked together by joints. There are three main types: fibrous, cartilaginous and synovial joints.

FIBROUS JOINTS

Fibrous joints knit the bones of the skull together. The bones fit tightly to each other and have fibrous tissue between them so that no movement is possible.

CARTILAGINOUS JOINTS

Cartilaginous joints are found only between the vertebrae of the spine and in the joint at the front of the pelvis (the pubic symphysis) that expands during childbirth to allow the baby to pass through the birth canal. In such joints, the bones are connected by a disc of fibrocartilage and there is no joint cavity. This arrangement enables a small amount of movement at each joint, but our ability to bend comes from the fact that in the spine a large number of cartilaginous joints are piled up, one on top of the other.

SYNOVIAL JOINTS

The vast majority of joints in the body are synovial joints. In these joints the articular surfaces of the bones are covered with friction-reducing cartilage. The joint is contained within a fibrous capsule that is lined on its inner side with a membrane and full of lubricating, shock-absorbing fluid. This is strengthened by ligaments that run between the bones. Synovial joints, their make up and the different forms they can take, are discussed in more detail over the next few pages.

Joints and movement

Synovial joints are divided into several different types, depending on their structure and so the range of movements that they allow. The degree of movement possible in a specific joint depends on various factors: the shape of the articulating surfaces; the amount of tension in the ligaments, joint capsule, muscles and tendons; and the age of an individual, since tissues tighten up with age.

Here I'm going to take a brief look at a typical synovial joint, the various types of synovial joint and the movements they allow. Later I will describe individual joints in more detail.

A SIMPLE SYNOVIAL JOINT

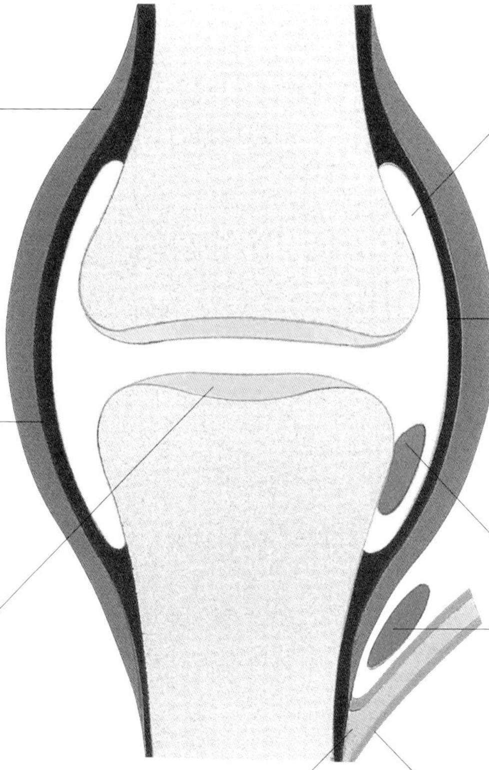

Ligament
A strong band of fibrous tissue that runs from one bone, or part of a bone, to another, to protect and reinforce a joint. Ligaments may also form part of the joint capsule (see below) surrounding a joint.

Joint capsule
A sealed layer of fibrous tissue that surrounds the area at which two bones meet, or 'articulate', in synovial joints.

Cartilage
There are three types of cartilage in the body: hyaline, elastic, and fibrocartilage. Hyaline cartilage, or gristle, (shown here) is hard, clear and tough, yet springy. It lines the articulating surfaces of joints and is one of the most friction-free substances known to science. Elastic cartilage is found in the ear and nose, and fibrocartilage forms the intervertebral discs in the spine and the cartilages in the knee.

Tendon
Also called a 'sinew', this is a fibrous cord that attaches a muscle to the bone (or the outer covering of the bone, known as the periosteum). The cord moves the bone when the muscle contracts. Often, tendons are encased in a sheath that helps them glide smoothly over other tendons and bones.

Synovial fluid
This fills the interior of the joint capsule, acting as a shock absorber and lubricating the movement of the joint. It has the thickness of motor oil, but looks like egg white.

Synovial membrane
The inner lining of a joint capsule in a synovial joint. It secretes synovial fluid, reabsorbs any excess fluid, and disposes of foreign bodies, such as bacteria, and dead red blood cells.

Bursa
A hollow area in fibrous tissue, lined with synovial membrane and containing synovial fluid, that reduces friction between tendons and bones. Sometimes a bursa is connected to a joint capsule.

Synovial sheath
A sleeve of tissue, lined on its inner side with synovial membrane and containing synovial fluid, which envelops some of the tendons of the hands and feet to ease movement.

Hinge joints

In the same way that a door hinge only allows movement in one plane, only one plane of movement – flexion and extension – is allowed by the hinge joints of the body. The main hinge joints are at the knee, ankle and elbow, and between the bones of the toes and fingers (this last group are called 'interphalangeal joints'). They are all synovial joints, and most of them are protected by strong ligaments designed to prevent any sideways movement. If too much sideways force is exerted on a hinge joint – as happens when you sprain your ankle, for example – the ligaments and joint capsule will give way, causing considerable pain and damage to the tissues.

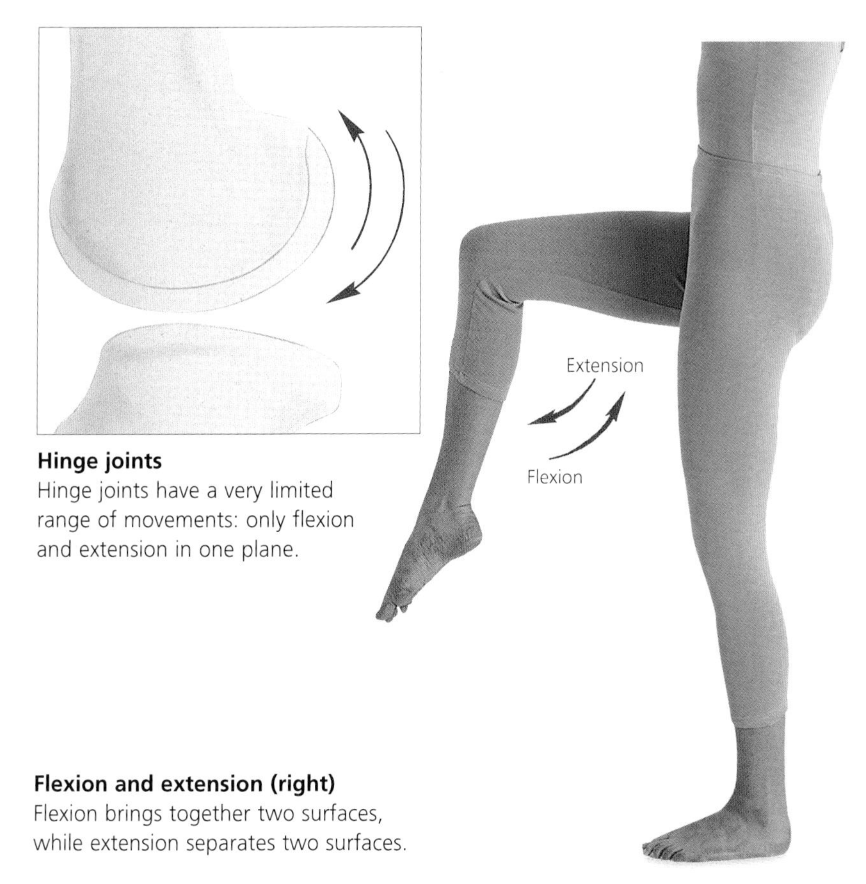

Hinge joints
Hinge joints have a very limited range of movements: only flexion and extension in one plane.

Flexion and extension (right)
Flexion brings together two surfaces, while extension separates two surfaces.

Pivot joints

There are two types of pivot joint: in the first, a pivot turns within a containing ring; in the second it is the ring that turns around the pivot. Both types allow rotation in one plane.

The joints in the elbow and wrist between the radius and ulna are pivot joints of the first type. The ulna and a ligament form the ring and the radius is the pivot that turns within it.

The other pivot joint in the body is of the second type. The ring (an arch and ligament of the atlas, the top vertebra in the neck) rotates around the pivot (part of the axis, the vertebra below it).

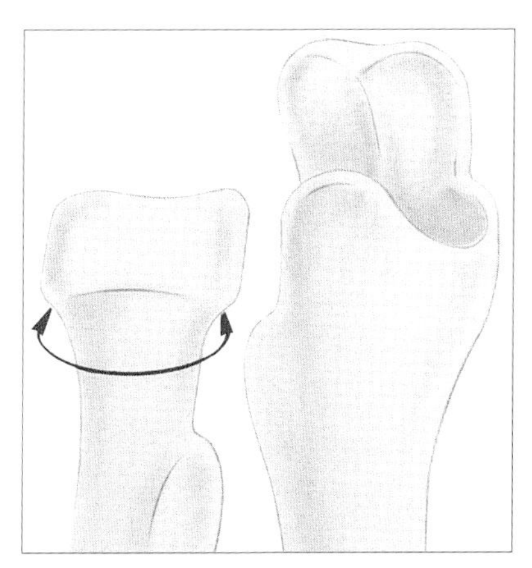

Pivot joints
At the elbow, the radius (left) pivots in the notch of the ulna (right).

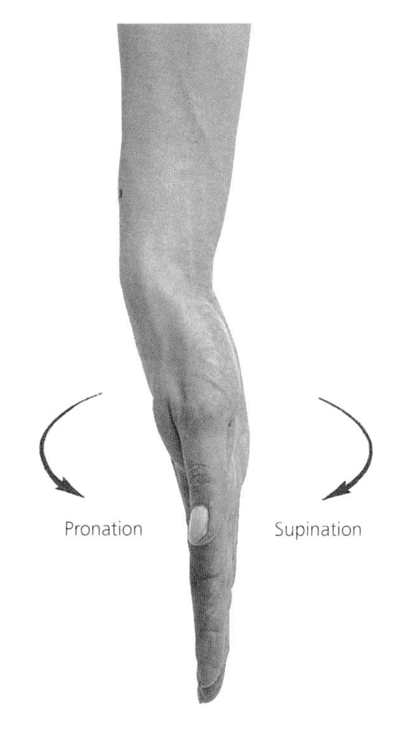

Supination and pronation (right)
The pivot joints in the elbow and wrist allow the forearm, and so the hand, to rotate. Outward rotation is known as supination; inward rotation is pronation.

Ball and socket joints

As the name suggests, a ball and socket joint is an articulation between two bones in which the ball-like head of one bone fits into a concave socket on another. This arrangement allows a considerable range of movement and is ideal for the shoulder and hip joints, which enable movement of the limbs. Ball and socket joints are synovial: that is, they are covered in a sealed capsule full of lubricating, pressure-absorbing synovial fluid and protected and stabilised by ligaments. The groups of short muscles that surround each joint are also important as stabilisers: these are the phasic muscles (see page 23) that are designed to hold the joints in their correct positions.

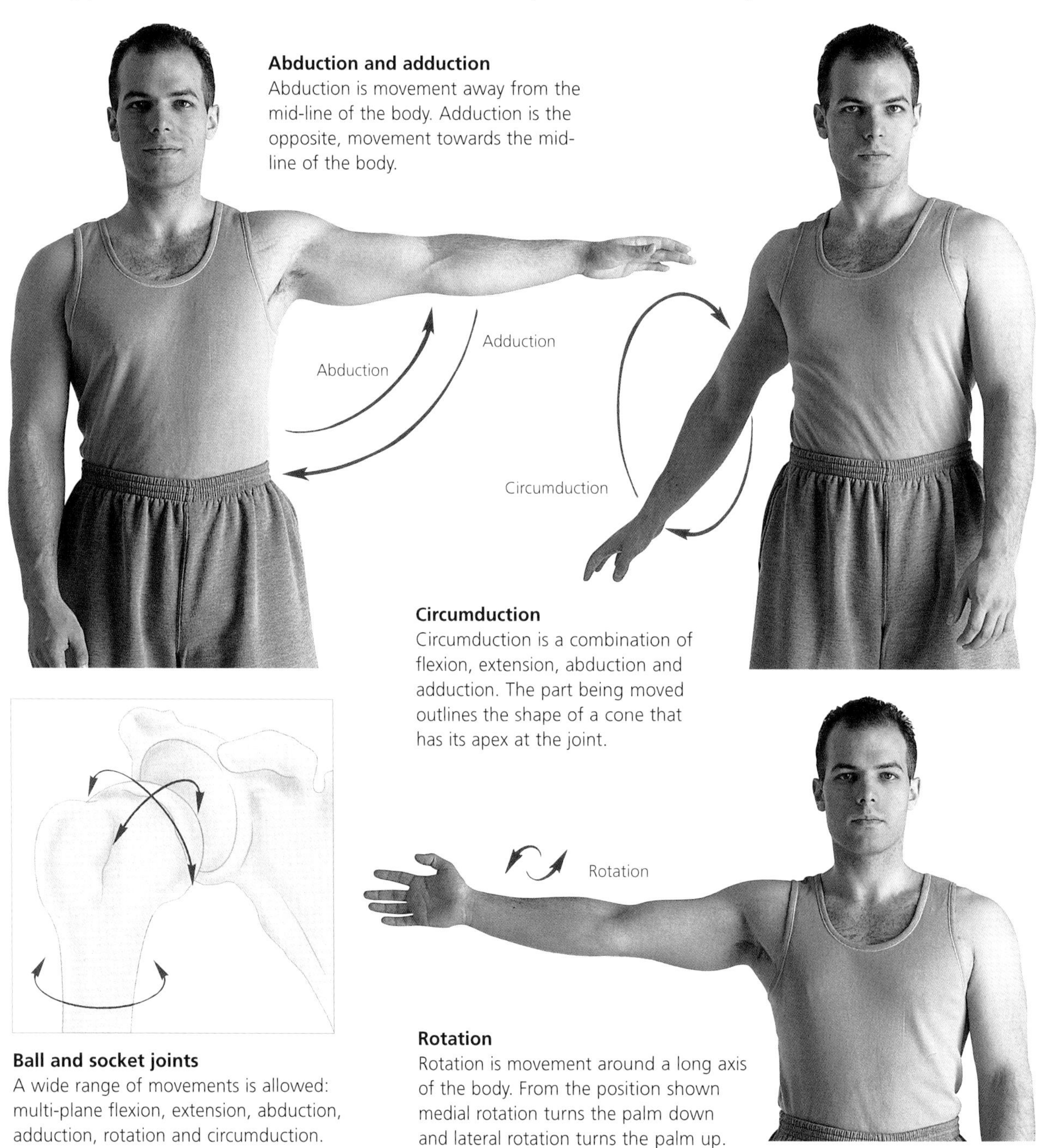

Abduction and adduction
Abduction is movement away from the mid-line of the body. Adduction is the opposite, movement towards the mid-line of the body.

Circumduction
Circumduction is a combination of flexion, extension, abduction and adduction. The part being moved outlines the shape of a cone that has its apex at the joint.

Ball and socket joints
A wide range of movements is allowed: multi-plane flexion, extension, abduction, adduction, rotation and circumduction.

Rotation
Rotation is movement around a long axis of the body. From the position shown medial rotation turns the palm down and lateral rotation turns the palm up.

Other types of joint in the body

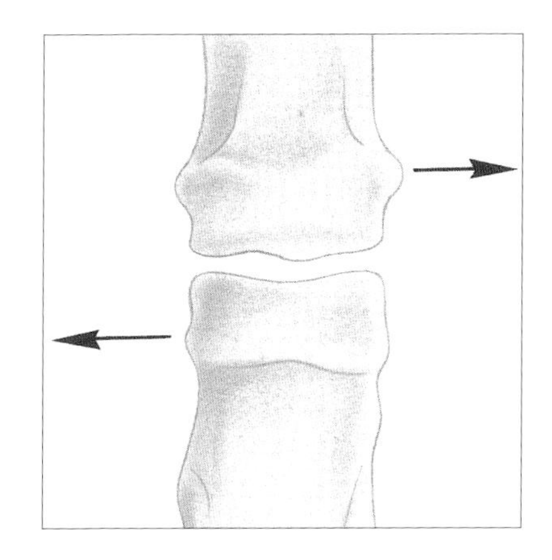

PLANE JOINTS

Plane joints (right) allow limited gliding movements in many different directions, as one bone slides over the other. They are found between the small carpal and tarsal bones of the hands and feet.

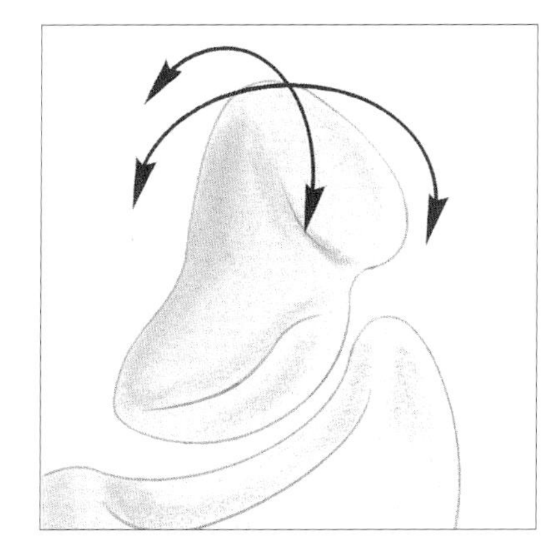

ELLIPSOID JOINTS

Ellipsoid joints (left) are found in the wrist, where the convex surfaces of the radius and ulna meet the concave surfaces of carpal bones, allowing flexion, extension, abduction, adduction and circumduction in two planes.

SADDLE JOINTS

A saddle joint (right) occurs in each thumb, allowing the wide range of movement available in the thumbs: multi-plane flexion, extension, abduction, adduction, rotation and circumduction.

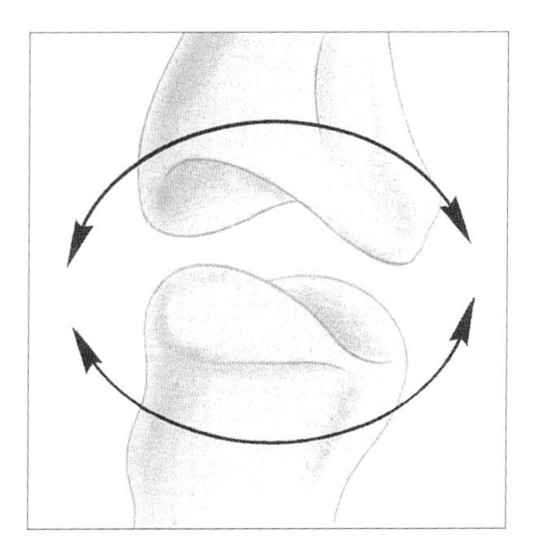

TYPES OF MOVEMENT THAT JOINTS ALLOW

You will find the vocabulary introduced here to describe individual movements useful when you want to work out what specific muscles do. This is because many muscles include the medical description of their activity in their name: *extensor digitorum*, for example, extends the finger.

Flexion bends a joint, reducing its angle, to bring the surfaces of the two bones closer together.

Extension increases the angle of a joint, increasing the distance between the surfaces of the bones.

Abduction moves a bone or limb away from the mid-line of the body or, in the case of extremities, away from the axis of a limb.

Adduction moves a bone or limb towards the mid-line of the body or towards the axis of a limb.

Rotation moves a body part along its axis (medial rotation is towards the body; lateral rotation is away from it).

Circumduction is all the above movements combined (with the exception of rotation).

Supination turns the palm of the hand up.

Pronation turns the palm of the hand down.

Inversion turns the sole of the foot inwards.

Eversion turns the sole of the foot outwards.

Elevation lifts the shoulder girdle and jaw.

How muscles cause movement

Muscles – the flesh of the body – have three functions: they contract and relax to make bones move through joints; they maintain posture; and their activity produces body heat.

A muscle contracts when triggered to do so by an impulse from the nerve that supplies it. 'Impulse' here is a shorthand for a complex interaction of chemical reactions that create and transmit an electrical signal.

Each muscle is made up of bundles of fibres, and each fibre consists of two types of filament: thicker myofilaments, made of one type of protein; and thinner myofilaments made of another. The thin myofilaments are anchored at the end of each cell, while the thicker myofilaments float unanchored, interleaved with the thinner ones. When a muscle is relaxed, there is some distance between the thin myofilaments anchored to the two opposing sides of the cell; when a nerve impulse is received, the two types of filament – and the two types of protein – slide in on each other, decreasing the length of the cell and so making the muscle contract.

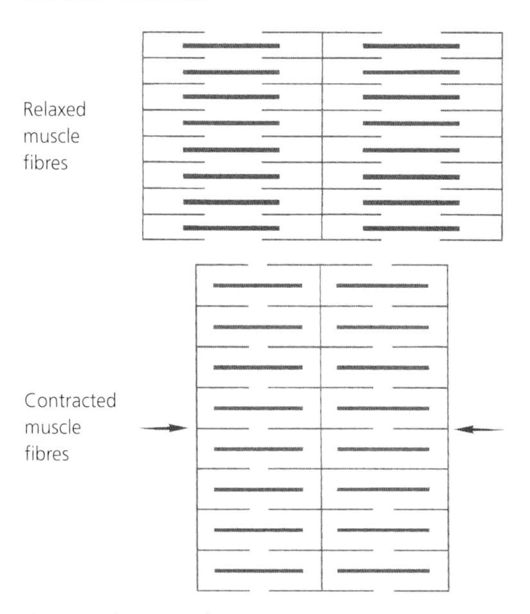

Contracting muscles
When a muscle contracts, the myofilaments in each cell of its fibres slide over each other to make it shorter and fatter.

Fast and slow twitch

The arrangement of bundles of fibres within an individual muscle depends on what function that muscle has. For example, *trapezius*, a muscle on the back that twists the body, has its fibres arranged in spirals; while in *deltoid*, a short, powerful muscle in the shoulder, the bundles are arranged in a pattern similar to that of the feathers on a bird's wing.

There are also two different types of fibre. Red, slow-twitch fibres contract slowly but repeatedly, sustaining tension over a period. These are predominant in muscles used over long periods – for example, to maintain posture (see pages 20–23) and during aerobic exercise (see pages 28–29). White, fast-twitch fibres, on the other hand, are predominant in muscles that contract rapidly and are used intermittently, in short bursts. Muscles driven by anaerobic exercise (see pages 28–29), which are used for sprints, fast movements or playing squash, are typical examples of these.

Human muscles contain both types of fibre in varying proportions, but this is not the case with all animals. The fibres of a chicken's muscle, for example, are much more differentiated: the dark meat of the leg muscles contrasts with the white meat of the breast – the legs are used all day, to maintain posture and to move, while the breast muscles are used intermittently to flap the wings.

Opposite actions

In terms of simple physics, a bone acts as a lever, a joint acts as the fulcrum between two or more bones, and a muscle pulls the lever to move the bone through the fulcrum. Unfortunately, however, human biomechanics are not quite as simple as that.

In order to move a bone, a muscle – known as the 'agonist' – must contract. But for every muscle that contracts there is a muscle that opposes the action. This is the 'antagonist'. So, for example, in order for *biceps* – the agonist – to raise the forearm towards the shoulder, *triceps* – the antagonist –

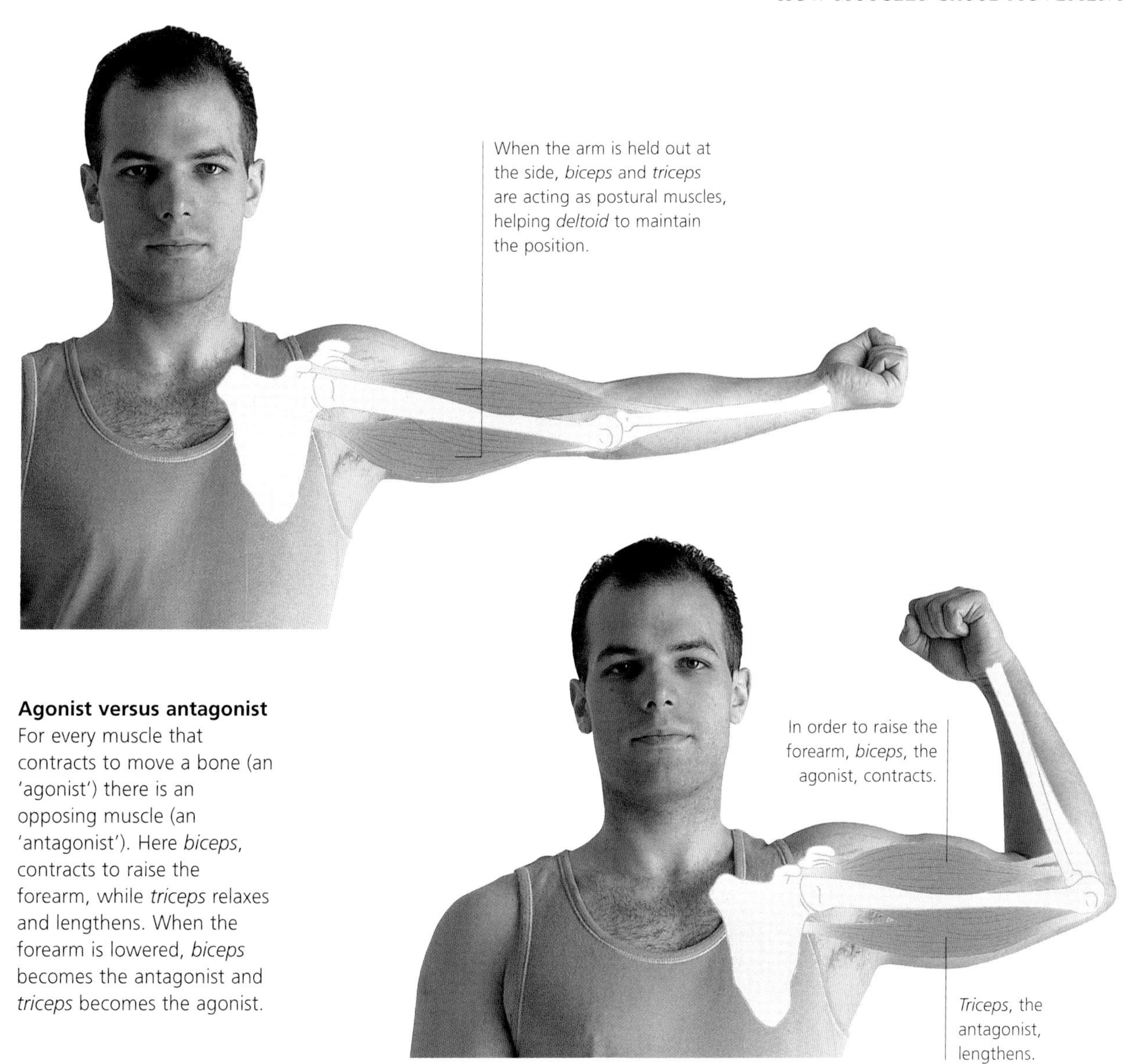

Agonist versus antagonist
For every muscle that contracts to move a bone (an 'agonist') there is an opposing muscle (an 'antagonist'). Here *biceps*, contracts to raise the forearm, while *triceps* relaxes and lengthens. When the forearm is lowered, *biceps* becomes the antagonist and *triceps* becomes the agonist.

must relax and lengthen; when the forearm is lowered, the process is reversed. The antagonist must relax rather than just do nothing, because at any one time both *triceps* and *biceps* are in a state of tension to greater or lesser degree in order to maintain the position of the forearm at the elbow joint. So, unless your arm is hanging loosely by your side, your *biceps* and *triceps* are acting as postural muscles (see page 23), even when they seem to be doing nothing.

But it is not just *biceps* and *triceps* that are involved when you raise your forearm, because the fulcrum must be held in the required position while the lever – the forearm – is moving. This means that the upper arm, into which the muscle that is pulling the lever attaches, must be kept still. This is done by the short muscles around the shoulder joint, which act as 'fixators' to the bone. Other small muscles, called 'synergists', improve the precision and accuracy of the movement. They ensure, for example, that if you raise your forearm to touch your nose, your finger will not miss it.

This complex system needs precise, coordinated control, and it is supplied by the nervous system and brain. But alcohol and some medicines can disrupt this control and so reduce coordination of the synergists – which is why a person who has drunk too much alcohol will miss his or her nose.

POSTURE Perfect posture

We are all familiar with the clichéd image of a soldier standing to attention: eyes front, shoulders back, stomach and backside in. But does it demonstrate good posture?

The answer to that question is 'No'. A guardsman standing to attention may look smart, and the various parts of his body are certainly in their correct positions. But his body is rigid and taut. And that breaks one of the prime rules of good posture: your body must always be loose and flexible, held in what is called a 'neutral' position.

Good posture means holding your body in such a way that pressures over joints are even and natural, and muscles are loose, not stretched or tensed. Anything else causes muscle tension and, in the long-term, muscle damage, and puts strain on the joints.

On these two pages we look at what good posture really means with a series of photographs and diagrams. On the next two pages you will find some common examples of bad posture and the damage it can do.

Your head should be in the same plane as your pelvis, neither jutting forwards nor back; a vertical line drawn through the crown of your head should pass through the middle of your pelvis.

Your shoulders should be back, but not rigidly so, like those of a guardsman on parade. They should also be level with each other and relaxed downwards, with no suggestion of hunching or rounding forwards.

Your bottom should be tucked in, so that the lower spine can follow its natural curve. Don't exaggerate this, though, so that you look like a cat-walk model – doing so puts strain on the lower spine.

Your knees should be straight, but not braced back rigidly.

Your weight should be distributed evenly over toes and heels. This can be difficult if you wear badly fitting or high-heeled shoes.

Benefits of good posture

By maintaining a good posture as described above you can:

- Reduce both physical and emotional tension and stress
- Lower the chances of suffering from headaches, neck pain, backaches and arm pain
- Make movements more precise and less stressful on muscles and joints
- Allow greater efficiency of breathing mechanisms, so increasing intake of oxygen and, therefore, boosting energy levels
- Give a positive, confident impression to others

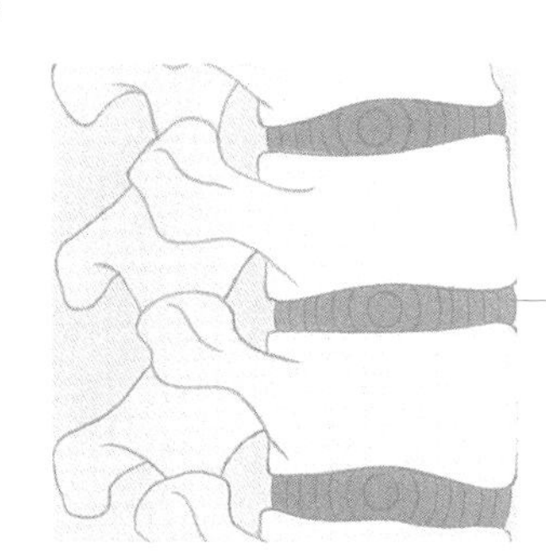

Even pressure

Your spine should be straight, in both planes. This evens out the pressure on the intervertebral discs. Any distortion to the spine increases the pressure on individual areas as well as stretching ligaments and making muscles either tense or stretch.

HOLD YOUR HEAD UP

The position of the head and neck provides the key to good posture. If your head is in the correct position, your shoulders tend to fall into place naturally and there is a feeling of balance and harmony. If your head is not in the correct position, the muscles of the neck and upper back have to stretch and tense constantly in an attempt to adapt to the position, and the result can be neck pain and headaches. You probably move your head more than any other part of your body, as you look at things and talk to people, so it's essential that you learn good habits and stick to them, even while your head is moving.

Such habits don't come easily, especially if you spend a lot of your time seated, staring at a fixed point – looking at a computer screen, for example, or keeping an eye on traffic while driving. It's all too easy to let your head sag and your neck twist. The only way to change your habits is to focus on the points listed to the right, and continue doing so until a correct head position becomes automatic.

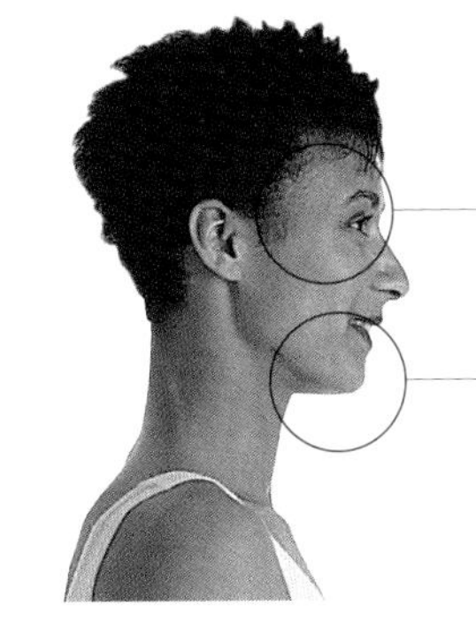

You should be looking straight ahead – neither up nor down.

Your chin should be in a straight, neutral position, not sticking up or tucked in.

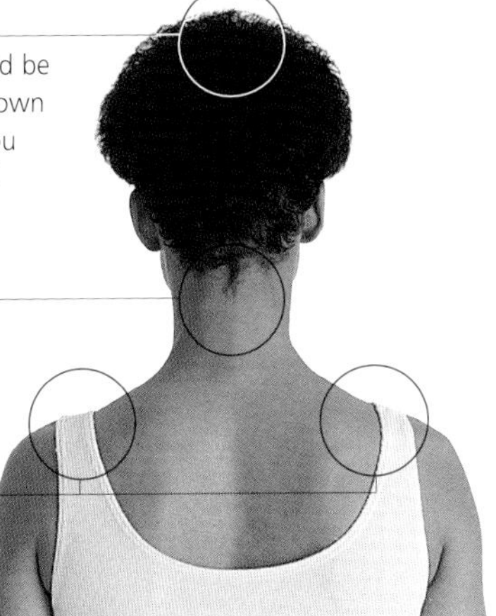

The crown of your head should be its highest point. Push your crown towards the ceiling, so that you elongate your neck, but avoid any tension.

Your neck should be straight – neither tilted to one side nor the other.

Your shoulders should be back and down, not hunched or rigid.

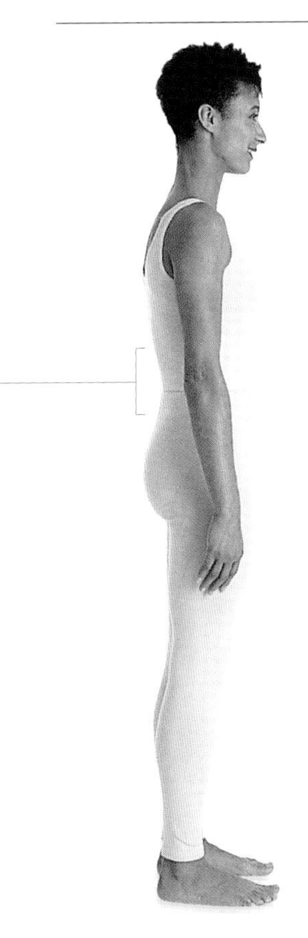

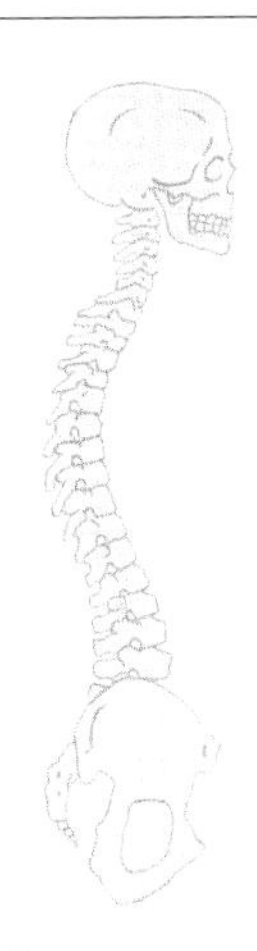

Natural curves
The spine has two natural curves to help absorb shock: one in the neck and one in the lower back. The aim of good posture is to maintain these natural curves, so that no more than the usual muscle tone is needed to keep the vertebrae in place and undue pressure is not put on joints and ligaments.

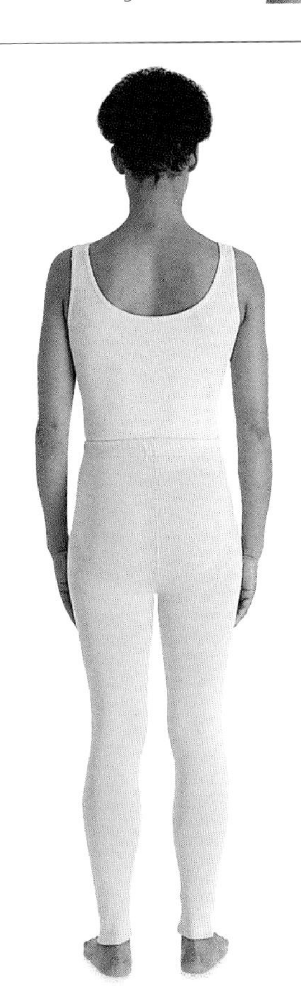

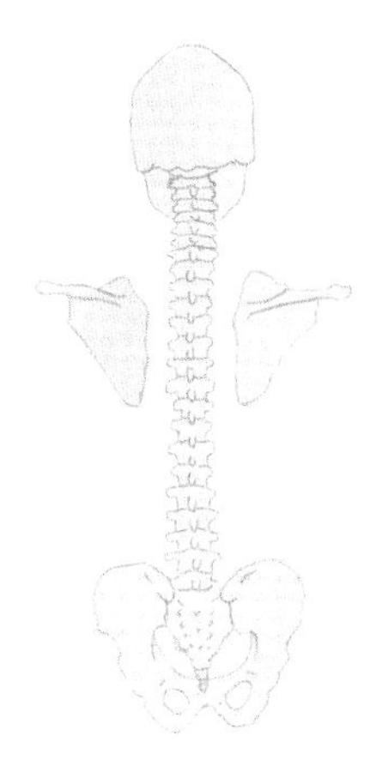

Body balance
Any variation of the spine from the vertical can cause great strain on joints and muscles. So make sure your body is balanced vertically: your shoulders and hips should be level, with your arms hanging loosely by your sides and your head balancing comfortably on your neck.

Check your posture

Strip down to your underclothes and stand in front of a long mirror. If you have long hair, pile it on top of your head so that you can see your shoulders and ear lobes. First of all, try to put your head in the correct position, as described on the previous page. Then ask yourself the following questions. (It is a good idea to ask a friend to help – it is all too easy to deceive yourself!)

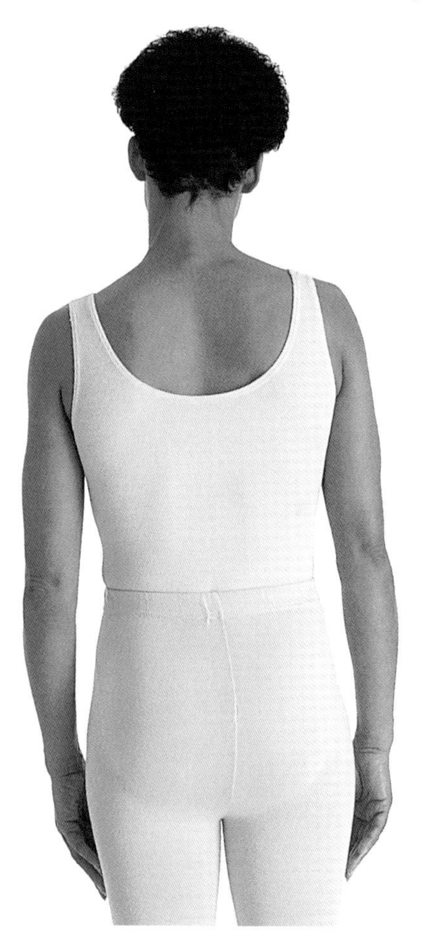

Is your head tilted or are your shoulders crooked?

If so (see left), your *trapezius* muscle will be too tight on one side and too stretched on the other. This may be a sign of scoliosis (see also kyphosis, page 49), a lateral curvature of the upper spine that strains all the muscles of the upper back. In some cases, a degree of scoliosis is inborn, but more often it is caused by poor posture, in which case it will disappear if you bend forwards. (See self-help exercises, pages 82–85.)

Are your shoulders hunched up and tense?

If so (see left), your neck muscles will almost certainly be tense as well, causing strain on the cervical spine and shoulder joints, and giving rise to tension headaches. (See self-help exercises, pages 78–79.)

Are your shoulders rounded and does your chest curve in?

If so (see right), you will notice that the palms of your hands face too far back. Your pectoral muscles will be too tight and your upper back muscles will be over-stretched. In women, breasts will sag. This imbalance can impair breathing efficiency, and so lower the amount of oxygen inhaled and carbon dioxide exhaled. (See self-help exercises, pages 82–85).

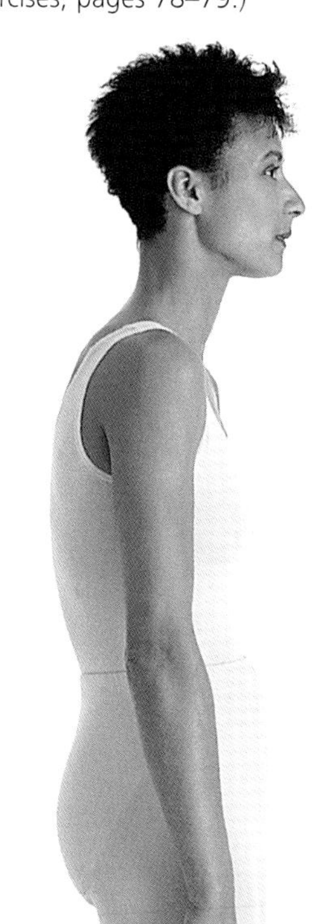

Are the tips of your hip bones crooked and pointing too far forwards or backwards?

If so, you may have a scoliosis of the spine. If the tips of your hip bones are too far forward (see above), you probably have a lordosis – an accentuated curve of your lumbar spine – that causes your back muscles to tighten, your abdominal muscles to become weaker and your bottom to stick out. If the tips are too far back (see left) you may suffer from the opposite problem, and have a flat back and, in some cases, a protruding stomach. Both these problems affect the way in which weight is transferred by the lumbar spine and put strain on the intervertebral joints, so causing low back pain. (See self-help exercises, pages 82–85.)

Are your kneecaps pointing outwards or inwards?

Your knees should be level and the kneecaps pointing forwards. If they point outwards (see far right) you may well suffer from bow-legs (genu varum); if inwards (see right), you may have knock knees (genu valgum). Both problems can affect the way in which weight is transferred down the leg and cause problems at the arches of the feet. (See self-help exercises, pages 110–11.)

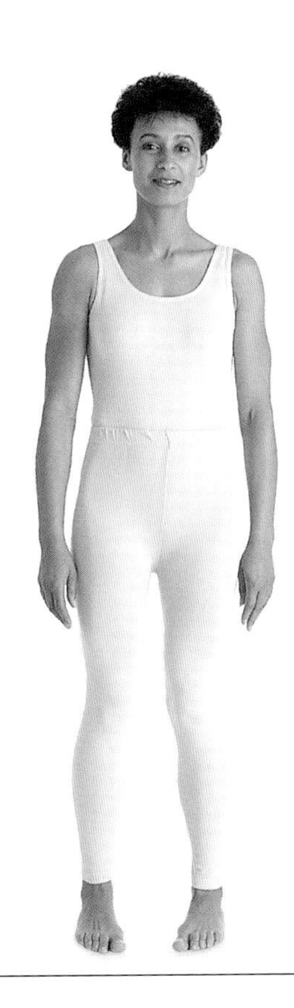

Do your feet point outwards or inwards?

People whose feet point out from the mid-line (see right) often suffer from a fallen medial arch, or flat feet. But foot problems are likely to be the result whether your feet point either inwards or outwards, because weight is no longer distributed efficiently through the foot when walking. (See self-help exercises, pages 110–11.)

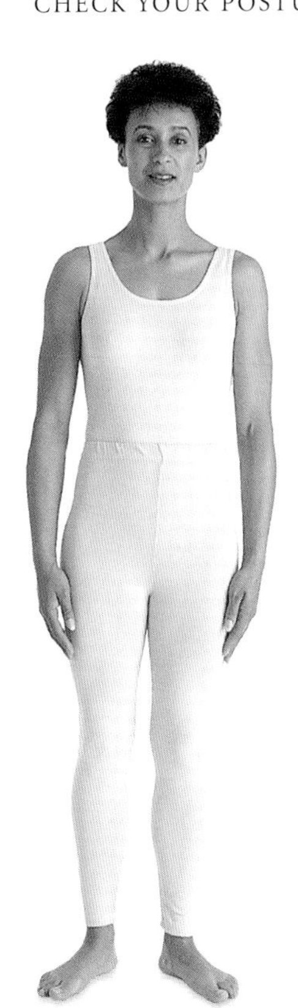

Why posture matters

As I've said, the key to good posture is that pressure over joints is even and natural and that muscles are loose, not tense or stretched. This is because there are two types of muscle: phasic and postural. Phasic muscles contain a high proportion of fast-twitch fibres (see page 18) and are the muscles you use to make a definite action. However, postural muscles, with a high proportion of slow-twitch fibres, are at work all the time, keeping the body upright and in its correct position.

If your posture is poor, and the various parts of your body are not positioned correctly relative to each other, one group of postural muscles will be taut and the opposing muscles will be over-stretched. As a result, neither group works efficiently, and with time the stretched muscles become weaker, leading to increased postural misalignment and, eventually, joint damage. For example, if your lumbar spine is too arched, your abdominal muscles will be over-stretched and their opposing muscles will shorten and become too tense.

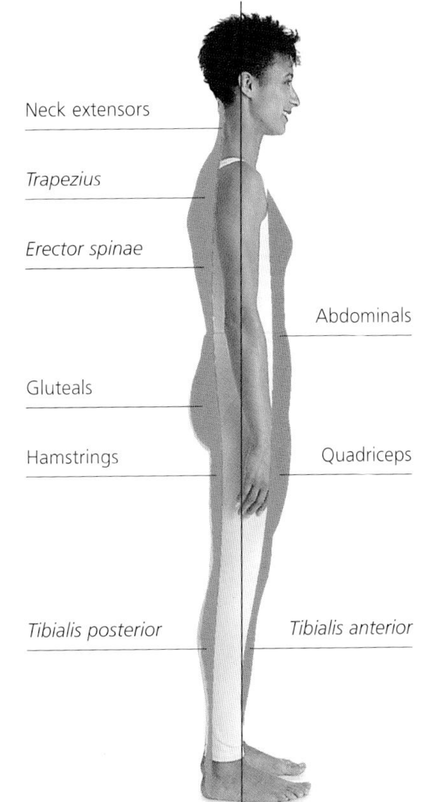

Postural muscles

The muscles that work all the time, keeping the body in its correct position, are known as postural muscles. They have a high proportion of slow-twitch fibres, as opposed to the phasic muscles, which are the ones you use when you make a positive movement.

Special postural problems

If you make a bit of an effort, it is not too difficult to keep posture in mind when you are walking from place to place or moving from task to task. The difficulty, and the danger, comes when you are stuck in one position for some time and concentrating on something else; or when you are carrying out a task that has unusual physical demands. Over the next four pages I will look at some special situations that put you at particular risk of developing problems as a result of bad posture: driving, sitting at a desk, doing housework, and lifting. Each has different areas of potential danger, but most can be avoided if you keep in mind these three watchpoints: choose the correct equipment; use the correct technique; and take regular breaks. (See also Alexander Technique, page 137.)

Car journeys

Whether you are a driver or a passenger, long car journeys can wreak havoc on your back. This is especially true if you tilt your seat back, when your lumbar spine has to bear too much of your body weight, which should be borne by your haunches. When you are stuck in one position for some time it is vital that you sit correctly, and it is easiest to do so if your seat is kept upright.

Choose a car with seats that help maintain this upright position. A car seat should be firm, adjustable and supportive. The base should not slope down at the back or too much weight will be borne by the base of your spine rather than by your thighs. Its back rest should be sufficiently high and wide to support your whole trunk.

Even if you have the correct type of car seat, immobility will cause an excessive build-up of tension in your postural muscles. The answer is to take frequent breaks on any long journey. Get out of your car, stretch and move around, and do some exercises to relieve any tension in your neck and shoulder muscles (see pages 78–79 and 88–89). If you start gripping the wheel tightly and tensing up in your car, breathe evenly and deeply for a few moments, allowing the tension to drain away and relaxing your shoulder muscles with each exhalation.

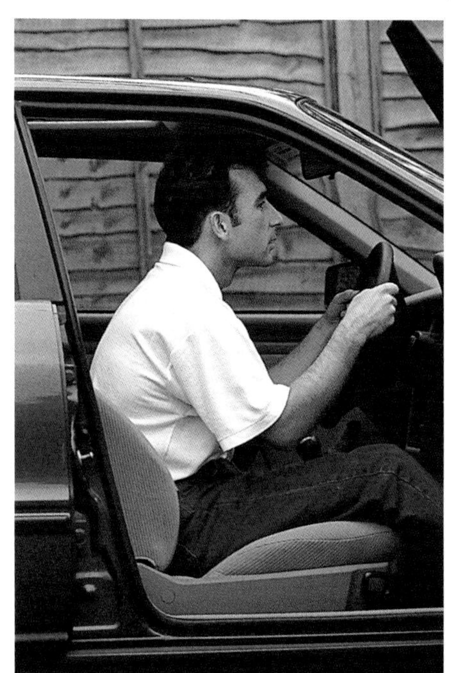

Behind the wheel
The lumbar spine bears too much of your weight when driving in an incorrect position (left). In the correct driving position (right), the back of your car seat should be upright, and the base should be positioned so that you can operate the pedals comfortably with your knees slightly bent. Some car seats are fitted with an adjustable lumbar roll that supports your lower back – if your car seat doesn't have one, buy a small cushion and fix it to the seat with a strap. And always wear flat shoes.

◀ Wrong Right ▶

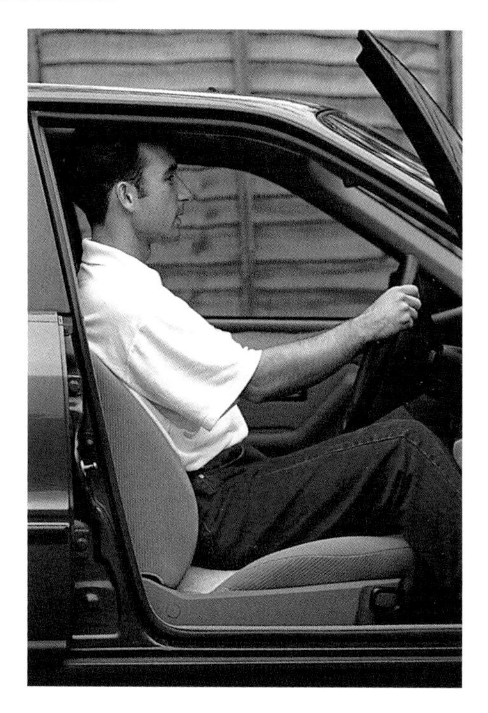

Working at a desk

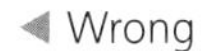

◄ Wrong

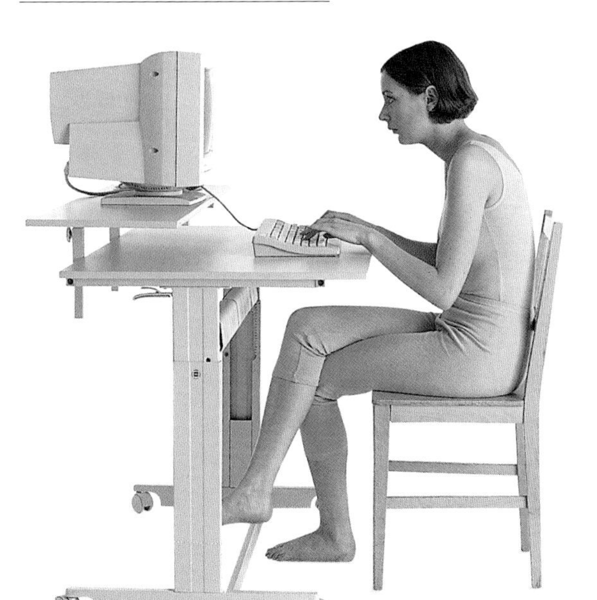

Right ►

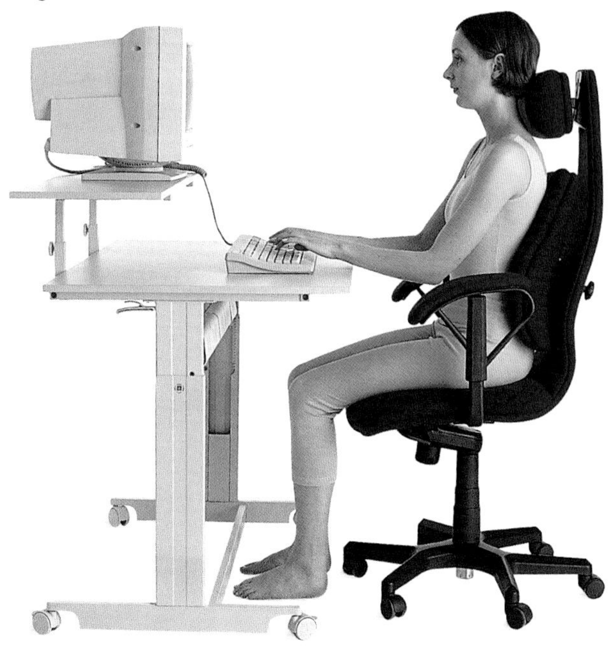

Computer work
In the correct position (above right), you should let your hands fall naturally onto the keyboard with your elbows and forearms supported, on armrests if necessary. This means that your chair has to be higher than if you were writing at a desk. You will probably need a chair that has a height-adjustment mechanism to make this possible – such chairs are more expensive than normal ones, but worth the investment.

I can tell you quite a lot about the problems working on a computer can cause. Of course authors do not always practise what they preach, so I have been known to work at my computer in the past while sitting on a kitchen chair: the results can be extremely painful, and I have now bought a specialist orthopaedic typing chair. You may not have to go this far – though I think that doing so is an extremely good investment – but you should not, under any circumstances, work in conditions that impose unnecessary strains on your body.

Computer work necessarily imposes a fair amount of strain on the back, neck and shoulder muscles, so it is vital that your chair helps to support these areas. The backrest of your chair should be adjustable, so that it can be manoeuvred to support the lumbar region of your spine, and any chair that has a full-length backrest should have an additional support area at this level.

Your chair should be deep enough from front to back to support the whole length of your thighs, and its seat should be tilted forwards and downwards to an angle of five degrees from the horizontal. This should allow your thighs to rest at 90 degrees when your feet are flat on the floor.

Your computer's monitor should be positioned so that you do not have to look downwards at it, because doing so puts strain on the extensor muscles of the neck (this also applies when you are reading for long periods, so you should use a reading stand if at all possible).

As with driving, it is important that you take frequent breaks from your computer. As well as easing any tension in your postural muscles, taking a break will also reduce the risk of strain injury (see page 58), upper limb disorders and eye strain. It is difficult to be precise about how frequent and how long such breaks should be, because the necessity for them varies according to the intensity with which you work. However, short, frequent breaks are to be recommended – I try to take off five minutes or so every half-hour, and walk around while I loosen my shoulders, roll my neck to release any tension and exercise my back.

Housework

A recent survey demonstrated that young mothers and housewives were fitter than women who exercised at a fitness club. This is probably because much housework involves bending, stretching, pushing and pulling. But this can also place considerable strain on your back and encourage poor posture. Here are a few pointers on how you can reduce the risk of developing postural problems.

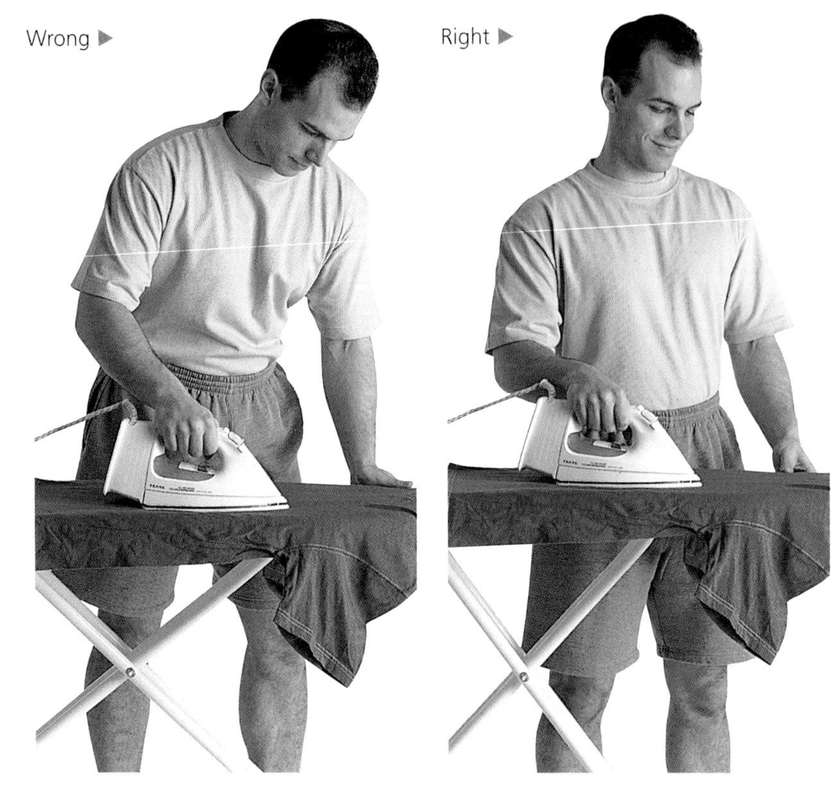

Ironing

Make sure you fix an ironing board at the correct height (far right): you should be able to stand straight with your upper arms relaxed by your side. Again, remember to take regular breaks.

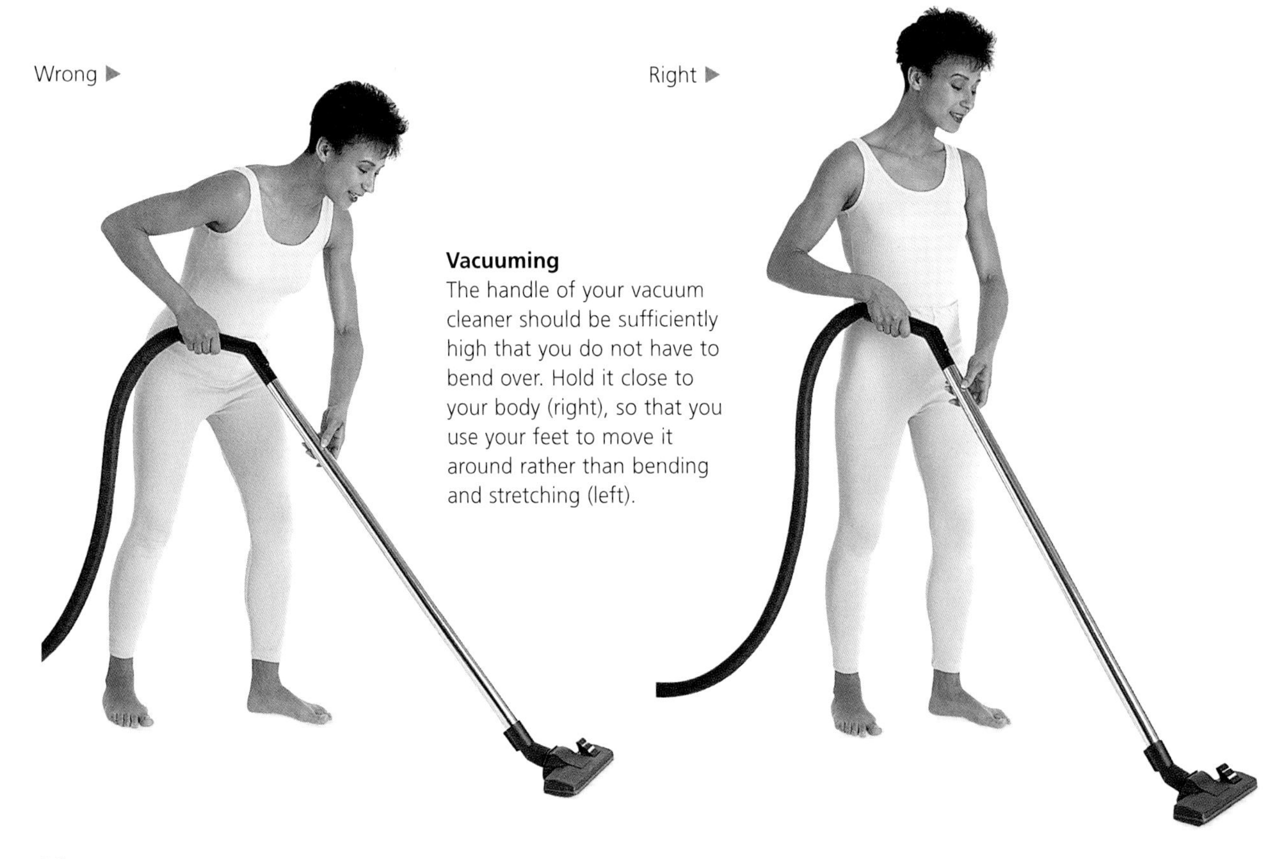

Vacuuming

The handle of your vacuum cleaner should be sufficiently high that you do not have to bend over. Hold it close to your body (right), so that you use your feet to move it around rather than bending and stretching (left).

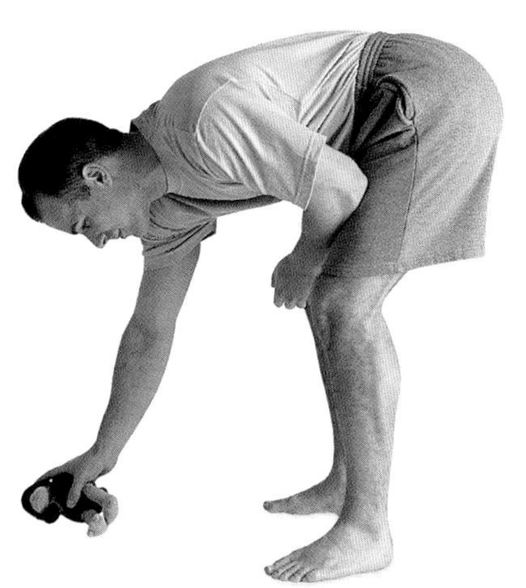

Bending down
When loading a washing machine, putting a dish in the oven, gardening or just picking up a toy from the floor, make sure that you bend your knees (right) rather than your back (left).

◀ Wrong Right ▶

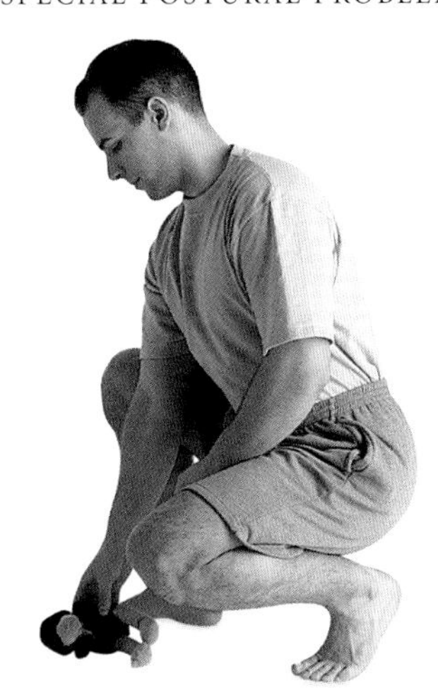

Lifting

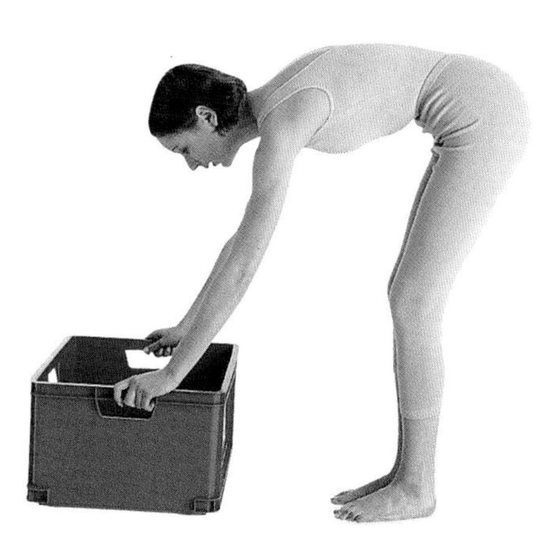

Incorrect lifting techniques can be dangerous, because you are using the postural muscles of your back to do work for which they are not designed. Instead, you should keep your back straight and use the phasic muscles of your legs. Place one hand underneath the object, if possible, and pull it into your body – a weight held at arm's length increases the stress on your spine by up to ten times that of the weight itself.

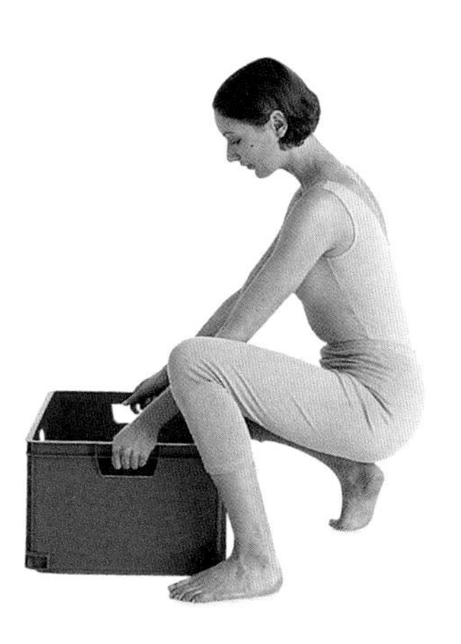

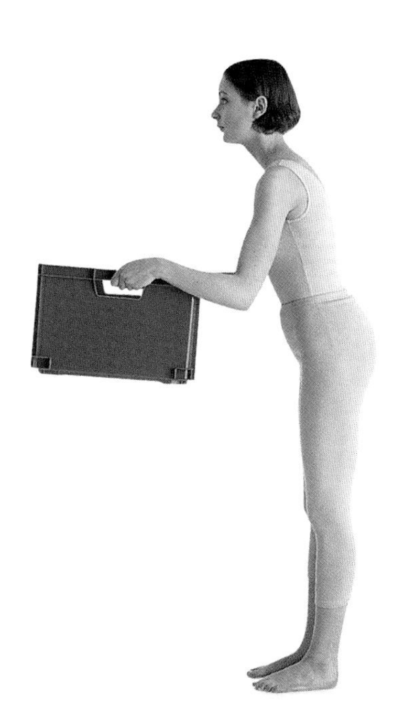

Heavy objects
It is a great temptation to just stoop down and grasp a heavy object in order to lift it (above left and left). But if you do this you are putting yourself at considerable risk of damaging your back.

Instead, stand with one foot slightly in front of the other as close as possible to the object to be lifted. If you can, keep both feet flat on the floor. Bend the knees and hips until you are low enough, keeping your back straight (above right). Straighten up in one smooth movement, using your leg muscles and keeping your back straight. Only start to move once you are standing erect (right).

◀ Wrong Right ▶

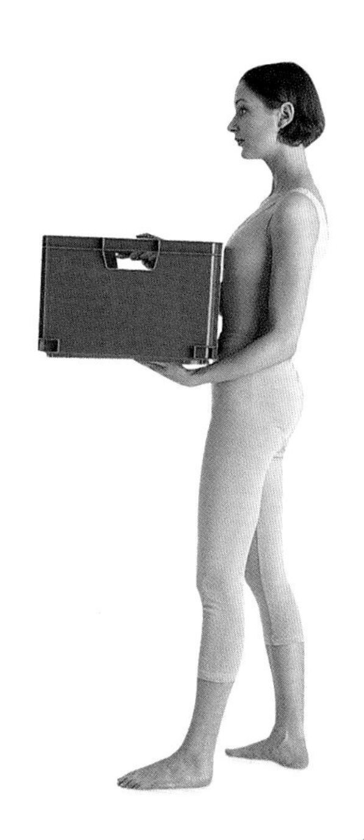

LIVING FOR MOBILITY Fit for life

Later in this book, I will introduce you to some maintenance exercises for specific muscle groups and joints (see pages 120–131). These are designed to help reduce the risk of damage to the tissues and to keep you fit and active. But there are other, more general, measures that help reduce the risks. Good posture is one of them, but regular exercise, control of your weight and the management of stress also play their parts in keeping your muscles and joints trouble-free, active and mobile – no matter what your age.

Bone idle?
Exercise is vital to the growth of bones during youth. But it is also the key to counteracting osteoporosis in old age, because collagen and calcium – building blocks of bone – are laid down in response to the physical stresses of activity, and blood supply is increased, too. Exercise is particularly important in the case of the upper femur (right) – the thigh bone – because the bone cavity is large here and the layer of bone is thin, making it vulnerable.

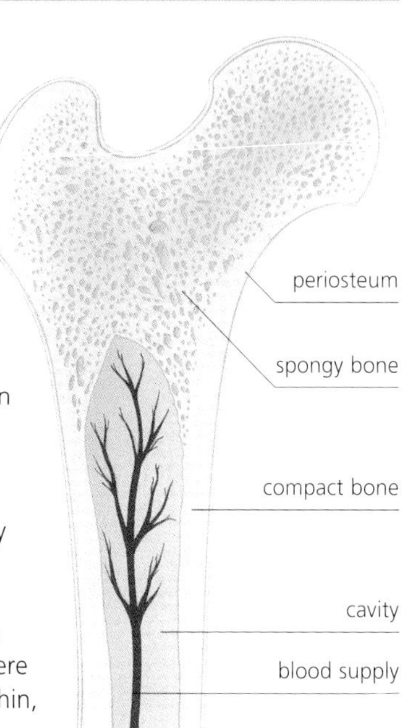

Exercise for strength and efficiency

Everyone knows that regular exercise is good for the heart and circulatory system, but it is not always appreciated that it also has an extremely beneficial effect on the musculo-skeletal system.

One reason for this is that exercise helps to develop strong bones in young children and guards against osteoporosis, or 'brittle bones', in older people – especially post-menopausal women. This is because bone reacts to the mechanical stress that exercise places on it by laying down more of the basic materials from which it is built: calcium and collagen. Collagen is a protein found throughout the body: in cartilage, the skin and even in the cornea of the eye. (Anyone who has made chicken stock will be familiar with it, too: heat turns the collagen in the chicken bones into the gelatine that makes the stock set.) Both the collagen and the calcium are deposited along the lines of pull in the bones, strengthening and enlarging them. So, as more calcium and collagen are built up, the bone gets stronger and larger – the ulna of the racket arm of a professional tennis player, for example, is larger than the one in his or her other arm.

Exercise also benefits muscles, and not just by increasing their bulk. It enlarges the size of the myofilaments (see page 18) so improving the muscles' ability to take up oxygen from the blood, and increases the size of the network of tiny blood vessels that supply them. As a result, the muscles' fuel supply is increased, and waste products are removed more quickly. Exercise also increases the tensile strength of the ligaments that support the joints and the tendons that connect the muscles to the bones. Finally, exercise improves the efficiency of the transmission of nerve impulses that control muscular action, making the muscles work more smoothly and quickly.

Aerobic versus anaerobic exercise

So the benefits of exercise are clear. However, muscles obtain the energy needed to initiate a movement in two different ways, making two distinct types of exercise. The first type is aerobic exercise, for which the energy comes from oxygen and the nutrients that you eat: carbohydrates, fats, and, on the rare occasions when these are not available (if you are starving, literally, for example), proteins. The basic ingredients of food are broken down by the process of digestion into glucose. This circulates in the blood and reacts with oxygen in the muscles to produce energy, carbon dioxide and water. (In fact, most of this energy is dissipated as heat, and only 20 to 25 per cent powers the muscle contractions.) The veins then carry the carbon dioxide back to the lungs, where it is expelled.

However, in certain circumstances, the second type of exercise – anaerobic – comes into play: when you make a quick sprint for a bus, for example, or play squash. Here, the heart and the respiratory system cannot keep up with the demand for oxygen, and the muscles do not relax for long enough to allow blood to flow through the fibres. In such cases, the muscles have to use stored glucose without oxygen, and a different waste product is produced. This is lactic acid, which collects in the muscle fibres causing tiredness, stiffness and cramp. Eventually it can build up to such a level that it prevents the muscle fibres from contracting. After the exercise stops, oxygen is needed to break down the lactic acid – the muscle is said to have an 'oxygen debt'.

Most sports involve both aerobic and anaerobic exercise. But for the average person, aerobic exercise is the better of the two types. This is because it benefits the muscles, heart and respiration without placing unnecessarily high demands on them. People of any age can take aerobic exercise – after all, a brisk walk comes into this category.

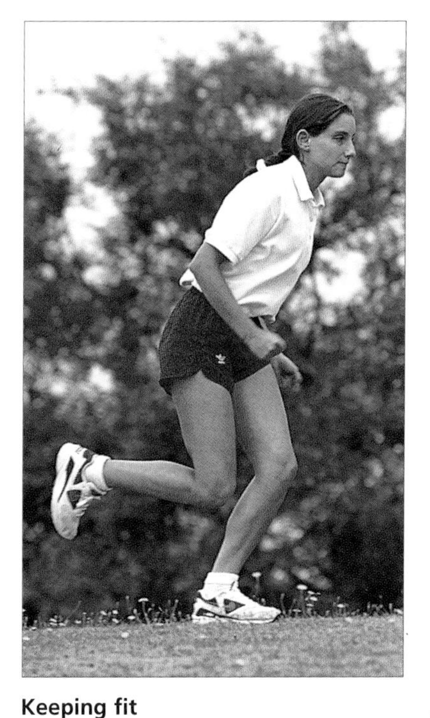

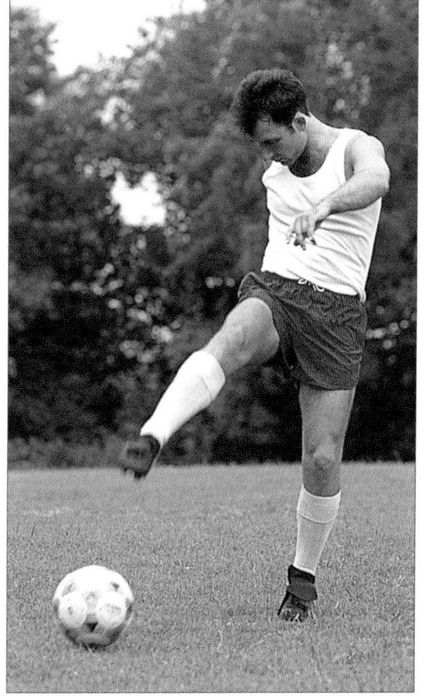

Repaying the oxygen debt
After anaerobic exercise, muscles are left with what is called an 'oxygen debt'. This is why you breathe heavily after sharp bursts of exercise and why a warm-down routine is so important. It keeps the rate of blood circulation high so that oxygen is pumped to the muscles more quickly, flushing waste products away.

▲ **Safety watchpoint** It is always advisable to consult your doctor before embarking on an exercise programme, especially if you have any medical condition or have previously led a sedentary life.

Keeping fit
Exercise benefits the body on many levels, and the general recommendation is that everyone should take at least three half-hour sessions of aerobic exercise each week, be it jogging, playing a game of football or tennis, or just taking a walk.

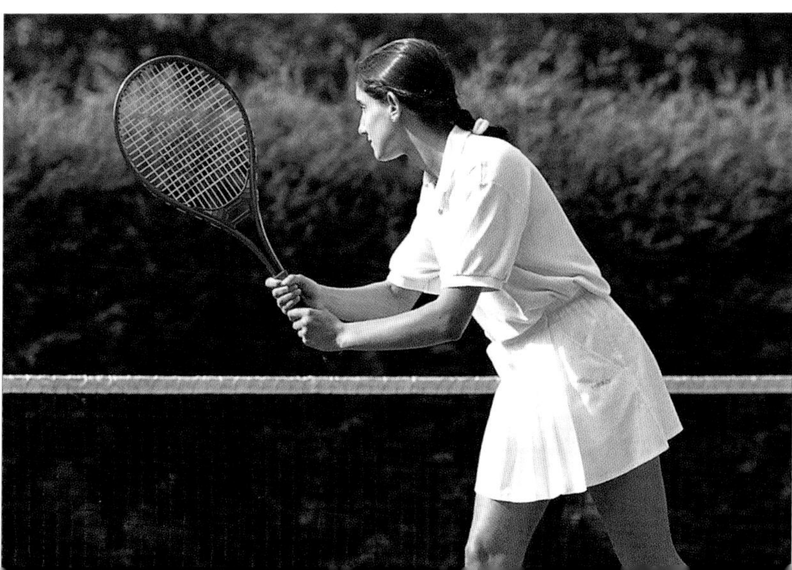

Controlling your weight

Obesity is becoming more and more of a problem in the Western world. It is responsible for much ill health and premature death as all of the body's systems have to work overtime in an attempt to cope with the extra physical mass. As far as we are concerned, it means the muscles receive an inadequate blood supply, and so not enough oxygen. And the sheer weight of fat deposits puts extra strain on joints and muscles. Of course, most people are not obese, but many are overweight – and that means they suffer from the same problems, though to a lesser degree.

The weight-bearing joints suffer first: the spine (the lower back in particular), the hips, the knees and the feet. Excess weight also increases wear and tear, so osteoarthritis tends to develop earlier. The hip is particularly vulnerable to this condition. To complete the vicious circle, people carrying extra weight are less inclined to exercise as it takes more effort. As a result, their metabolic rate – the speed they convert food to energy – will be slow, hence fewer nutrients are used and more fat is stored. So, check the chart below to see whether you are overweight. If you are – do something about it.

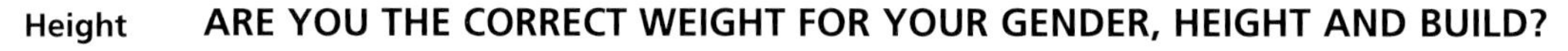

ARE YOU THE CORRECT WEIGHT FOR YOUR GENDER, HEIGHT AND BUILD?

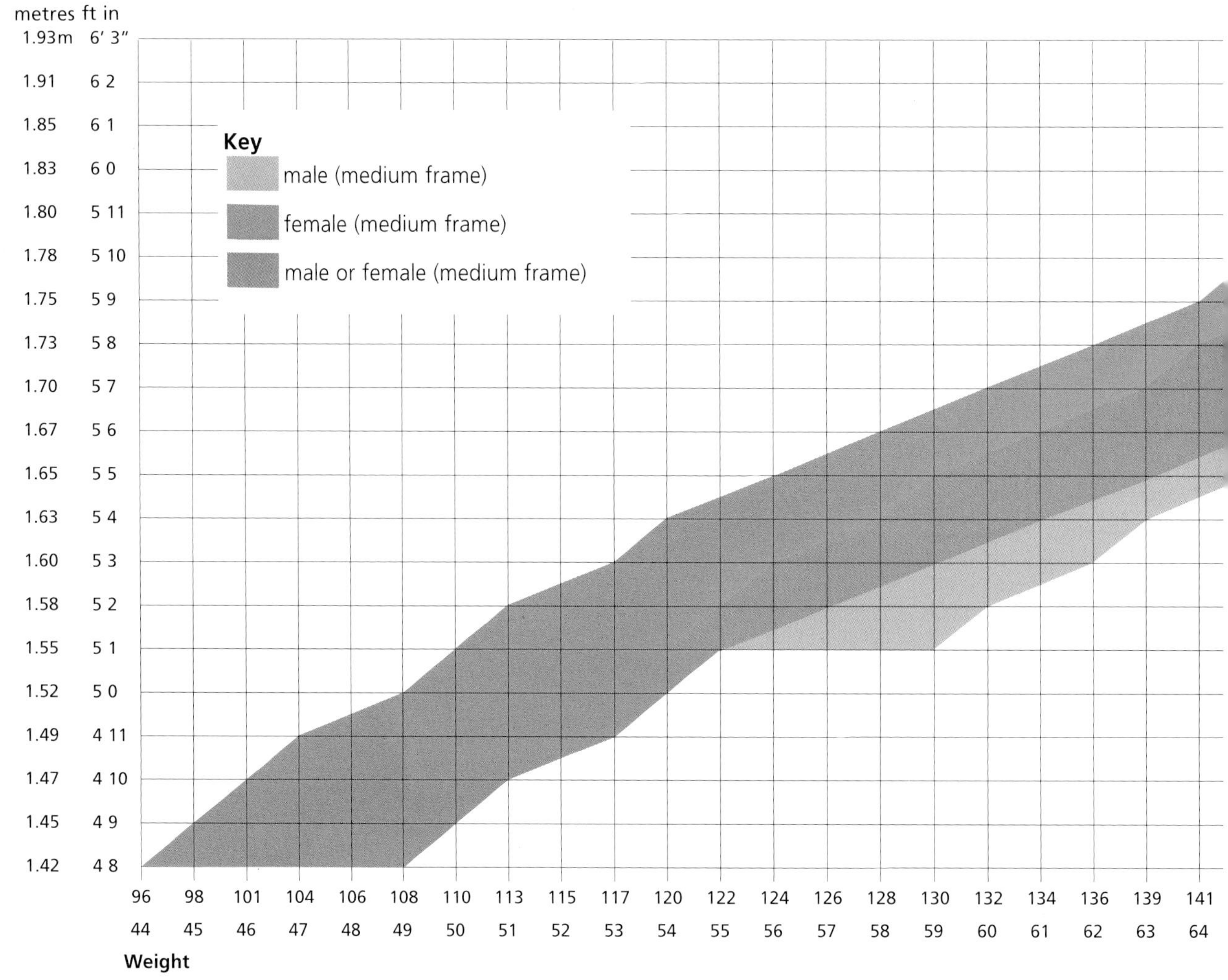

But crash dieting is not the answer, for two reasons. First, it can be dangerous to your health; second, it doesn't work. A crash diet slows all the body's systems down in an attempt to prolong survival – so the less you eat, the less your body uses.

There is only one way to lose weight: reduce your intake of fats and unnecessary extras, such as alcohol, and increase your metabolic rate by means of regular exercise. If you do this, you will take in fewer energy supplies than the body requires, so the body's fat stores will be broken down to provide energy. Over time your weight will stabilise and you can then increase your food intake to match your energy output. It is often helpful to join a reputable slimming club – but not one that combines evangelical fervour with public humiliation.

SKIN-FOLD CALLIPERS

The ratio of fat to muscle in your body gives a more accurate guide to whether you are overweight than your overall weight, because body fat weighs less than muscle tissue. This ratio can be worked out using skin-fold callipers; most doctors, dieticians and health experts use them, but some health stores also stock them. Many different types are available, but most are pincers with which to measure the thickness of fat at various sites: the stomach, buttocks, upper thighs and upper arms. The fat to body-weight ratio is calculated from these measurements: normally it is 20 to 30 per cent in women and around 20 per cent in men. Any higher result means that you should probably consult your doctor about a diet.

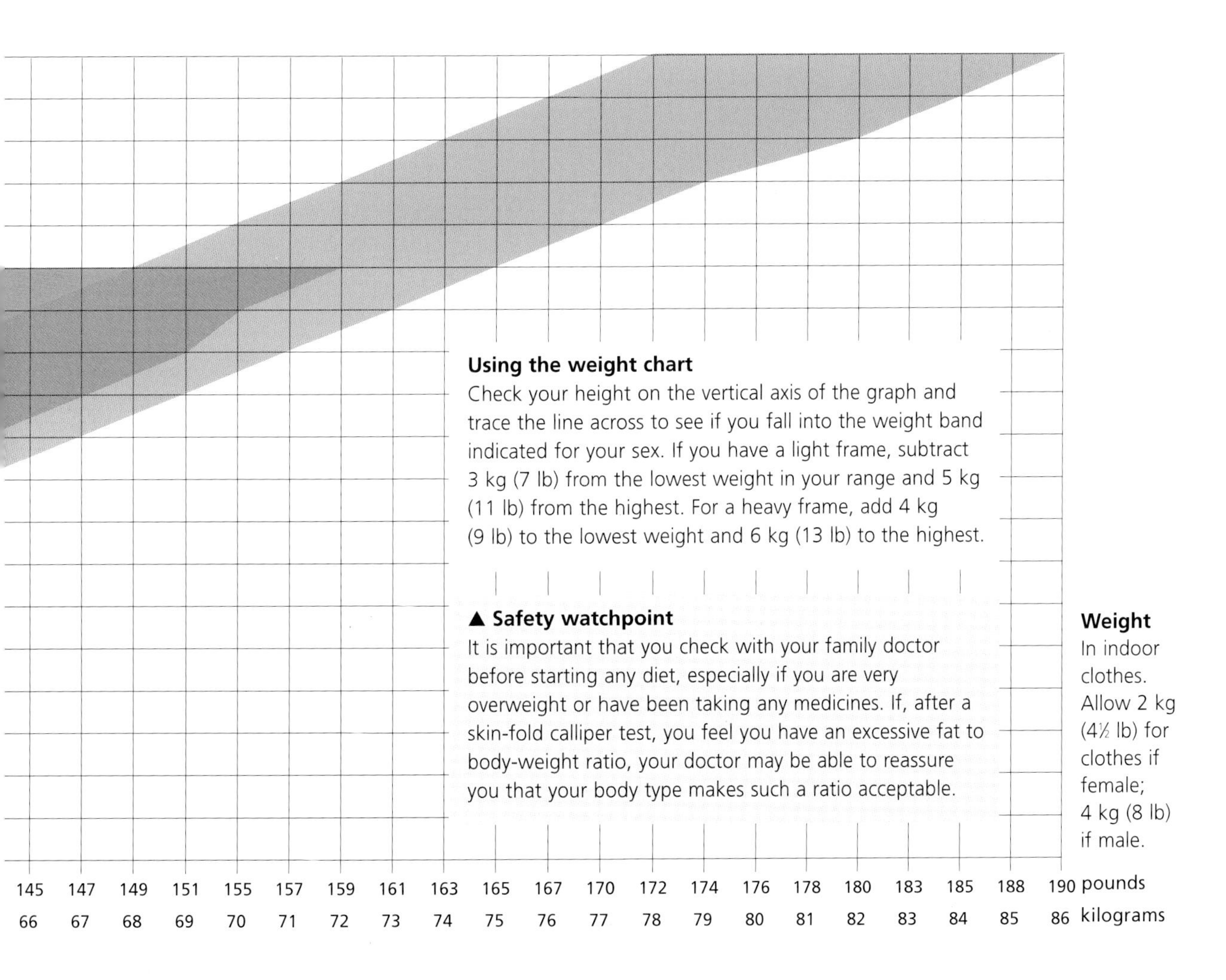

Using the weight chart

Check your height on the vertical axis of the graph and trace the line across to see if you fall into the weight band indicated for your sex. If you have a light frame, subtract 3 kg (7 lb) from the lowest weight in your range and 5 kg (11 lb) from the highest. For a heavy frame, add 4 kg (9 lb) to the lowest weight and 6 kg (13 lb) to the highest.

▲ Safety watchpoint

It is important that you check with your family doctor before starting any diet, especially if you are very overweight or have been taking any medicines. If, after a skin-fold calliper test, you feel you have an excessive fat to body-weight ratio, your doctor may be able to reassure you that your body type makes such a ratio acceptable.

Managing stress

Many people believe that the word 'stress' is rather over-used these days, and it is true that it does seem to have changed its meaning to encompass anything from minor irritations upwards. But the word has a more precise medical meaning, too, that refers to a definite physiological response – one that is very primitive and instinctive.

FIGHT OR FLIGHT

The very word 'stress' is taken from the language of engineering, in which a structure is put under pressure. In our case, what puts the body and mind under pressure is a perceived threat, and our response is known as 'fight or flight', which means that the body prepares itself either to fight for survival or to run away from the danger as fast as possible. It does this by flooding its systems with chemical messengers, called hormones, that trigger physical changes: the rate of breathing increases; blood pressure is raised; energy supplies are diverted to the muscles; and the body is tensed, ready for action.

This response was very useful in the days when a sabre-toothed tiger might lurk around any corner. Primitive humans would run away or – less sensibly – fight, after which their bodies would return to normal. Today, though, it is not so simple. You cannot hit your boss when your position is under threat; and you cannot fight for the last loaf of bread on a supermarket shelf. So, having been pumped up ready for action, your body has no method of release. As a result, the state of being physically, emotionally and physiologically prepared for decisive action can become almost permanent.

Stress can affect individuals in many different ways, both physical and psychological. Here, we are concerned with muscles and joints, and the one

Relaxation exercise

The essence of relaxation is to cut the outside world out of your mind and to focus on yourself, so that you become sensitive to the tensions within your body. You might find this technique tricky to master at first, but persevere and you will notice the benefit. Don't worry if your mind wanders – just concentrate on your breathing and you will soon get your focus back. After a while you will become sensitive to any abnormal tensions and strains in your body and find that it becomes second nature to relax in this way. In fact, many people find that they become so relaxed that they fall asleep at the end of a session.

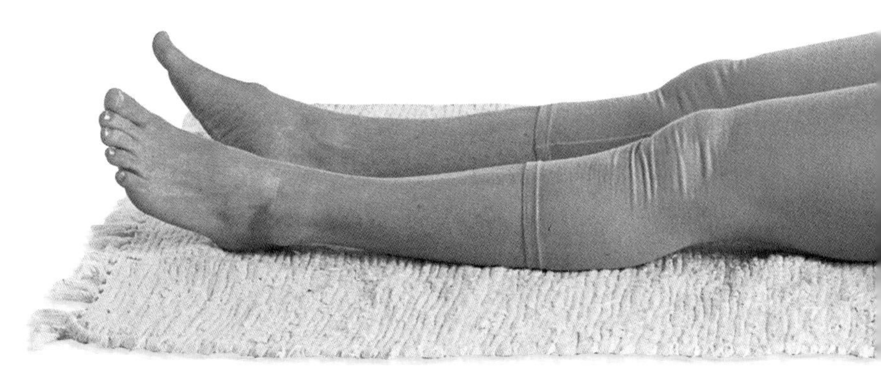

1 Lie on your back on a firm bed in a quiet, warm, dark room, so that there are no physical distractions. If you find it more comfortable, put one cushion under your head and another under your knees.

2 Let your mind go blank and take two deep breaths, letting the air out gradually.

3 Focus on your right foot. Tense all the muscles in it and let go after a few seconds, so that it feels floppy. Do the same with your right calf, then move on to the thigh – if your leg does not feel sufficiently relaxed, raise it in the air and hold until the position becomes uncomfortable before letting it relax again. Repeat the process with your other leg.

common factor is that stress tenses muscles: they become tight and knotted and lose the ability to relax fully and lengthen. This means that the postural muscles lose their effectiveness – and this, in turn, means other muscles have to work too hard to compensate for them. The result is that posture suffers, and joint damage follows.

This is not a book about lifestyles, so I will not advise you on how to avoid stress or how to deal with it by means of psychological techniques. But I can show you how to reduce the effects of stress on muscles by means of some simple relaxation exercises and breathing techniques. Try them when you feel the onset of muscular tension or have a headache – one of the prime causes of headaches is tension in the neck muscles – or fit them in as part of a bedtime routine.

▲ Safety watchpoint

If you start to feel faint while following the breathing techniques – a rush of oxygen to the brain can cause this feeling – relax and breathe naturally for a while. Then try again, but do not hold your breath.

Breathing technique

As we have seen, muscles produce waste products when they burn up energy. Stress makes muscles tense in a state of permanent semi-contraction, so that waste products build up. Oxygen is needed to break them down and help the muscles to relax once more. This breathing technique increases the flow of oxygen to the muscles and speeds up relaxation.

1 Ideally, lie on your back on a firm bed, wearing loose, comfortable clothes, and try to relax completely. Once you have mastered the technique, however, you can use it anywhere – at your office desk, for example.

2 Place your hands on the lower border of your rib cage and breathe in slowly and deeply through your nose. You will feel your hands rise as your diaphragm and ribcage expand.

3 Hold the breath for three seconds, then exhale gently. Do not force the air out of your lungs, but try to empty them completely.

4 Repeat the deep breaths four times, then relax and breathe naturally for a while.

5 Start the sequence again, and repeat four times.

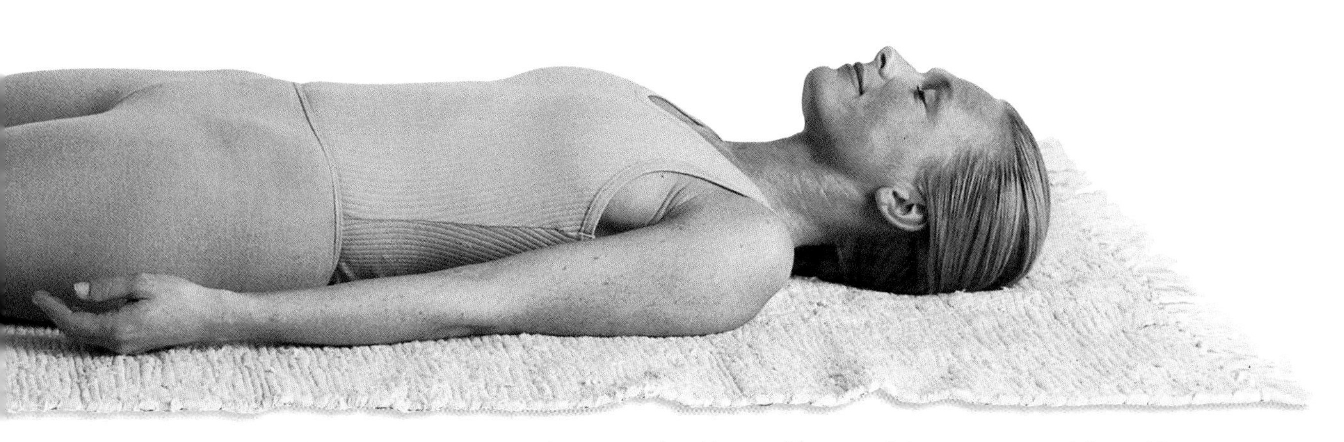

4 Remembering to keep breathing deeply and evenly, move up your body and repeat the process, tightening and relaxing the muscles of your buttocks and stomach. Work on one hand and arm, then the other.

5 Hunch up your shoulders and let go, then lift them off the ground towards the ceiling. There is often so much tension in this area that you may have to repeat this exercise a few times.

6 Loosen your neck by rocking your head slowly from side to side. Open your mouth and yawn as widely as you can, purse your lips, raise your eyebrows, and then relax.

7 All the muscles in your body should now be limp, warm and floppy. Stay in this position for about 15 minutes, breathing deeply and evenly.

SECTION TWO

WHAT'S THE PROBLEM?

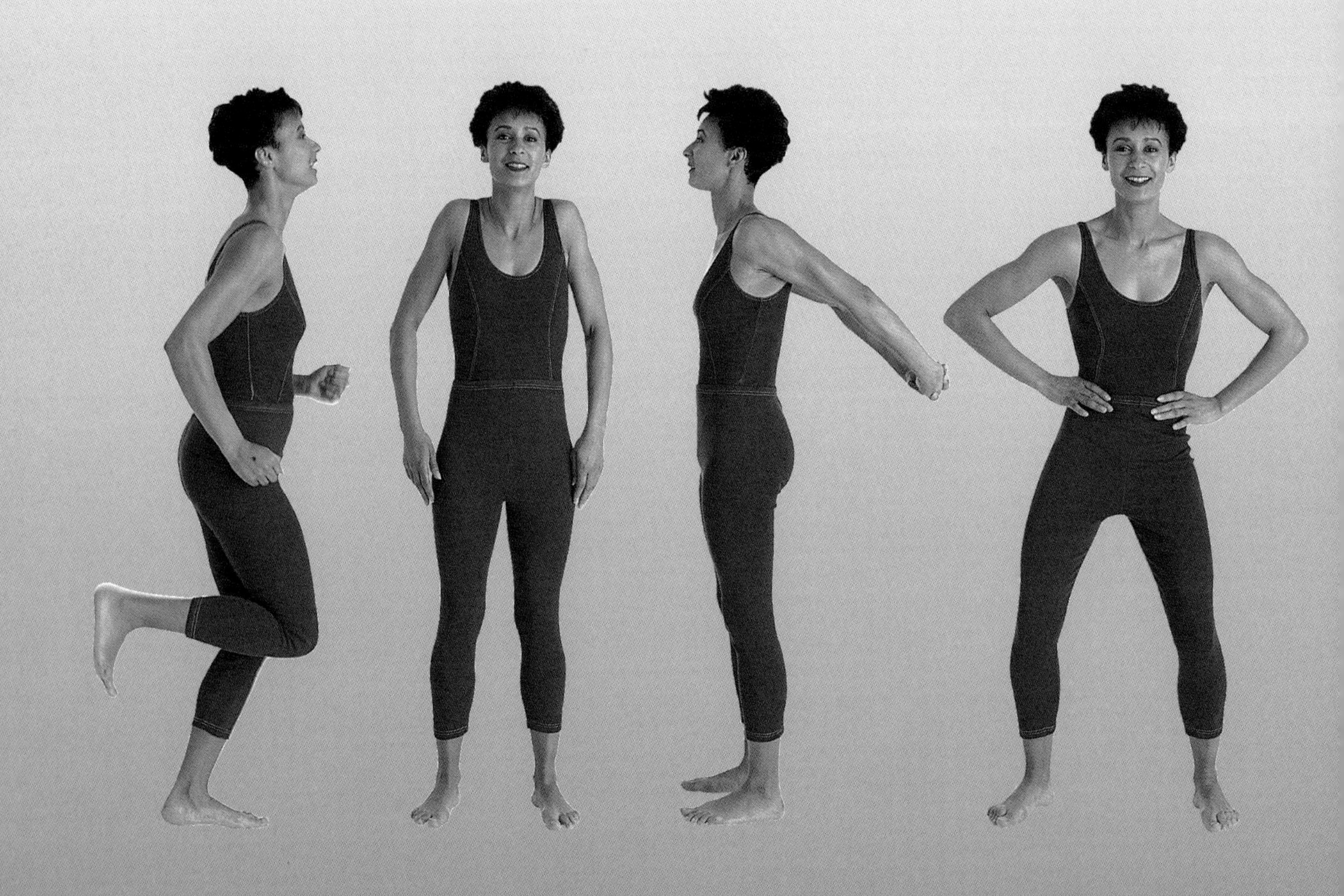

The first section of this book showed you how the musculo-skeletal system is designed to work in conjunction with the other systems of the body. I described how its various components function, in principle; but in practice, of course, things do not always work as they should.

This section of the book addresses what can go wrong and how various types of damage to this intricate system can manifest themselves as pain in the muscles and joints – and even as pain far away from the site of the problem. It also gives you a pain-analysis questionnaire that helps you to describe the nature of any pain you may have and to see how well you are coping with it.

Then I go on to take a closer look at each area of the body in turn, examining the muscles and joints and discussing a range of common complaints, from frozen shoulder to fallen arches, that can affect each area. Special features allow you to view each problem 'at-a-glance', note possible causes, learn how to avoid them, and cross-refer to remedial exercises and preventive measures described elsewhere in the book.

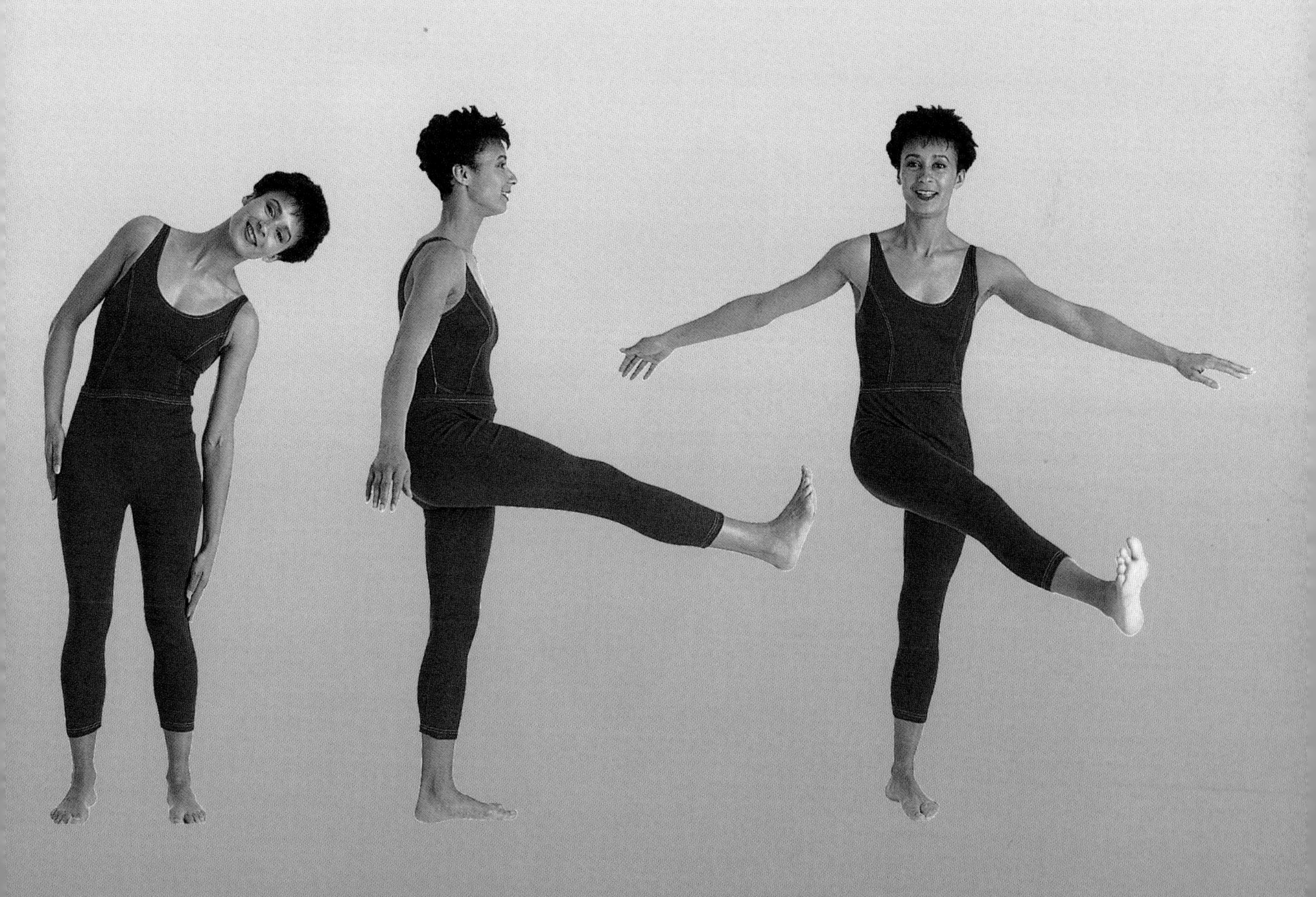

PAIN The nature of pain

'Pain is the body's warning system,' some people say. But that is only half the story, because there are two different types of pain. If you slip with a knife and cut your finger, for example, you will feel the sharp, intense stabbing sensation of acute pain. It has a purpose, in that you will immediately move your hand away from the knife and will know that the tissues have been damaged. The acute pain wears off fairly quickly, but it is followed by the second type of pain: the dull, nagging ache of chronic pain.

Pathways for pain

The two types of pain can be clearly differentiated in terms of how they are treated by the nervous system. Acute pain is triggered by any event that damages or threatens to damage the body's tissues, be it mechanically, or by means of chemicals or heat. The pain is detected by receptors, which are free nerve endings found close to the surface of the skin, and in muscles, tendons and joints, as well as in some organs, such as the heart and liver. These transmit nerve impulses through sensory pathways to the brain, composed of special 'A-delta fibres' which have myelin sheaths that speed the pain impulses to the brain in a tiny fraction of a second. The brain assesses the information, and sends motor nerve impulses to the appropriate area so that the muscles act to withdraw your body from the danger: in our example, you pull away from the knife.

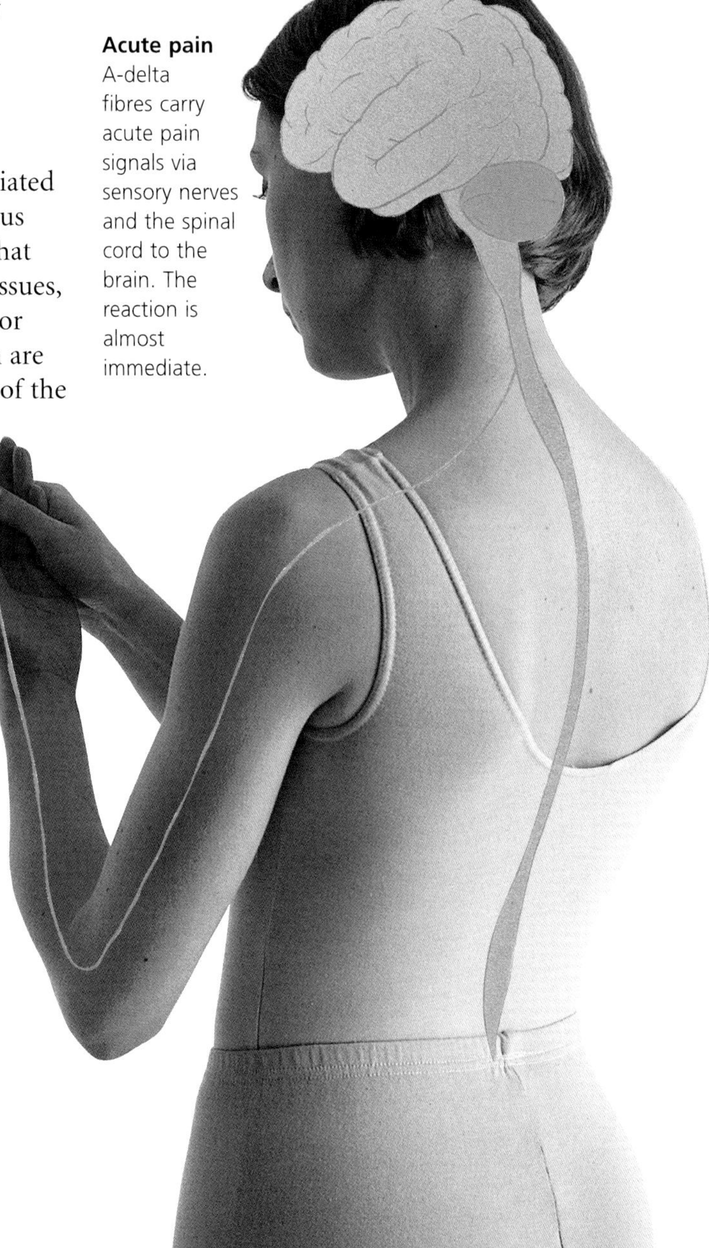

Acute pain
A-delta fibres carry acute pain signals via sensory nerves and the spinal cord to the brain. The reaction is almost immediate.

A CROSS-SECTION OF THE SURFACE OF THE SKIN

A-delta fibres (red) link to receptors near the skin surface and transmit acute pain impulses ten times faster than C fibres.

C fibres (blue) link to deeper receptors and transmit chronic pain impulses slowly.

Hair follicle

Sweat gland

Epidermis

Dermis

However, there is a second sensory pathway made up of 'C fibres'. This pathway is linked to receptors lying deeper in the tissues, and its fibres transmit impulses at about a tenth of the speed of the A-delta fibres. The result is that, after the acute pain subsides, you become aware of a pain that is variously described as being dull, aching, tender, gnawing, throbbing, nagging and sore: a chronic pain, in short, which persists.

How gate theory works

A gate is a junction between nerves in the spinal cord. Large numbers of acute pain impulses open it, blocking C fibre impulses until they cease.

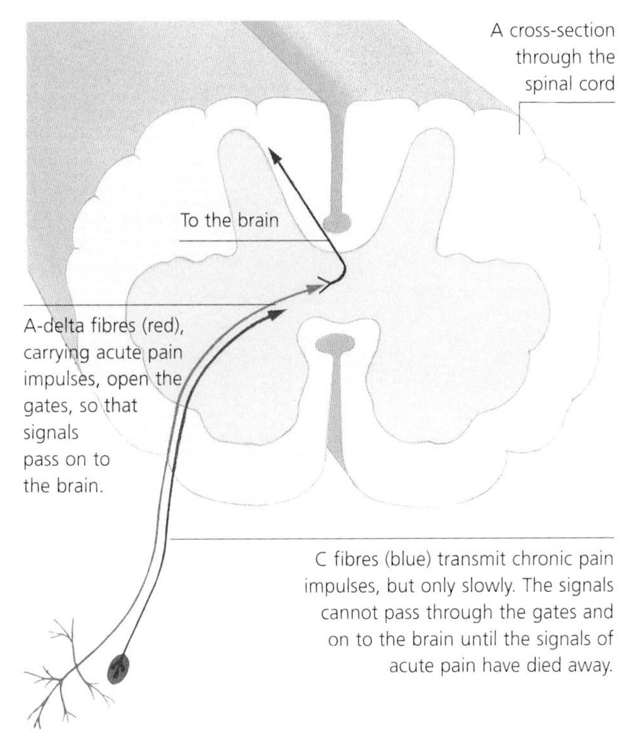

Spinal reflexes

It is not just the impulses of acute pain received by the brain that move your hand away from the kitchen knife, because a simpler, more direct system also exists. This is a spinal reflex, in which specific stimuli produce a direct motor response as soon as they reach the spinal column – information is still relayed to the brain, but action is taken independently of it.

The knee jerk is one example of a spinal reflex: doctors tap the tendon of the patella, just below the knee, to see if the lower leg kicks forwards and so discover whether the nervous system is in good working order.

Blocking pain

It is by no means certain that all the impulses generated by pain receptors reach the higher levels of the brain, because the sensory pathways that carry them contain three junctions, and at least some of the pain impulses can be blocked at each one. The first junction is in the spinal column, where two nerves join at a 'synapse'. The second nerve carries the impulse up the spinal cord to the brain.

Neurologists have developed something they call 'gate theory' to explain how this works: they see the synapse as a gate that is normally shut, but can be broken open by a large number of strong pain impulses – as in acute pain. However, the gate can only be open to one type of pathway at a time, and as the impulses transmitted by the A-delta fibres travel more quickly than those carried by the C fibres they reach the gates first and take precedence over them. But as the pain becomes less acute, and A-delta fibre impulses die away, the C fibre impulses of chronic pain can pass through the gates that have already been opened.

This means that the chronic pain carried by the C fibres can be blocked off at the gates and prevented from reaching the brain if the gates are occupied by other impulses that reach the gates first. Such impulses can be generated by applying pressure around the area that has been hurt. The pressure triggers receptors linked to large, fast fibres – called A-alpha fibres – to fire off impulses, and since these travel faster than the C fibre impulses that carry chronic pain, they reach the gates first and block them. So mother really did know best: 'rubbing it better' works!

Shutting the gate

Gate theory is utilised in a method of pain relief called TENS (Transcutaneous Electrical Nerve Stimulation) that is very effective in relieving chronic pain (see Physiotherapy Aids, page 72). A TENS machine stimulates the pressure receptors by means of a small electrical charge. The receptors then fire off impulses that block the gate in the spinal column to pain impulses. Some scientists think that acupuncture may rely on the same principle, since it, too, stimulates the pressure receptors.

Natural painkillers

In addition to the spinal 'gate', there are two more junctions at which pain impulses can be reduced. These are in the brain, but they are below the level at which conscious thought takes place. The first is in part of the brain stem, the oldest and most primitive section of the brain; and the second is in the thalamus, a relay station and coordinating centre for sensory impulses.

Again, the impulses of acute pain generally pass directly through these junctions and are received by the cortex of the brain. There are exceptions, however. It is now known that electrical stimulation of some areas of the brain makes animals oblivious to pain, and that, in extreme circumstances, impulses can be sent from the brain stem down the spine to block pain impulses off at the first junction – or 'gate' – in the spinal column. The latter phenomenon explains, for example, how soldiers can continue to fight after suffering terrible injuries.

In less extreme circumstances, however, a group of substances known as the endorphins comes into play. The body's natural painkillers, these can block pain impulses in the brain stem and thalamus, and can also help block them at the junction in the spinal cord, though to a smaller degree. One type in particular – encephalin – blocks pain impulses by linking with a receptor at the junctions to shut them down. Such receptors are known as 'opiate receptors', because opium and its derivatives, such as morphine and heroin, also block them. It is the endorphins that are responsible for the 'runner's high', to which some people who over-exercise become addicted.

So why do we feel pain at all? The answer is that the level of endorphins in the body varies considerably. Exercise increases the levels of endorphins, as does relaxation, feelings of happiness and calm, sleep, a positive mental outlook, and being prepared for a 'fight or flight' reaction (see page 32). On the other hand, tension, fear, depression, anxiety and concentrating on the pain all decrease endorphin levels. And without sufficient endorphins, more pain impulses will get through the junctions, so you will feel more pain.

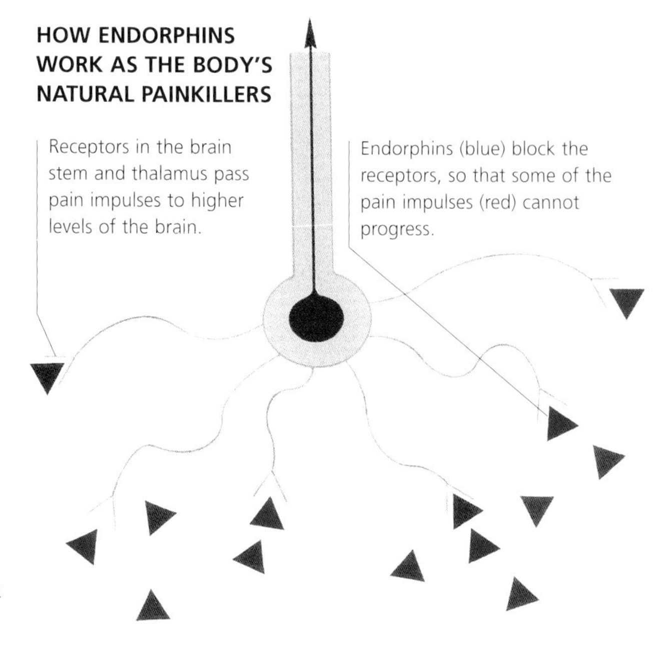

Vicious circle

One of the dangers of using painkillers regularly over a long period of time is that their action mimics that of your body's own painkillers, the endorphins. As a result, the body stops manufacturing its own painkillers, because it becomes unnecessary to do so. This means that not only will you need to take more painkillers to achieve the same effect, but also that the pain will be worse when you stop taking them.

Analyse your pain

It's far from easy to define the nature of a pain you are experiencing, but doing so can be of great help in working out the nature of the problem. This fact was recognised by Canadian, Ronald Melzak, Professor of Psychiatry at McGill University in Montreal (and one of the experts who developed gate theory). He devised the questionnaire opposite that is now used internationally to measure pain: it is known as the 'McGill Questionnaire'.

Some of the questions focus on the effect of the pain, rather than the pain itself, so that the amount of psychological distress being caused can be evaluated. Use the questionnaire opposite to identify the type of pain from which you are suffering, and then look below it to see the significance of your answers.

THE McGILL QUESTIONNAIRE

If any word in one of the groups describes your pain, circle it, but do not circle more than one word in any group – if more than one word applies, circle only the most relevant one. If none of the words in a group applies to you, ignore the group. Refer to the box below for analysis.

1.
Flickering
Quivering
Pulsing
Throbbing
Beating
Pounding

2.
Jumping
Flashing
Shooting

3.
Pricking
Boring
Drilling
Stabbing
Lancing

4.
Sharp
Cutting
Lacerating

5.
Pinching
Pressing
Gnawing
Cramping
Crushing

6.
Tugging
Pulling
Wrenching

7.
Hot
Burning
Scalding
Searing

8.
Tingling
Itchy
Smarting
Stinging

9.
Dull
Sore
Hurting
Aching
Heavy

10.
Tender
Taut
Rasping
Splitting

11.
Tiring
Exhausting

12.
Sickening
Suffocating

13.
Fearful
Frightful
Terrifying

14.
Punishing
Gruelling
Cruel
Vicious
Killing

15.
Wretched
Binding

16.
Annoying
Troublesome
Miserable
Intense
Unbearable

17.
Spreading
Radiating
Penetrating
Piercing

18.
Tight
Numb
Drawing
Squeezing
Tearing

19.
Cool
Cold
Freezing

20.
Nagging
Nauseating
Agonising
Dreadful
Torturing

Your pain analysis results

The questionnaire is designed so that the groups of words you choose give a broad indication of how well you are coping with your pain in psychological terms. The position of the word you circle in the group is important, too: the lower in the group, the more significant the feeling is to you.

If you circle more words in groups 11, 12, 13, 14, 15, 16 and 20 than in others, you are probably not coping adequately with your pain and are in some psychological distress. Consult your doctor and show him or her your completed questionnaire.

Otherwise, keep the results of this questionnaire, and use them to help you find out the nature of your problem by referring to the problem solvers in section three (pages 68–111). Run through the questionnaire again after a course of the appropriate self-help treatment to keep a track of how effective it has been. Keep the results as your doctor or physiotherapist may wish to see them.

Where's the problem?

Generally, the brain is remarkably adept at pinpointing where in the body acute pain is being felt and can identify the point of origin of acute pain impulses extremely precisely. This is a skill learned in the first six months or so of life: if given an injection, for example, a baby that has not yet developed the skill will scream, curl up and react as if its whole body has been hurt, because it cannot identify the site of the pin prick.

It is a different story, however, with the slower C fibres that transmit chronic pain. You may feel puzzled if a doctor whom you consult about a pain in the back of your thigh and your calf examines your back instead of the areas where you feel the pain. But there is method behind what might appear to be madness. In fact, it is quite common to feel pain at a site in the body some distance from the place in which it is being caused. This phenomenon is known as 'referred pain' and can result from any one of three different causes: the first involving nerve damage, and the second and third being due to embryology – that is, how we all develop from a single-cell embryo in the womb.

The lower part of the neck and shoulders is particularly susceptible to problems, often as a result of pressure being put on the nerves in the area by taut, knotted muscles.

The nervous system
Apart from the head, whose nerves come directly from the brain, the whole body is supplied with nerves that branch off the spinal column. Each muscle has a sensory nerve, which relays information to the brain, and a motor nerve, which transmits impulses controlling it in response.

Nerve damage

The first reason why pain is referred is that some part of a nerve has been damaged, with the result that pain is felt in all the areas that it supplies. For example, if a problem in the lower back leads to swelling and distortion of the tissues near the spine, the sciatic nerve may be compressed. This is the longest nerve in the body and travels down through the buttock, the thigh and the lower leg to the foot. So, damage to the nerve near the spine may cause a stabbing, hot, intermittent but chronic pain along the line of its route (see sciatica, pages 50–51). The same applies to the motor nerves that leave the spine to travel down through the arm to supply its muscles.

Phantom limbs

A good example both of the brain's ability to judge the site of acute pain and the ease with which it can become confused as a result of nerve damage can be seen in people who have had a limb amputated. If the nerves at the stump of the amputated limb are stimulated, the brain assumes that the stimulus comes from the point lower down in the limb to which they once went: this feeling is known as having a 'phantom limb'.

Common origins

The second cause of referred pain is a function of our embryological development. Well before the embryo has become recognisably human in shape, its tissues differentiate in respect of their function and their association with the various spinal vertebrae. So when the body has completely developed, it is inevitable that there will be some overlap. What this means in practice is that fibres from two different areas – which may have been close together in the embryo – meet at the same relay cells in the spine and trigger these relays when there are a large number of strong pain impulses from one area of them. For example, pain from an internal organ is often felt in a different region: the chronic heart pain of angina is felt in the left arm and left jaw.

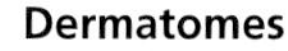

Dermatomes
As the embryo grows, areas of skin that were once close together are pulled out of their original shape. But the same spinal nerve still supplies the whole of each area, making it difficult to know the exact origin of any pain.

Pain from the hip can often be felt in the skin above the knee.

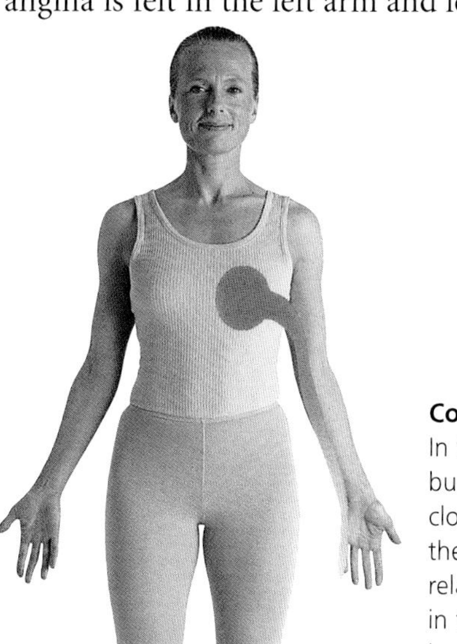

Common relays
In the embryo, the limb bud for the left arm is close to the heart and the two share spinal relays. As a result, pain in the heart can be felt in the left arm.

Skin patterns

Embryology also lies behind the third reason for referred pain. In the embryo, a nerve from each vertebra supplies the area of skin directly by it. As the embryo develops, and arms and legs grow, these areas of skin become stretched into elongated shapes. These shapes are called dermatomes, and are still supplied by the same spinal nerve. Because of this 'stretched' pattern in the adult, pain from joints or other deep tissues may be felt in the skin, but not always at the site of its cause.

▲ Safety watchpoint
The diagrams on this page are not intended as a guide to self-diagnosis, because a number of complex factors are involved in establishing whether pain is referred from somewhere else or comes from the site at which it is felt. They are merely intended to give you a sense of the possibility of referred pain and to explain why doctors and physiotherapists examine you in the way that they do.

GENERAL COMPLAINTS

DEFINITIONS

Here are definitions of some of the terms that are used to describe the effects of muscle and joint damage in the sections that follow.

Inflammation

This includes any condition ending in 'itis', such as tendinitis, bursitis and synovitis. Inflammation is a localised reaction of the tissues to trauma or disease: the affected area becomes swollen and painful as blood vessels expand and leak and, in a joint, more synovial fluid is produced; pain results from compression of the tissues by this fluid and from general irritation.

Rupture

This is a tear to a ligament, muscle or tendon. A rupture may be either complete or partial, and the amount of damage, and so pain, depends on the degree of rupture. Generally, though not always, a complete rupture causes bleeding, swelling and severe pain; in less severe cases an intramuscular haematoma (bruise) may form inside a muscle, causing pain, tenderness and a restriction in movement (see Achilles tendon rupture, page 66).

Spasm

This is an over-tight contraction. A muscle may go into spasm for a variety of reasons: as a result of a lack of oxygen; because of an excessive build-up of lactic acid (see page 29); or in order to protect an injured part, as, for example, when a bone has been fractured. In some cases only a few fibres are affected, but if a whole muscle is involved the result is cramp.

Fracture

A crack in the material of a bone may be the result of an accident, a stress injury or osteoporosis ('brittle bones', see page 43). It causes inflammation, considerable pain at the site and muscle spasms.

Wear and tear

Also known as osteoarthritis (see osteoarthritis of the hip, page 62), this is caused either by the natural and inevitable process of ageing, a repetitive movement, poor posture or a combination of all these factors. It results in the thinning of the cartilage covering the articulating ends of bones, the formation of bony spurs within a joint and the lack of adequate production of synovial fluid. This damage, which is irreversible, causes joint stiffness, pain and a restriction of mobility.

In the next four pages I will show you how to recognise and avoid a number of common problems affecting the musculo-skeletal system in general – and what you can do if you don't manage to avoid them. Cross-references will lead you to the self-help steps in section three and to the preventive measures described in section four. Later in this section I will look at complaints common to specific areas of the body.

A number of diseases can cause damage to the musculo-skeletal system. However, most of them are rare, so are not described here – the least rare being rheumatoid arthritis (see below), gout, connective tissue disorders, ankylosing spondylitis, osteomyelitis, tumours and osteochondritis dessicans. Osteoporosis (see page 43) is included because its onset can, to a certain extent, be prevented or delayed by self-help measures.

ARTHRITIS AND RHEUMATISM

I have only included 'rheumatism' because I know that many people will expect to see it here – but no such condition exists! The term is used as a catch-all phrase to cover any pain involving muscles and joints. It is often confused with arthritis, a condition that exists in two main forms: osteoarthritis and rheumatoid arthritis.

Osteoarthritis is a condition in which the structure of cartilage and bone changes, generally as a result of wear and tear. While a certain amount of osteoarthritis is inevitable in old age, its symptoms can be considerably reduced and its effects on mobility lessened by preventive measures (see osteoarthritis of the hip, page 62).

Rheumatoid arthritis, on the other hand, is thought to be a disease, and one to which sufferers have an inherited predisposition. Its cause is not yet completely understood, but it results in chronic inflammation of the synovial linings of the body. While a number of the exercises described in section three may be of help to sufferers, the condition is one that requires specialist treatment, and so is outside the scope of this book.

Osteoporosis

Although it is also known as brittle bone disease, osteoporosis is not so much a disease as a disorder that to some degree forms part of the natural process of ageing. It involves the leaching of calcium and bone fibre into the blood, with the effect that the bones become less dense and more prone to fracture as they become unable to bear the stresses and strains of everyday life. The condition affects the inner, porous layers of bone more than the outer, more compact ones, so the bones with the most porous material are the first to suffer: these include the hips, spine and wrists.

Under normal circumstances, the bones start to become weaker very gradually from about the age of 30. However, diseases that cause overactivity of the adrenal glands or the parathyroid glands, as well as long-term treatment with corticosteroid drugs, can accelerate the condition, with the result that osteoporosis sets in during middle age. The female hormone oestrogen has a preventive effect against the disorder, so osteoporosis is a particular hazard for post-menopausal women, as well as women who have had a hysterectomy before the menopause. A diet that is low in calcium, a high intake of alcohol, heavy smoking and a lack of exercise also predispose towards the development of osteoporosis. However, a balanced diet, adequate exercise (especially during youth, when bone mass is built up) and – in the case of post-menopausal women – hormone replacement therapy (HRT), can all help to ward off the problem.

AT A GLANCE: Osteoporosis
Cause: loss of calcium and bone fibre due to low calcium intake, the menopause and certain glandular problems
Medical treatment: bone density scan for diagnosis, then medication such as HRT
Physiotherapy: weight-bearing exercises; advice on posture and diet
Self-help: good posture; exercise; a diet rich in calcium (e.g. milk, cheese, nuts, oily fish, figs and apricots)
Avoidance: exercise; not smoking; a low intake of alcohol
Prognosis: good with early detection, as the loss of bone density can be slowed or halted; there are new drugs at research stage that may help bones to reabsorb bone fibre and calcium and reverse the problem

Cramp

The causes of cramp – a sudden painful spasm of a muscle – are not completely understood, though the problem is thought to be the result of a chemical imbalance within the muscle. This may be caused by loss of salt through excessive exercise, sweating or diarrhoea, or by a disorder affecting the circulation of the blood. As a result, there is no specific treatment for cramp, other than stretching and massaging the muscle, though a drink of slightly salted water may help relieve cramp or prevent it from developing. Warming up and warming down before and after exercise (see pages 114–19) also help prevent cramp from developing. You should consult your doctor if you experience cramp frequently, as your cramps may be a sign of a circulatory or other disorder.

AT A GLANCE: Cramp
Cause: chemical imbalance in muscle, often caused by excessive sweating during exercise
Medical treatment: none – see your doctor if you experience cramp frequently
Physiotherapy: muscle stretching and massage
Self-help: warm-up and warm-down (see pages 114–19)
Avoidance: drink slightly salted water if you are likely to exercise sufficiently to sweat a lot
Prognosis: good, unless cramp occurs frequently

Pulled muscles or tendons

A variety of factors can be responsible for a muscle or its tendon becoming strained, or 'pulled', and the damage involved can run from an over-stretching of the fibres to a partial tear in them. The most common cause is an excessive demand placed on the tissues, as when a hamstring muscle is pulled while playing sport. However, such injuries can also be caused by a sudden movement when the muscles and joints are not correctly aligned to deal with the load that is placed on them – when you bend forwards and jerk a heavy shopping bag from the boot of a car, for example. Another common cause is an unexpected demand for muscle activity after a period of inaction – playing three sets of tennis, for example, after months of inactivity.

A muscle either contracts when it has been strained or goes into spasm, which has the effect of protecting damaged fibres. However, it also restricts blood flow, and this may lead not only to a chemical imbalance in the muscles, causing pain, but also to a painful build-up of pressure since the fluid in any swelling cannot disperse.

The risk of pulling a muscle is much reduced if sudden, jerky movements are kept to a minimum and warm-up and warm-down routines (see pages 114–19) are carried out before and after any exercise.

AT A GLANCE: Pulled muscles or tendons
Cause: sudden, jerky movements or excessive, unaccustomed exercise
Medical treatment: if pain continues for more than two weeks after physiotherapy treatment, it may be necessary to consult a doctor to rule out other problems, such as a deep-lying abscess
Physiotherapy: ultrasound, massage and friction techniques; specific exercises depending on the muscle or muscles involved
Self-help: RICE (see pages 74–75); self-massage (see page 73); exercises (see pages 78–111)
Avoidance: maintain correct posture (see pages 20–27); avoid jerky movements; warm-up and warm-down (see pages 114–19)
Prognosis: good – minor strains usually clear up in two weeks

Sprains

Ligaments act as stabilisers to joints, so when a joint is forced to allow movement outside its normal range the ligaments stabilising that joint are likely to be stretched or torn: the result is a sprain.

Most people have sprained an ankle at some time. Usually, the ankle twists inwards and in doing so wrenches the three ligaments that stabilise the joint where the fibula joins the talus (see page 64). The fibres of the ligaments are torn, or sometimes completely ruptured, and in severe cases the ligaments inside the joint may be damaged as well. The result is bleeding and inflammation around the joint, and the muscles of the ankle strap go into spasm to protect the ankle and prevent it moving.

Unfortunately, movement is necessary if the joint is to disperse swelling efficiently and prevent the formation of scar tissue. And if the swelling is not fully dispersed, and the muscles do not relax completely, the joint will lose some of its range of movements – especially inward movement (inversion) in the case of the ankle.

For a sprained ankle, this, in turn, reduces the flexibility of the foot, so that any irregularity in the surface on which you walk will cause pain, tenderness and more swelling. Each time this happens, the ankle becomes a little weaker and more likely to turn over once more – further reducing the range of movements.

The way out of this vicious circle is to take appropriate steps to relieve the swelling and help it disperse as quickly as possible, and to embark on an exercise regime that will strengthen the muscles.

AT A GLANCE: Sprains
Cause: torn or ruptured ligaments as a result of wrenching
Medical treatment: X-ray to exclude possibility of fracture; rarely, surgical suture of a torn ligament
Physiotherapy: ice and air splints; ultrasound treatment; for ankle: balancing exercises
Self-help: ice (see page 70); elastic support for 48 hours; for ankle: balancing exercises (see page 73); walk barefoot as much as possible
Avoidance: maintenance exercises (see pages 130–31); correct posture (see pages 20–27); sensible shoes
Prognosis: good, with treatment

Bruises

If blood vessels beneath the skin are ruptured by a blow or by pressure, but the skin does not break, blood collects in the tissues to form a bruise. The colour of the bruise changes as the blood loses its oxygen content and is broken down: at first it is red, then purplish, then brown, and, finally, yellow. A blow to a bone may cause the periosteum that lines it to be lifted from it and blood to accumulate beneath it. A bruise that appears a few days after a fall may indicate that a bone has been fractured: if you are unsure, consult a doctor.

Normally, a bruise is obvious to the eye, but sometimes bruising can occur deep in the tissue of a muscle or inside a joint. In this case the bruise is known as a 'haematoma', and in serious cases it may be necessary for a doctor to aspirate the blood – to remove it by means of a syringe – to relieve pressure and ease pain. Medical intervention may also be necessary if superficial bruising occurs in those who are particularly prone to difficulty in stopping bleeding: the elderly, and sufferers from scurvy or haemophilia (a blood-clotting disorder).

Generally, however, the amount of bleeding – and, therefore, bruising – can be limited by compression and by packing ice around the area.

AT A GLANCE: Bruises
Cause: a blow or pressure
Medical treatment: rarely needed, though aspiration of blood may be necessary in some cases
Physiotherapy: compression and ice treatment followed by exercises for the muscles in the affected area. In cases of intra-muscular haematoma, deep friction may be used to break down clots and aid reabsorption
Self-help: RICE (see pages 74–75)
Avoidance: difficult. If you know that your blood does not clot easily, take advice from a doctor and try to avoid everyday bumps and knocks
Prognosis: good – most bruises clear up in a few days, though the precise length of time depends on the extent of the bleeding

Fibrositis

When there is unexplained pain and tenderness in muscles – especially those in the upper back – the problem is often referred to as 'fibrositis'. This is a catch-all phrase that does not refer to any specific condition, but to a set of symptoms that may have some connection with psychological stress, though they may also be attributable to conditions such as a thoracic kyphosis (see page 49). As such, there is no specific treatment for fibrositis, other than exercises and, sometimes, anti-inflammatory drugs.

AT A GLANCE: Fibrositis
Cause: varies; may be connected to psychological stress
Medical treatment: anti-inflammatory drugs
Physiotherapy: exercising the affected area
Self-help: exercise affected area (see pages 78–111)
Avoidance: correct posture (see pages 20–27); manage stress (see pages 32–33)
Prognosis: good, if the root cause is dealt with

Tendinitis and tenosynovitis

When the outer sheath of a muscle's tendon becomes inflamed as a result of an unusual or repeated movement that puts strain on it, the condition is known as 'tendinitis'. However, when the synovial lining of the tendon's sheath becomes inflamed too, the condition is called 'tenosynovitis'.

AT A GLANCE: Tendinitis
(see also *supraspinatus* tendinitis, page 54)
Cause: unusual action inflaming outer sheath of tendon
Medical treatment: hydrocortisone injection around tendon at painful spot – sometimes this is curative
Physiotherapy: gentle traction, friction and graduated stretching exercises to ease the inflammation
Self-help: exercise affected area (see pages 78–111)
Avoidance: maintenance exercises for area affected
Prognosis: good

AT A GLANCE: Tenosynovitis
(see also acute frictional tenosynovitis, page 58)
Cause: unaccustomed repetitive movements inflaming synovial lining of tendon sheath
Medical treatment: injection of steroid anti-inflammatories into the tendon sheath; anti-inflammatory drugs
Physiotherapy: ice and immobilisation; graduated stretching exercises to ease inflammation
Self-help: ice or splint (see pages 74–75); exercises (see pages 78–111)
Avoidance: warm-up; take breaks during repetitive work and move the joints involved through their range
Prognosis: good

Bursitis

Any inflammation within a bursa (see page 14) is known as 'bursitis'. The condition is generally the result of excessive pressure or strain on the bursa.

AT A GLANCE: Bursitis
(see also housemaid's knee, page 63)
Cause: excessive pressure on a bursa
Medical treatment: aspirating fluid; steroid injections; anti-inflammatory drugs; surgical removal of the bursa
Physiotherapy: RICE; ultrasound; graded exercises
Self-help: RICE (see pages 74–75)
Avoidance: limit time of any undue pressure on area
Prognosis: good

THE NECK AND BACK

The spine is the most complex of all the elements of the skeleton, both in terms of structure and function. In fact, the demands that we place on our spines are such that it would be impossible for a single joint to accommodate them: the spine must be sufficiently strong to hold the head upright, level and balanced, and strong enough, too, to anchor the muscles that contract to move the lower limbs; yet at the same time, it must be flexible enough to allow the ribs to rise as we breathe in, and to make twisting and bending possible. And it must also protect the spinal canal, which carries the nerves that link the brain to the rest of the body.

The solution to this design problem is an elegant one. Flexibility and strength are combined in a spinal column that comprises 33 individual bones, or vertebrae. Each joint between them allows only limited movement, but together the movements give the spine considerable flexibility without sacrificing strength. There are five groups of vertebrae: cervical, in the neck; thoracic, in the chest; lumbar, in the low back; sacral, between the buttocks; and coccygeal, at the spine's base.

Spinal joints

The flexibility of the spine is further enhanced by the nature of the joint between each vertebra. In fact, I should say 'joints', because each vertebra is connected to the one above it – and below it, too – by three separate joints. First, there is the intervertebral joint. A layer of cartilage – called the 'annulus fibrosus' – links each vertebra. Its centre is full of a viscous, gel-like substance – rather like a chewy centre in a boiled sweet – that is 85 per cent water. This central area acts not only as a shock absorber, but as a ball bearing that allows the spine to bend and twist. (The water content reduces with age, so limiting the amount of movement that is possible.)

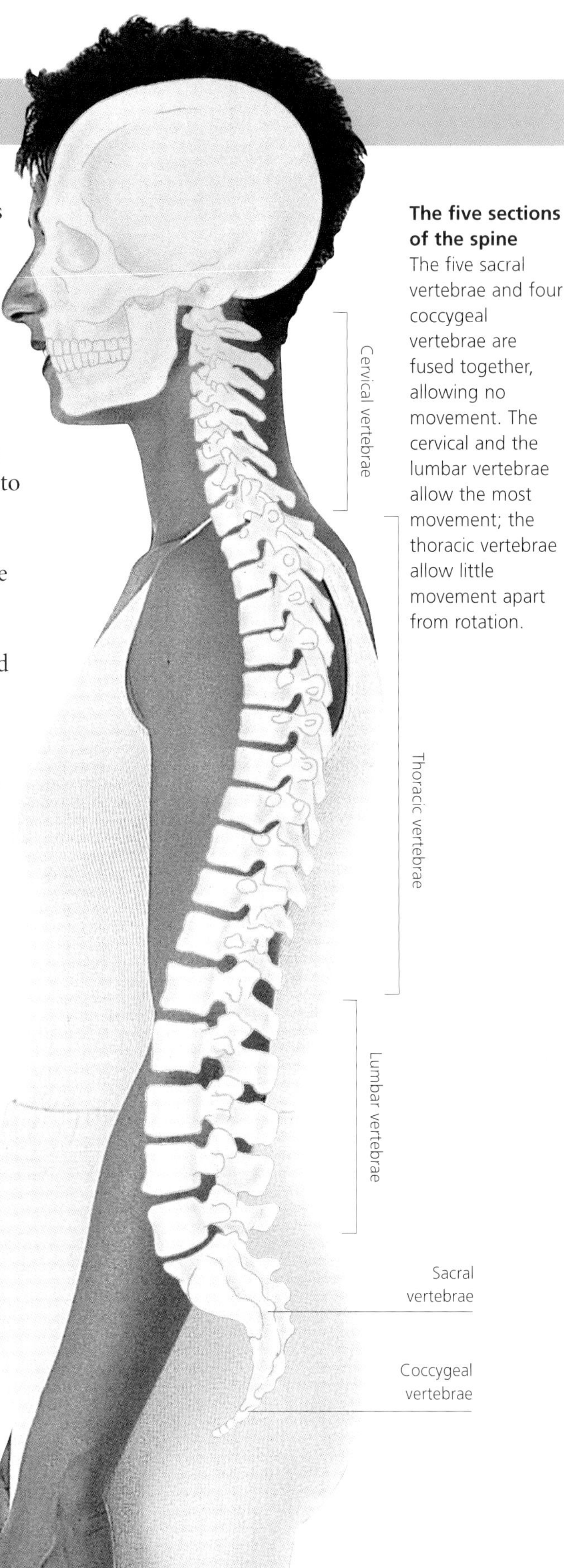

The five sections of the spine The five sacral vertebrae and four coccygeal vertebrae are fused together, allowing no movement. The cervical and the lumbar vertebrae allow the most movement; the thoracic vertebrae allow little movement apart from rotation.

Then there are two synovial plane joints (see page 17) – called 'facet joints', because they have smooth, even surfaces like the facets of a diamond – above and below each vertebra. They form bony catches that link the vertebrae together in a chain, preventing each one from slipping off the next. Strength and stability are also provided by a network of small ligaments that runs between the vertebrae, and by two long, strong ligaments that run the length of the spine at the front and back of the body.

The thoracic vertebrae also have two other simple plane joints, between the vertebrae and the ribs. These only allow a limited range of gliding movements when breathing in and out.

The atlas is joined to the axis by a pivot joint: the atlas swivels on the central peg (dotted) of the axis to rotate the head.

The axis, atlas and skull
The joints between the first and second vertebra (the atlas and axis) and between the atlas and the skull are different from the other spinal joints. The first, the joint between the atlas and the skull, is condylar, and allows the head to rock backwards and forwards, in a nodding action; the second (above) is a pivot joint.

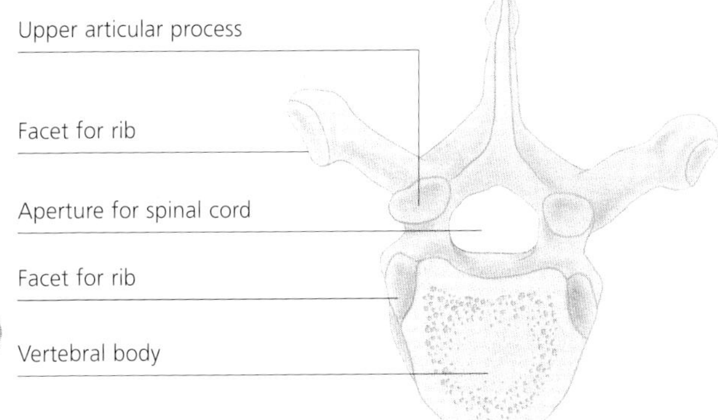

Plane joints
This cross-section of a thoracic vertebra shows the two upper articular processes, which are linked to the lower articular processes of the next vertebra up by plane joints. Below them are the facets where the ribs are joined to the vertebra by simple plane joints. Both types only allow a limited range of gliding movement.

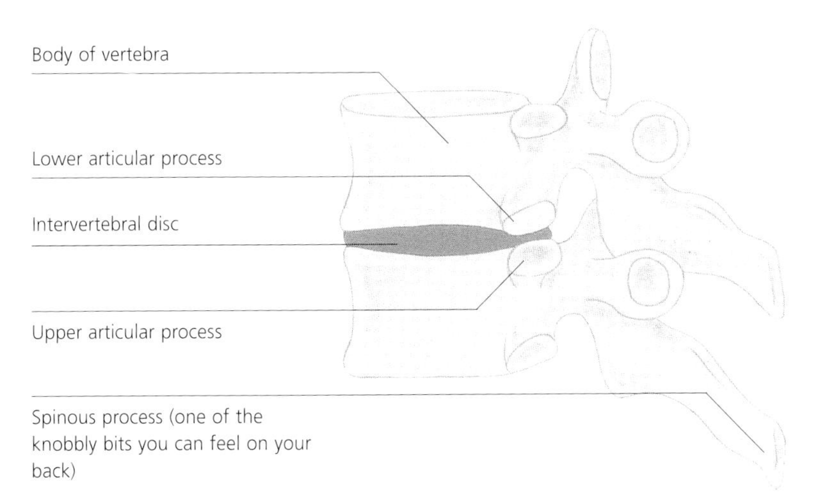

Vertebral joints
Each vertebra is joined to the one above and below it by three separate joints. A layer of cartilage – the disc – joins the cartilage lined surfaces of each vertebra to form the intervertebral joint. Then plane joints link the upper articular processes of each vertebra with the lower articular processes of the next one. And, in the case of thoracic vertebra, plane joints link the ribs to the vertebral body.

Growing overnight
The weight of the body on the intervertebral discs exerts such pressure that each disc can shrink by as much as ten per cent during the day. However, the discs take up water and nutrients during sleep and expand overnight to their full height once more. That is why you can wake up about an inch taller than when you went to bed!

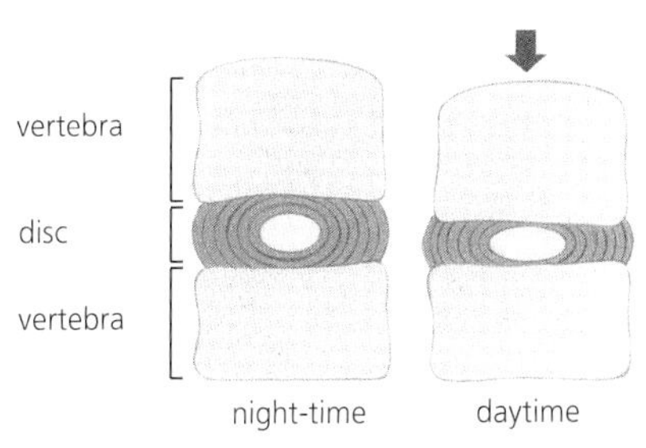

Neck and back complaints

Acute neck pain

With age, pregnancy or poor posture from muscular tension (see pages 20–27), the ligaments surrounding the cervical vertebrae in the neck become looser and have more give in them. This reduction in their stabilising power means that any sudden movement – it may be as simple as brushing your hair or as obvious as a whiplash injury – can disturb one of a vertebra's facet joints. When this happens, the surrounding muscles knot up in a spasm in order to protect the area: it feels as if your neck is 'locked' and unable to move. The main muscles involved are the extensors at the back and sides of the neck, but the small muscles that run from vertebra to vertebra also go into spasm. The condition, known as acute neck pain, causes considerable discomfort, with a deep ache and a feeling that your head is so heavy that it could fall off.

If an intervertebral disc has also been wrenched, the condition is even more painful and less movement is possible. There may also be some swelling; this may impinge on a nerve, causing pins and needles or shooting pains down its course. If the ligaments are strained, too, there is likely to be a dull ache when at rest, but any movement made to ease the ache will cause acute twinges across the shoulders, into the head or down the back.

Without proper treatment, the joint involved is unlikely to recover its full range of small movements and will always be an unstable link in the neck, which may lock at the slightest excuse.

▲ **MEDICAL ALERT** The course of the vertebral arteries as they run up the cervical spine to supply the brain lies just in front of the facet joints. This means that any arthritic changes to the joints (such as swelling or the growth of bony protrusions) may impinge on the arteries. The result can be transient blackouts, dizziness and blurred vision, particularly when looking up or moving suddenly. Do not attempt to mobilise the neck muscles if any such symptoms are felt. See your doctor without delay.

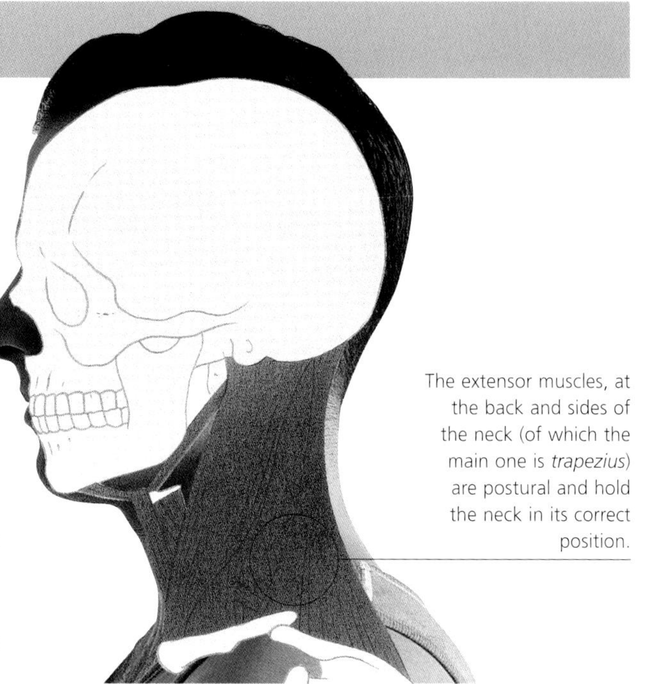

The extensor muscles, at the back and sides of the neck (of which the main one is *trapezius*) are postural and hold the neck in its correct position.

Why the neck locks
Looseness of the ligaments stabilising the cervical vertebra – often due to poor posture – allows facet joints to be disturbed. In response to tissue damage the muscles go into spasm to protect the affected area: inflammation increases and the neck locks.

The problem is compounded by the natural compression of the cervical spine during movement, which increases inflammation by jamming any affected joints together.

AT A GLANCE: Acute neck pain
Cause: a strain or rupture of cervical ligaments and misalignment of facet joints between vertebrae as a result of a sudden, unprotected movement of the neck
Medical treatment: X-ray to check for fracture; injection of steroids to reduce inflammation; rarely, sclerosant therapy (injection of a fibrous tissue irritant into the ligament near the bone junction to thicken and strengthen the ligament)
Physiotherapy: rest; soft collar; traction; posture correction; lifting instruction; neck exercises
Self-help: wear a soft collar (see page 70); mobilise gently with neck exercises (see pages 78–79); in acute stage, avoid gardening, housework, DIY tasks and driving
Avoidance: maintain flexibility of neck and thorax; maintain correct posture (see pages 20–27); ease neck tension using relaxation techniques (see pages 32–33)
Prognosis: good, unless the problem recurs frequently

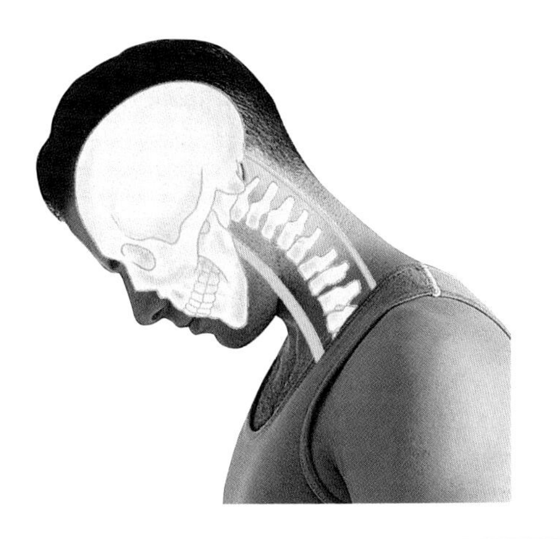

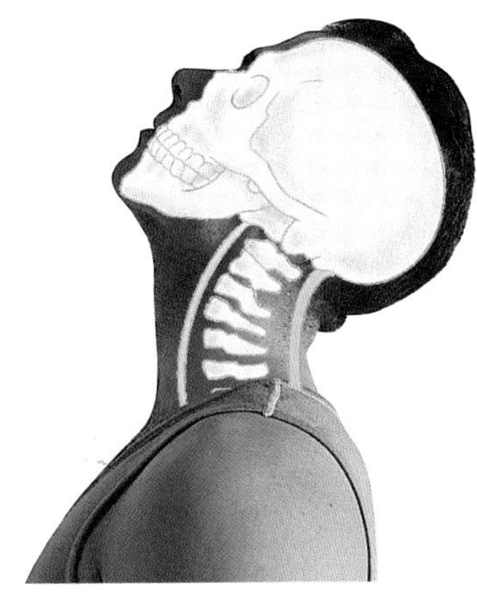

Whiplash injuries
Sudden, unexpected movement of the head forwards and then back can cause damage ranging from strained ligaments to broken cervical vertebrae.

▲ **MEDICAL ALERT** Typically caused by a head-on car crash, whiplash is a serious injury. As with any back injury, it is vital that the victim is not moved until the situation has been assessed by medical staff. Call an ambulance.

Thoracic kyphosis

The spine has a natural outward curve in its thoracic region (where the ribs connect to it), both to allow room for the lungs and chest and to make it more efficient at absorbing the stresses of movement. If this curve becomes excessive, giving a humpback and a sunken chest, it is said to be a 'kyphosis'. Occasionally a kyphosis is present from birth, and sometimes it is caused by a condition such as ankylosing spondylitis (see page 80) or osteoporosis (see page 43). The most common cause, however, is poor posture (see pages 20–27).

A kyphosis is usually associated with drooping, rounded shoulders and a head that is held too far forwards. (The condition is linked with obesity, because excess weight moves the body's centre of gravity forwards, making it easier to allow the head and shoulders to move forwards.) The weight of the head is such that the *trapezius* muscles of the upper back are in a constant state of mild contraction as they try to prevent the head falling further forwards and to pull it back into alignment with the shoulders.

In time, particular areas – trigger points – in the muscles go into spasm and become knotted and painful (see fibrositis, page 45). In severe cases, breathing may become less efficient. The intervertebral discs are affected, too, because the incorrect positioning of the cervical and thoracic vertebrae exposes them to wear and tear. The result can be the early onset of osteoarthritis (see page 42) and, without treatment, permanent damage.

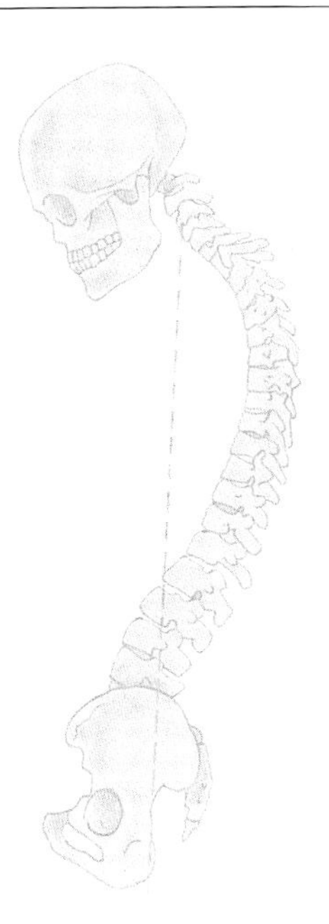

'Dowager's hump'
The excessive outward curvature of the spine in thoracic kyphosis increases wear and tear on the vertebrae, makes muscles go into spasm and impedes breathing. The most common cause is poor posture, though the condition can be the result of osteoporosis – especially in elderly women, when it is known as 'dowager's hump'.

AT A GLANCE: Thoracic kyphosis
Cause: poor posture (see pages 20–27)
Medical treatment: injections of hydrocortisone and painkillers into the painful areas of the spine – generally the facet joints – and advice on weight loss and posture; surgery is sometimes an option
Physiotherapy: deep friction massage to trigger points and posture correction and re-education
Self-help: correct posture (see pages 20–27); back exercises (see pages 82–85); shoulder exercises (see pages 88–89); lose weight if appropriate (see pages 30–31)
Avoidance: maintain correct posture (see pages 20–27); adequate exercise
Prognosis: good if a diagnosis is made early, but there may be permanent damage to the joints if this is delayed

Sciatica and slipped disc

This may seem a strange heading, but there is so much confusion about what exactly sciatica and a slipped disc are that it makes much more sense to deal with them together.

'Slipped disc' is a misleading term that is often used to describe a problem that does not involve an intervertebral disc at all, such as damage to the soft tissues. In a true slipped disc, the gelatinous core of an intervertebral disc – rather than the disc itself – protrudes through its fibrous outer covering; the disc does not move. Sometimes this causes pressure on a spinal nerve. If it does, there will be pain along the course of the nerve. On other occasions there is no pressure on any nerve, and there is only mild local pain. Sometimes, however, it impinges on the spinal cord, in which case there is acute pain in that area of the spine. If a pain is felt suddenly after a fall it is sensible to assume that a disc has 'slipped' in the third of these ways, and to seek medical advice.

Sciatica, on the other hand, is not a condition but a set of symptoms caused by pressure on a spinal nerve – in this case the sciatic nerve, the longest nerve in the body. This pressure can have a number of causes. One is a protrusion of the core of the disc between the vertebrae from which the roots of the sciatic nerve emerge (the lowest two lumbar vertebrae and the first three sacral ones). But more often the pressure on the nerve comes from inflammation of the facet joints of the vertebrae. Other possible causes for the pressure are pregnancy – the intervertebral joints are made less stable by a hormone of pregnancy that causes ligaments to relax – osteoarthritis of the lumbar spine, and a narrowing of the spinal canal.

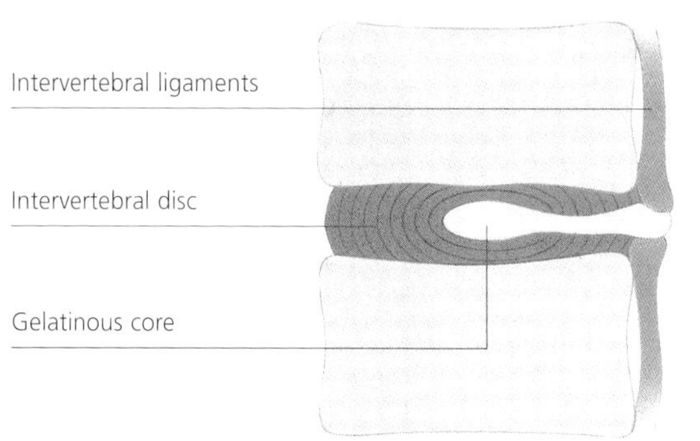

Slipped disc
The intervertebral disc itself does not 'slip' in a slipped disc: its core protrudes through its outer covering to put pressure on the nearby tissues – the intervertebral ligaments here, causing mild local pain.

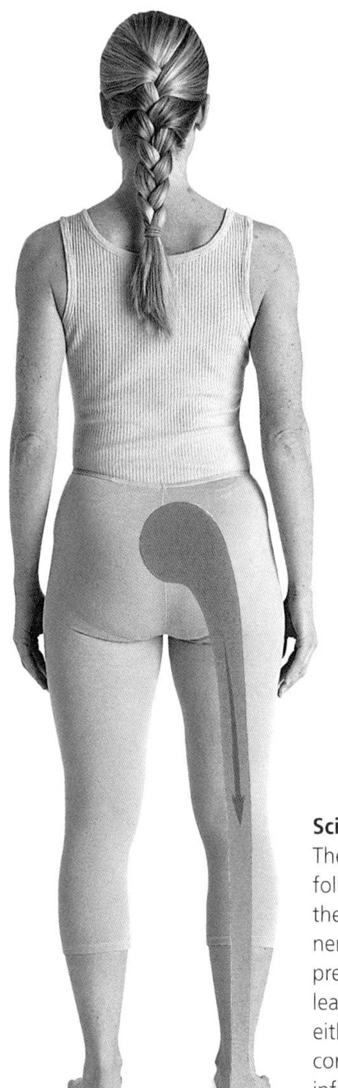

Sciatica
The pain of sciatica can follow the whole course of the sciatic nerve, the longest nerve in the body. Its cause is pressure on the nerve as it leaves the spinal cord – either from the protruding core of a disc, or from inflammation of the facet joints of the vertebrae.

The result is an acute, severe pain down the course of the area served by the nerve. This pain is often unrelenting, whatever your position, and may be accompanied by numbness or pins and needles in the associated area of skin (see skin patterns, page 41). How far the pain extends depends on which part of the nerve root is pinched, and how much pressure is involved. At its worst, the pain can radiate through the hip and buttocks, down the back of the thigh and calf and into the foot.

Whether caused by a slipped disc or an inflammation of a facet joint, the majority of cases of sciatica clear up on their own within a few weeks: the gelatinous disc is reabsorbed or the inflammation goes down. Basic treatment can hasten this, and is the same for both causes: bed rest for at least 24 hours in acute cases, followed by gentle mobilisation to prevent the problem from becoming chronic. If the disc is not reabsorbed, manipulation and traction or surgery may be necessary; if the inflammation does not reduce, it may be necessary to inject anti-inflammatory steroids and painkillers into the facet joint.

The root causes of both sciatica and a slipped disc are poor posture, poor lifting techniques and strenuous activity without adequate maintenance of the musculo-skeletal system and direct preparation for the activity.

AT A GLANCE: Sciatica and slipped disc
Cause: poor posture; incorrect lifting techniques; unusual arduous activity (such as gardening, squash, aerobics)
Medical treatment: local injection of steroid anti-inflammatories and painkillers; rarely, surgical fusion of intervertebral joints or removal of bony outgrowths or disc protrusion
Physiotherapy: traction and manipulation; posture re-education; mobilising exercises; back exercises
Self-help: correct posture (see pages 20–27); exercises to increase range and strength of muscles (see pages 82–85)
Avoidance: carry out warm-up and warm-down routines (see pages 114–19); maintain correct posture (see pages 20–27); back maintenance exercises (see pages 126–27)
Prognosis: good unless the condition becomes chronic, when orthopaedic surgery may be required

Chronic low back pain

Even though back pain accounts for more working days lost in the industrialised world than any other medical disorder, its cause can often not be established. And the continuous nagging ache of a bad back seems even more frustrating when nothing can be found to account for it. The reason for this diagnostic difficulty is that the spine is such a complex mechanism. The lumbar region in particular has to cope with considerable stress and strain that can adversely affect the muscles, tendons, ligaments, joints and nerves. It only requires minor damage to this area to cause low back pain.

The most common cause of chronic low back pain is compression of the lumbar vertebrae. As a result, the intervertebral discs shrink and the facet joints (see page 47) become jammed together causing the joints to become inflamed. Sometimes the edges of the vertebral bodies wear away, too, or grow bony spurs called osteophytes (see page 62).

Compression of the vertebrae can result from muscular imbalance or a weakness of the muscles – especially the abdominal ones, since these act as a support for the front of the spine – which may, in turn, result from poor posture. Sitting for extended periods also causes disc compression, and wearing high heels places unnatural stresses on the spinal muscles and ligaments. With age, too, the intervertebral discs naturally lose some of their water content and their fibrous outer rings become more brittle and may develop cracks from which the inner fluid can leak out. If this fluid presses on any nerve tissue, a ligament, the sheath of the spinal cord or a joint, pain will be the result.

The danger is that any sudden strain to an area of the back that has already suffered some damage can cause an attack of acute back pain (see sciatica and slipped disc, opposite).

▲ **MEDICAL ALERT** If low back pain is sufficiently severe during the night to wake you up or to prevent you from going to sleep, consult your doctor so that he or she can rule out the possibility that a disorder that is not musculo-skeletal is responsible.

AT A GLANCE: Chronic low back pain
Cause: poor posture; weak muscles; incorrect lifting; osteoarthritis; degenerative disc disease; often unknown
Medical treatment: painkillers; referral to a physiotherapist; X-ray
Physiotherapy: exercises to increase muscle strength and flexibility; lifting and carrying instruction; posture correction
Self-help: correct posture (see pages 20–27); exercises (see pages 82–85); learn to lift (see page 27); see an osteopath or chiropractor
Avoidance: keep fit; always warm up (see pages 114–17) before strenuous exercise – especially gardening or DIY tasks; avoid high heels; avoid taking too many painkillers
Prognosis: treatment and a maintenance programme can reduce length and frequency of attacks

THE ARM

The range of movements available to our arms is a reflection of the vital role they play in our survival. However, as you will see, this flexibility is only achieved at the expense of some stability.

The shoulder joint

The shoulder joint is surrounded by a circle of bones known as the shoulder girdle. This comprises the shoulder joints themselves, between the arms and the shoulder-blades (scapulae); the joints between each collar bone (clavicle) and the end (acromion) of each scapula; and the joints between each clavicle and the breastbone (sternum). However, the shoulder girdle is not just made up of bone and joints, because the shoulder-blades do not attach directly to the spine at the back, but are connected to the rib cage by muscles. This increases the range of movements that the shoulder-blade and arm can make.

All the joints of the shoulder girdle play their part in enabling movement of the arm through a system of checks and counter-balances in which the short, postural muscles play the major part. The most important joint is the ball and socket joint between the arm and the shoulder-blade. However, it has several key weaknesses. For example, the socket into which the upper arm bone (humerus) fits – called the glenoid cavity – is very shallow and relatively small. Rather than cupping the ball of the humerus, it is saucer-shaped and little larger than a bottle cap. And its rim, made of fibrous and

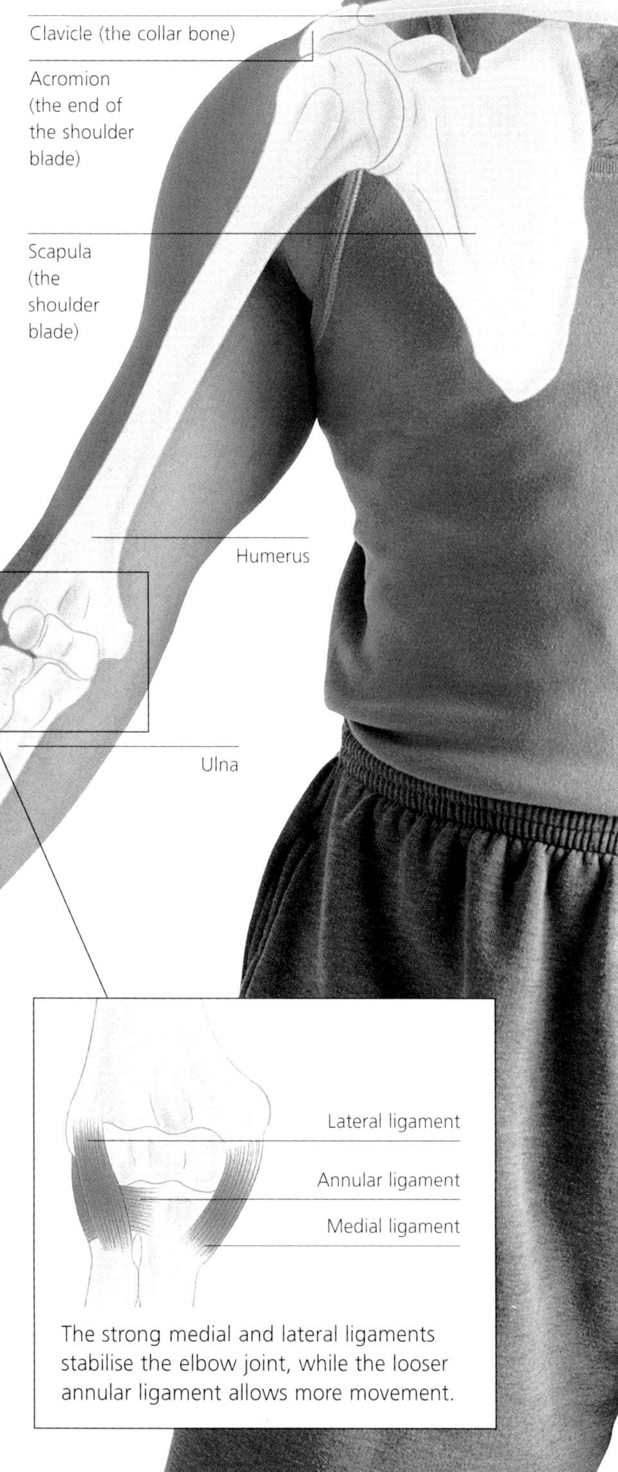

The strong medial and lateral ligaments stabilise the elbow joint, while the looser annular ligament allows more movement.

cartilaginous tissue, is also weak compared to that of the hip joint. In addition, the three short ligaments that protect the joint are somewhat inefficient and unstable. As a result, the joint's stability relies to a great extent on its short, protective muscles – the rotator cuff muscles – which are phasic rather than postural (see page 23), and so are easily damaged.

This all means that the joint is not only prone to dislocation, but also to malfunction as a result of weakening or tearing of the rotator cuff muscles.

The elbow joint

A simple synovial hinge joint that, like all hinge joints, only allows movement in one plane, connects the humerus, the bone of the upper arm, and the radius and ulna, the two bones of the forearm. In this case it allows the elbow to bend (flex) and stretch (extend). However, the simplicity of this arrangement is complicated by the presence of another joint: a pivot joint that shares the same joint capsule and allows the radius to revolve around the ulna to turn the hand palm-up – supination – and palm-down – pronation – (see page 15).

The elbow is given considerable stability by its surrounding muscles and by a strong ligament that runs on each side of it, but this stability is at the expense of some flexibility – there is little 'give' in the joint. By contrast, the annular ligament around the pivot joint, which is attached to the ulna and forms a ring within which the radius can swivel, is more flexible. However, this can sometimes tighten up, especially after any blow or strain to the area, and so cause a loss of the ability to rotate the arm. This inhibits pronation and supination, which are necessary, for example, for many hand movements.

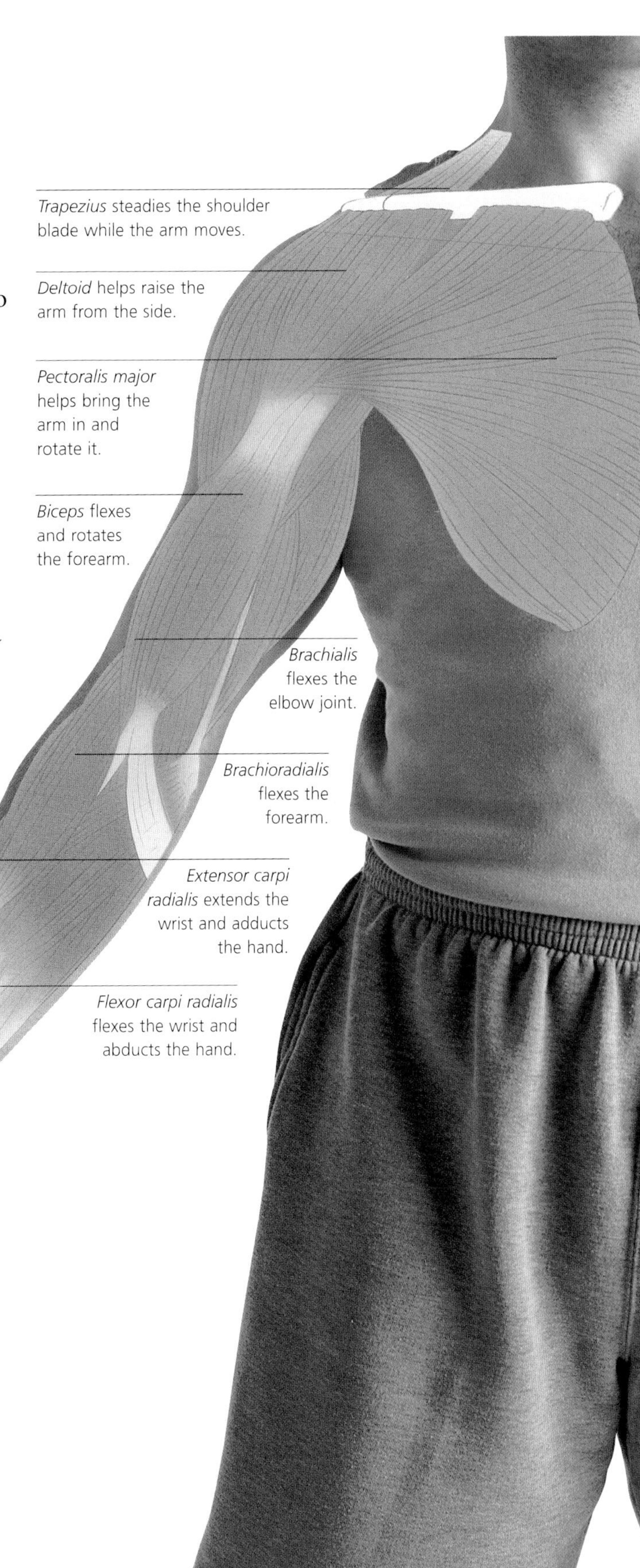

Trapezius steadies the shoulder blade while the arm moves.

Deltoid helps raise the arm from the side.

Pectoralis major helps bring the arm in and rotate it.

Biceps flexes and rotates the forearm.

Brachialis flexes the elbow joint.

Brachioradialis flexes the forearm.

Extensor carpi radialis extends the wrist and adducts the hand.

Flexor carpi radialis flexes the wrist and abducts the hand.

Arm complaints

Painful arc syndrome

Also known as '*supraspinatus* tendinitis', painful arc syndrome is caused by inflammation of the tendon of the muscle *supraspinatus*. This is one of the rotator cuff muscles (see below right) whose flattened tendons stabilise the shoulder joint; it also works with *deltoid* to lift the arm straight out to the side.

Intrinsic design weaknesses make this muscle vulnerable: it has little power, and can easily be strained by unaccustomed repetitive actions, a sudden wrench or a blow. If this happens, it will not work fluently and its tendon will be chafed by the collar bone, causing inflammation and soreness. And once the problem has set in, any activity that involves lifting your arm can result in a shooting pain.

It is easy to tell if you have *supraspinatus* tendinitis: raise your arm directly out from the side, palm down. If you feel pain between 60 and 120 degrees, the *supraspinatus* tendon is inflamed. Repeat the manoeuvre, palm up: there will not be any pain – unless the condition is advanced – as the tendon does not now slide over the shoulder blade.

It is vital that you seek medical treatment for painful arc syndrome, because you are likely to make awkward movements in an attempt to avoid the pain. These may, in turn, cause problems in the other muscles of the rotator cuff that may require surgical repair, and, before long, you may well have a frozen shoulder (see below).

AT A GLANCE: Painful arc syndrome (*Supraspinatus* tendinitis)
Cause: strain of *supraspinatus* muscle, followed by chafing on upper part of collar bone
Medical treatment: hydrocortisone injection into bursa around tendon at painful spot
Physiotherapy: aims to ease inflammation by means of gentle traction, friction and graduated stretching exercises
Self-help: exercises (see pages 88–89)
Avoidance: exercises (see pages 120–21)
Prognosis: good

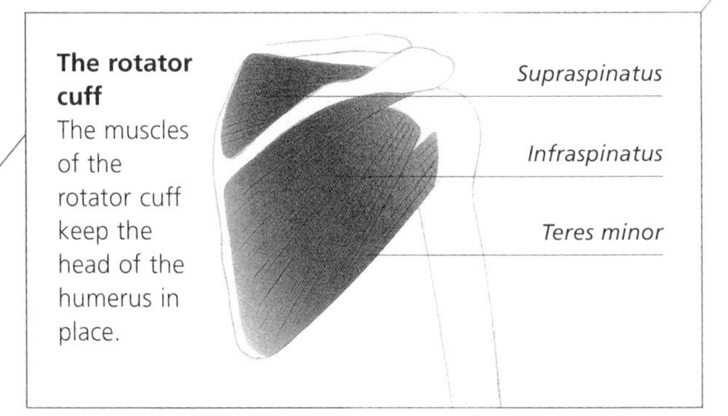

The rotator cuff
The muscles of the rotator cuff keep the head of the humerus in place.

Frozen shoulder

Also known as 'adhesive capsulitis', a frozen shoulder is the most common problem to affect the shoulder joint, and is a particular risk for those over 50. It can be triggered by *supraspinatus* tendinitis, or by frequent, and often tiny, strains to the rotator cuff muscles, causing inflammation of the capsule of the shoulder joint and severe pain.

Little or no movement of the joint is possible. So, instead of trying to move the joint, those affected tend to hunch their shoulders in an attempt to use the muscles attached to the shoulder blade; there is pain in the upper third of the outer arm, too. Lying on the arm is uncomfortable, with the result that those affected wake frequently during the night. Sudden, unguarded movement can send a shooting pain down the arm, and this often leads sufferers to believe that they have a muscular problem in the upper arm rather than in the shoulder. Unfortunately, trying to push through the pain barrier to achieve full mobility only exacerbates the problem. Seek advice from your doctor, though treatment tends to be effective only in relieving pain and preventing further damage rather than curative.

AT A GLANCE: Frozen shoulder
Cause: *supraspinatus* tendinitis; or frequent small strains of the rotator cuff muscles from using these muscles to help with carrying heavy items
Medical treatment: hydrocortisone injection into tendons at painful spots; in persistent cases, muscles and tendons are manipulated under a general anaesthetic to increase mobility, and tissue adhesions are cut away
Physiotherapy: gentle traction, friction and graduated stretching exercises aimed to increase mobility of the joint
Self-help: exercises (see pages 88–89)
Avoidance: exercises (see pages 120–21)
Prognosis: most cases recover naturally within 12–18 months, with or without treatment

Tennis elbow

Despite its name, tennis elbow is far more likely to be caused by ironing or polishing than playing tennis. It is caused by unaccustomed repetitive movements of the forearm and the elbow joint when the wrist is held up – as when playing a backhand tennis stroke or ironing. The tendons of the wrist and finger extensors – the muscles that raise the back of the hand – tear where they attach to the elbow. Acute pain is felt around the outer bony knob at the lower end of the humerus and a dulling, nagging pain is felt along a broad band down the forearm. It can become painful to carry anything heavier than a sheet of paper, and activities such as shaking hands or turning a door knob become impossibly painful.

AT A GLANCE: Tennis elbow
Cause: repetitive movements of forearm with the wrist held up
Medical treatment: hydrocortisone injection into tendon at painful spot
Physiotherapy: gentle traction, friction and graduated stretching exercises to increase mobility
Self-help: exercises (see pages 92–93)
Avoidance: exercises (see pages 122–23)
Prognosis: tends to recur unless the root cause is avoided

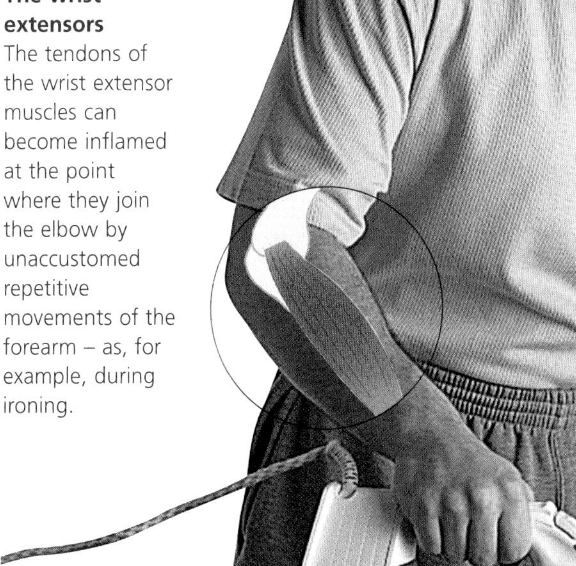

The wrist extensors
The tendons of the wrist extensor muscles can become inflamed at the point where they join the elbow by unaccustomed repetitive movements of the forearm – as, for example, during ironing.

THE WRIST AND HAND

Our hands are designed to carry out a variety of highly specialised tasks, so it is hardly surprising that they contain some of the most complex, interlinked sequences of joints in the body. The hands are not only capable of transmitting considerable force, but also of undertaking extremely fine, delicate movements with great precision.

The wrist joint

The first part of the wrist joint is the lower of the two joints between the radius and ulna – the upper one being part of the elbow joint. The two bones are linked by a synovial pivot joint (see page 15) that allows the radius to pivot around the ulna, in order to rotate the hand palm down (pronation) and palm up (supination).

The bottom of this joint is sealed with a disc of fibrocartilage that forms the upper border of the wrist joint proper, that links with the cartilage lining the base of the radius. The wrist joint is a synovial ellipsoid joint (see page 17) – the only other such joints in the body being in the knuckles. Its lower border is made up of three small carpal bones and the ligaments that join them, and these are linked to other small bones by further joints. This arrangement makes a wide range of movements possible, and all of them are controlled by the tension of opposing muscles and by ligaments that link the bones together.

All the joints that make up the wrist are protected and stabilised by strong ligaments. This means that a fall on an outstretched hand is more likely to result in a fracture of the end of the radius or the scaphoid bone than damage to a joint.

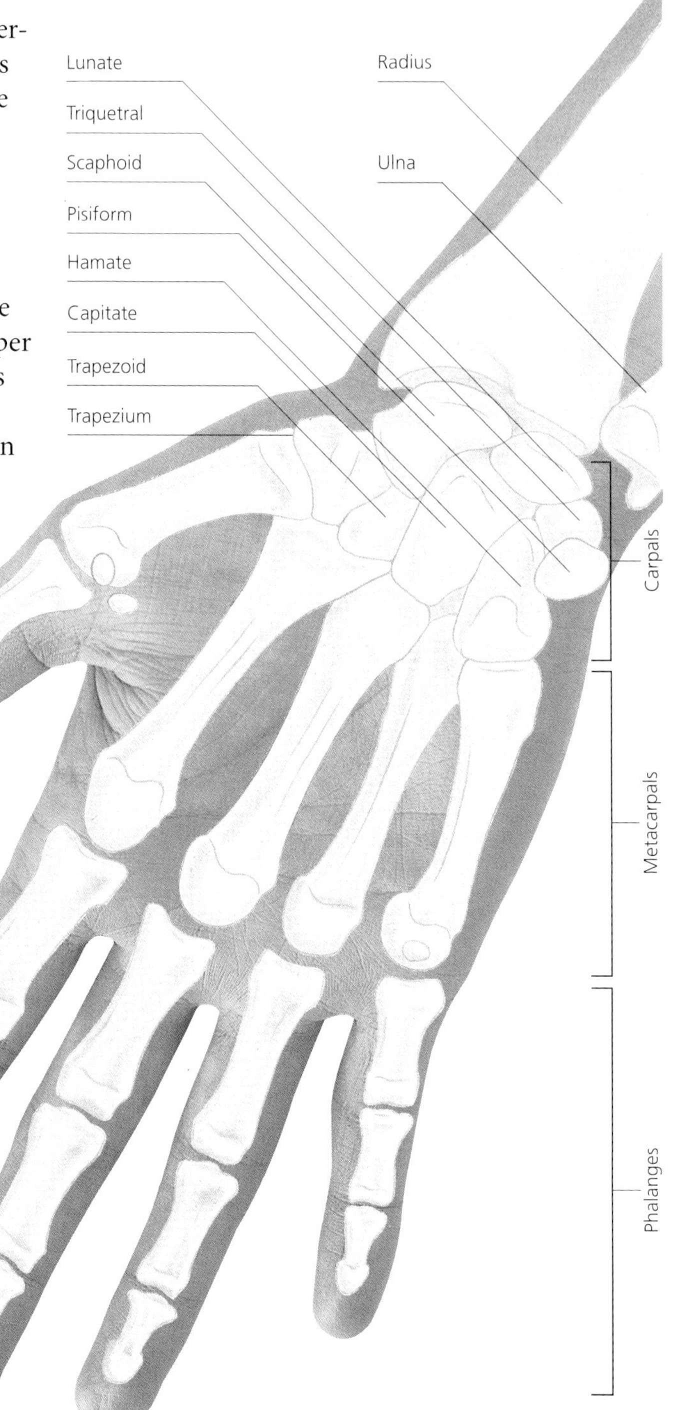

Twisting movements

The supinators are the muscles that rotate the hand palm up, and the pronators are the muscles that rotate the hand palm down. The supinators are stronger than the pronators, which means that a right-handed person can turn his or her wrist to the right with more force than to the left. This is why screws are traditionally manufactured with a right-hand thread.

Cracking your fingers

Each finger (and toe) is made up of three small bones that articulate with each other in simple hinge joints – interphalangeal joints – that allow flexion and extension and are stabilised by ligaments on either side. Purely because of the small size of these joints, little force is needed to stretch the synovial capsule: the resulting vacuum attracts the synovial fluid, and the noise you hear is caused by the fluid being sucked into the newly enlarged capsule. Much as children – and some adults – love to crack their fingers, it is not advisable to do so. The joint is being damaged each time it is cracked, and you could be storing up trouble for your old age.

The thumb and knuckles

The first carpo-metacarpal joint (the thumb joint) is a synovial saddle joint (see page 17). It is the only joint of this type in the body, and is unique to humans. In fact, the development of the saddle joint was vital to the process of human evolution, because it allows a range of movement that makes delicate, fine actions possible – grasping one piece of flint to fashion a tool out of another, for example.

There is a full range of movement in the joint, including flexion and extension, abduction and adduction, circumduction and a small amount of rotation, but the most important is the combination of movements that results in 'opposition' – unique to humans – in which the thumb moves across the palm to meet the fingers. It is made possible by the shape of the bones and the position of the surrounding ligaments. The thumb only produces one half of the movement, and so one side of a precise grip; the other half comes from the fingers.

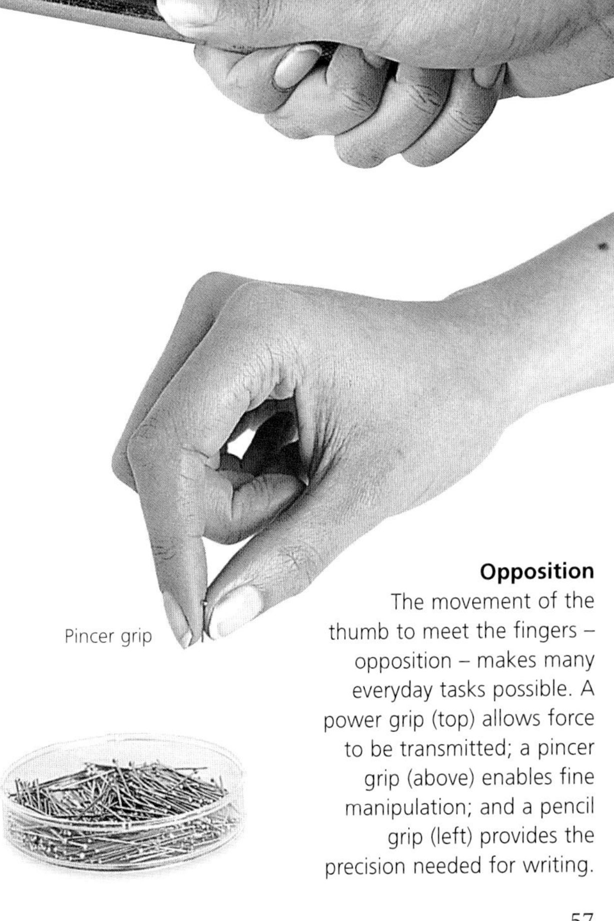

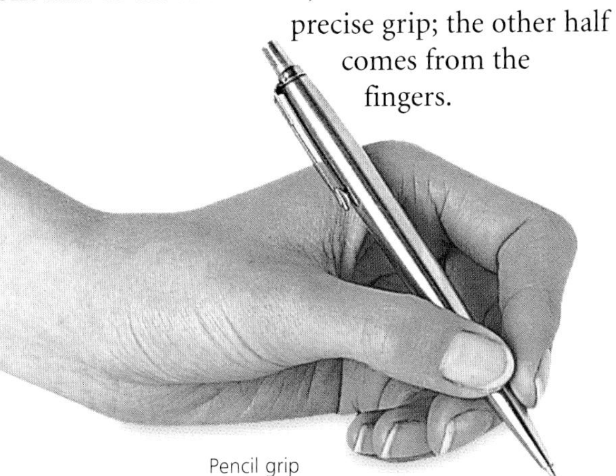

Opposition
The movement of the thumb to meet the fingers – opposition – makes many everyday tasks possible. A power grip (top) allows force to be transmitted; a pincer grip (above) enables fine manipulation; and a pencil grip (left) provides the precision needed for writing.

Wrist and hand complaints

Acute frictional tenosynovitis (AFT)

AFT has been recognised for some time, but it has recently become more widely known in Britain as repetitive strain injury (RSI) and in North America as cumulative trauma disorder (CTD). In this guise, it has become a blanket term used to cover not only AFT but also other symptoms that are more vague and subjective. All, however, tend to affect the hands and wrists of those who make frequent movements over a long period of time: keyboard operators, for example.

The variability of the symptoms of RSI/CTD makes it impossible to define the condition with any accuracy, especially as many of the more diffuse symptoms are thought to have strong psychological overtones, with few physical manifestations.

AFT, however, or 'true RSI', is an acute inflammation of the synovial sheaths of the numerous tendons that criss-cross the wrist. This is the result of holding the wrist in a fixed position while using the fingers over a long period when you are not used to doing so. When you are typing, for example, or playing the piano, the wrist is extended to an angle of about 20 degrees and kept still while the fingers tap the keys. However, the muscles that extend the wrist – the extensors – are phasic muscles, rather than postural ones (see page 23), so they are not designed to hold a position for any length of time.

The 12 tendons of the extensor muscles pass beneath a thick ligament – rather like a sweat band – on the wrist, and are protected from any friction as they do so by synovial sheaths that are full of fluid.

However, as the wrist muscles are not contracting and relaxing, but holding a position, less fluid is produced. The result is inflammation of the synovial sheaths – tenosynovitis – that can cause a shooting, burning pain when the tendon is moved. In fact, it is sometimes possible for those affected to feel the tendon grating within its sheath when they move their wrist.

AFT can be treated by injections, exercises and immobilisation, but it is best to prevent the problem from arising by training and taking frequent breaks from typing or other repetitive movements – individual cases vary, but five minutes or so, every half-an-hour is about right.

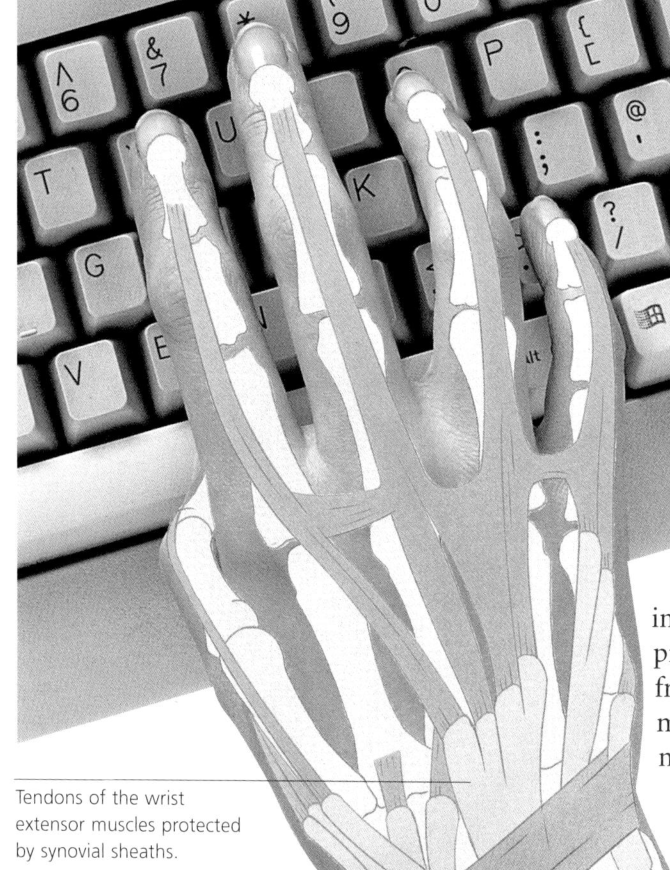

Tendons of the wrist extensor muscles protected by synovial sheaths.

Thick band of ligament (extensor retinaculum) across back of wrist.

How AFT develops

Synovial fluid within tendon sheaths protects them from friction, but its production depends on a full range of movements. Less is produced if an unaccustomed position is held for long periods, causing inflammation and pain.

AT A GLANCE: Acute frictional tenosynovitis (CTD/RSI)
Cause: unaccustomed repetitive movements of the hands and wrist
Medical treatment: injection of steroid anti-inflammatories into the tendon sheath; immobilisation by means of a splint for three weeks
Physiotherapy: ice and immobilisation for a few days; stretching exercises
Self-help: ice or splint (see page 70); exercises (see pages 96–97)
Avoidance: training; take frequent breaks during any repetitive work and move the joints through their whole range; improve work environment
Prognosis: good with adequate adjustment of working conditions

Carpal tunnel syndrome

On its way to the fingers the median nerve passes through a tunnel formed by the first row of carpal bones in the wrist and a ligament stretching across them. This is the carpal tunnel, and in carpal tunnel syndrome the nerve becomes compressed within it. Often there is no identifiable cause, although sometimes osteoarthritis of the wrist or chronic inflammation of the tendon sheaths (which also pass through the tunnel) may be responsible.

The syndrome can develop at any time during adulthood, but is more common in women than men. Certain factors predispose towards it: obesity (because of the extra weight of flesh in the area); pregnancy and diabetes (as a result of increased fluid retention); and prolonged activities using the hands and wrists that may cause inflammation affecting the tendons.

The first sign of the syndrome is a dull, numbing pain in the hand, which may wake you up at night or be felt in the morning, and pins and needles in the fingers (with the exception of the little finger); sometimes there is also pain in the arm and it may become difficult to push the thumb against the little finger. Sufferers often complain that their hands feel clumsy.

AT A GLANCE: Carpal tunnel syndrome
Cause: compression of the median nerve as it passes through the carpal tunnel of the wrist
Medical treatment: steroid injection into the carpal tunnel; a wrist splint; decompression by means of surgery
Physiotherapy: ice; exercises to stretch wrist flexors
Self-help: lose weight; work the wrist joint through its full range after carrying our repetitive movements (see pages 96–97)
Avoidance: maintain correct weight; stretch the wrist flexors (see pages 124–25); keep to a diet that discourages water retention
Prognosis: good if the problem is recognised early

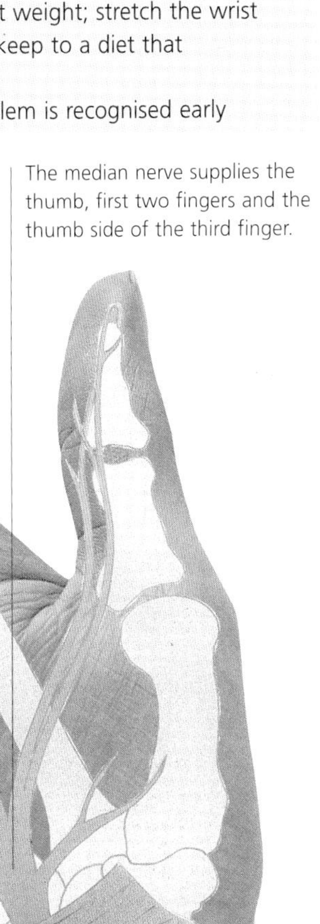

The median nerve supplies the thumb, first two fingers and the thumb side of the third finger.

The ulnar nerve supplies the last two fingers, but does not pass through the carpal tunnel.

The carpal tunnel is formed by the first row of carpal bones in the wrist and a ligament (flexor retinaculum) that stretches across and over them.

THE LEG

The hip joint

The pelvic girdle forms a solid mass of bone around the hips, knitted together at the front by a pad of cartilage at the pubic symphysis. The hip joint is more stable than the shoulder joint and, as a result, allows fewer movements.

In part, this stability derives from the depth of the cup-shaped socket – the acetabulum – of the hip bone and the large, spherical head of the thigh bone (femur), which is supported by a long shaft (or 'neck').

Then the capsule surrounding the joint is further strengthened by three ligaments: two at the front and one behind. The most important of these is the iliofemoral ligament. It is very strong, and, together with the short muscles around the joint, helps counteract the pull of gravity – if you draw the line of gravity through the body, it falls just behind the hip joint.

This level of protection for the joint means that, inevitably, its range of movement is reduced. So, while the leg can be bent forwards from the hip (flexion) to 120 degrees, it can only be extended backwards to 20 degrees, on average. This rigidity can cause problems. In the West, for instance, we tend to use a very limited range of hip movements. This seems to predispose us towards arthritis; certainly arthritis is less common in Asia, where people often sit cross-legged.

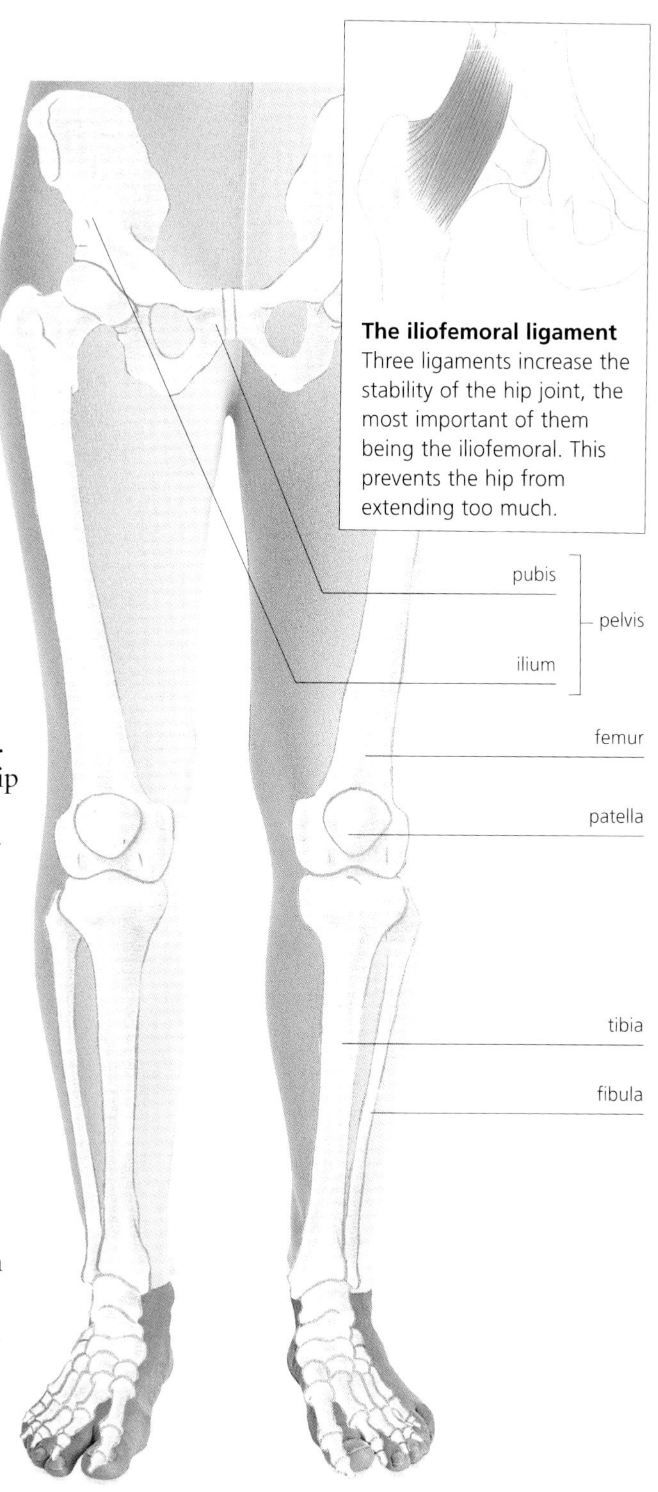

The iliofemoral ligament
Three ligaments increase the stability of the hip joint, the most important of them being the iliofemoral. This prevents the hip from extending too much.

The knee joint

Though three bones meet at the knee – the thigh bone, or femur, and the tibia and fibula in the lower leg – only the tibia and femur form part of the knee joint itself. The fibula, the slight bone on the outside of the leg, only acts as a point of attachment for some of the muscles of the foot; it does not take any part in weight-bearing.

The bottom of the femur looks rather like a downwards-pointing fist. Its two knuckle-like protuberances at each side – the condyles – fit into matching depressions in the head of the tibia, but are separated from them on each side by pieces of cartilage called the menisci.

The first level of protection for the knee is provided by two ligaments (called cruciate ligaments) running diagonally from each protuberance on the femur to the opposite depression in the tibia. These are often torn in sports injuries. Stability is also provided by the strong ligaments either side of the joint and by the muscles running over the joint. A different type of protection is offered by the kneecap, or patella.

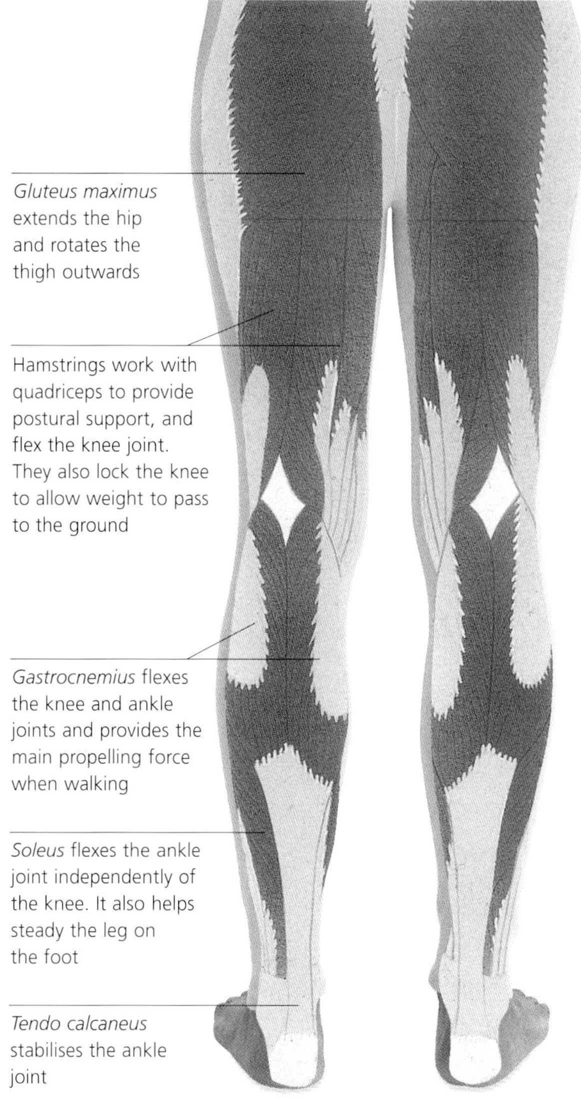

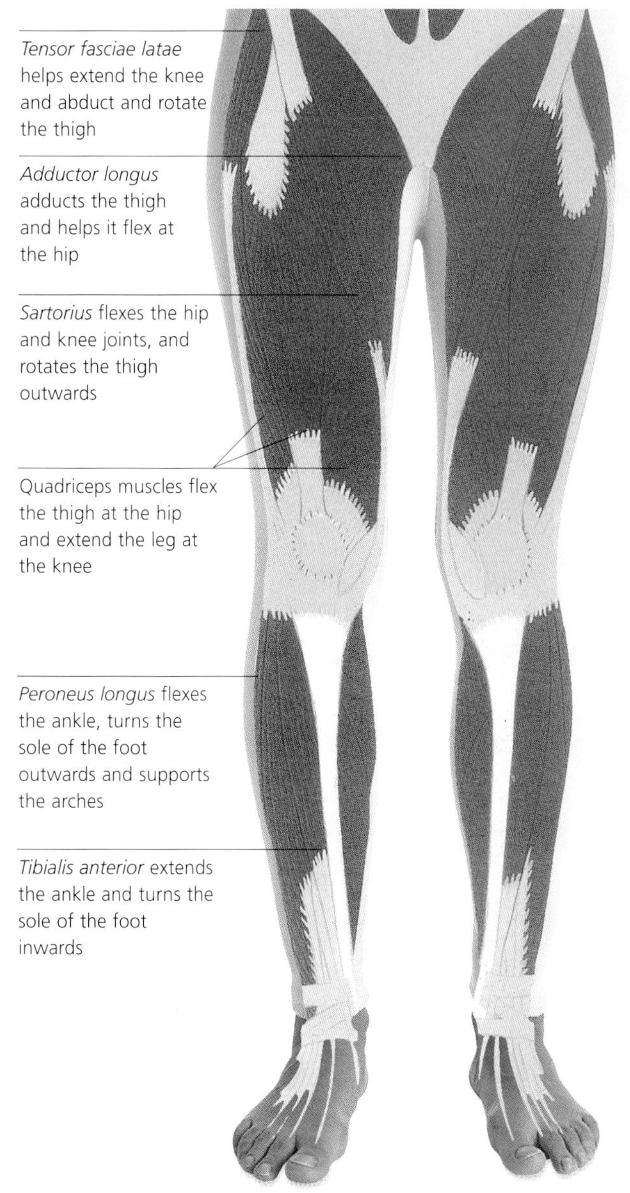

This is a small, cartilage-covered bone, embedded in the quadriceps tendon and connected to the tibia by the patellar tendon. It reduces friction by gliding over the edge of the joint, and prevents the quadriceps tendon from becoming frayed by what would otherwise be a continual sawing motion as the leg is bent and straightened.

The knee joint should properly be called a 'modified hinge joint', since the presence of the two menisci allows a slight degree of rotation in the joint. This enables us to turn corners, twist and even dance, but it also completes the locking movement of the knees – if you brace your knees you will see that they rotate inwards slightly – and makes the joint more robust when in this state.

Leg complaints

Osteoarthritis of the hip

The hip joint has a fairly limited range of movements and a relatively poor blood supply. Taken together, these two facts mean that it is vital for the hip to be moved regularly through its full range of movements, otherwise the synovial membranes surrounding the joint fail to secrete sufficient synovial lubricating fluid. A reduction in the synovial fluid leads to inflammation and damage to the cartilage in the joint, and so a reduction of the space within it, as well as the formation of osteophytes: bony, hook-like growths at the edges of the articulating bones. The result is the condition known as osteoarthritis of the hip.

The first signs that osteoarthritis is developing are stiffness and pain, sometimes in the joint itself, but more often in the groin and down the front of the thigh to just above the knee; occasionally the pain is referred only to the area just above the kneecap. The stiffness increases over time, until it becomes difficult to perform certain movements, such as doing up shoelaces or climbing steep stairs. As wear and tear continues, the head of the femur may be worn down to such an extent that one leg becomes shorter than the other. The first movement to suffer is usually extension (moving the leg backwards), though often this is not noticed by those affected; and then abduction (moving the leg out to the side) and lateral (outward) rotation start to become difficult.

The damage caused by osteoarthritis is not reversible, so prevention should be your watchword. Regular exercise is vital to maintain the levels of synovial fluid, but – rather unfairly – excessive exercise can make you as prone to osteoarthritis as a sedentary lifestyle. Sports that involve twisting, turning and placing stress on the hip, such as football, squash, running and dancing, all increase wear and tear – though good, specially designed sports shoes will help to absorb these stresses. Obesity and poor posture also increase the likelihood of osteoarthritis, since they increase the pressure on what is one of the main weight-bearing joints of the body.

How osteoarthritis develops
The hip joint is rarely put through its full range of movements, so synovial fluid production falls off.

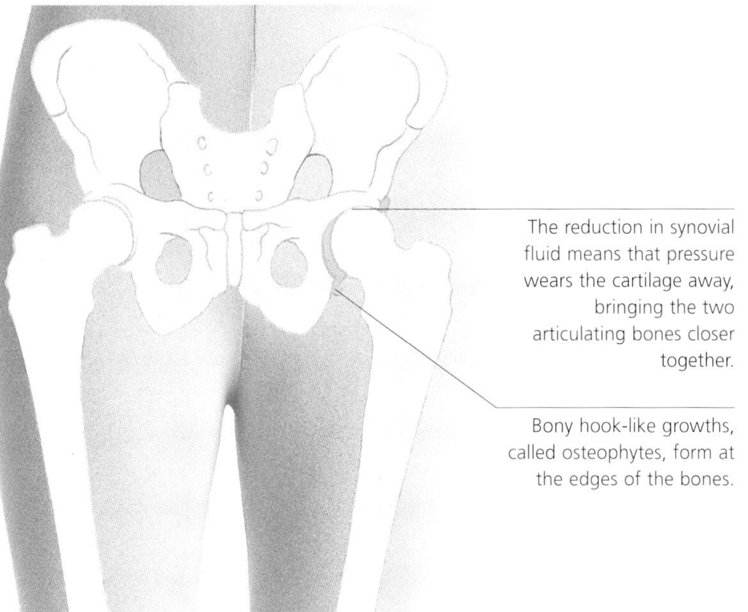

AT A GLANCE: Osteoarthritis of the hip
Cause: wear and tear on the joint; a sedentary lifestyle; excessive load bearing, as in over-exercise, lifting weights or some sports; poor posture; obesity
Medical treatment: painkillers; surgical hip replacement
Physiotherapy: stretching exercises and exercises that do not involve weight-bearing
Self-help: lose weight; correct posture (see pages 20–27); avoid excessive weight-bearing exercise
Avoidance: maintain correct weight and posture; take regular exercise; wear well-fitting sports shoes
Prognosis: avoidance is the best option, since osteoarthritis is not reversible; hip replacements are common and generally successful operations

Housemaid's knee

The pre-patellar bursa (see page 14) is sited over the kneecap (patella) that protects the knee joint. Inflammation of this particular bursa is known as 'housemaid's knee', but inflammation can affect a number of other bursae in the body. When it does, the condition tends to be named after those whose occupation makes them likely to suffer from it: 'clergyman's knee', for example, where another bursa in the knee – in total, there are ten bursae in the knee joint – is affected by kneeling at prayer; and 'dustman's shoulder', which affects a bursa in the shoulder.

Whichever bursa is involved, a chronic inflammation usually results from repeated pressure, while an acute inflammation is likely to be caused by an injury, such as a kick received while playing football. Housemaid's knee can be either acute or chronic, though its name reflects the chronic form of the condition, caused by the pressure of kneeling on the bursa. It can be differentiated from an inflammation *within* the knee joint itself as housemaid's knee should not affect flexion or extension at the joint. If there is limitation of movement or any pain after movement, you should seek medical advice, because the problem may lie inside the joint – with the cruciate ligament, for example.

AT A GLANCE: Housemaid's knee
Cause: kneeling for long periods; a blow above the kneecap; trauma to the front of the knee
Medical treatment: aspirating excess fluid with a syringe; steroid injections to reduce inflammation; anti-inflammatory drugs; in extreme cases, surgical removal of the bursa
Physiotherapy: RICE; ultrasound treatment; graded exercises to ensure full range of movements
Self-help: RICE (see pages 74–75); avoid putting any pressure on the knee; wear loose trousers
Avoidance: if you have to kneel for long periods, wear kneepads and alter your position frequently
Prognosis: good

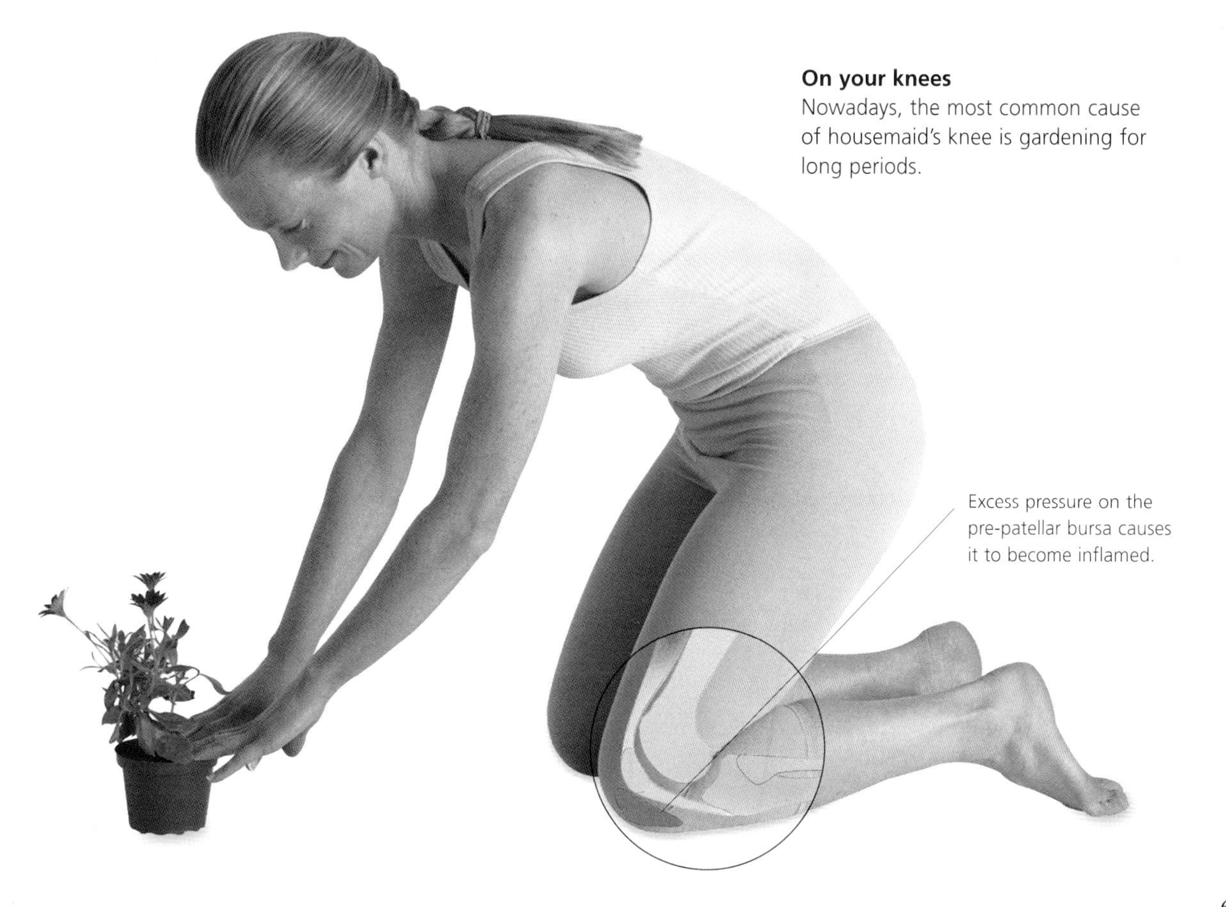

On your knees
Nowadays, the most common cause of housemaid's knee is gardening for long periods.

THE ANKLE AND FOOT

At first sight, you might think that the ankle and foot have a similar range of movements to those of the hand and wrist – after all, we walked on all fours at one point in our evolutionary history. But, in fact, the wrist and finger joints have developed considerably since those days, while the ankle joints have stayed much the same. Although it may seem as if there is a wide range of movements at the ankle, most of them are not controlled at the ankle joint, but by the muscles that work over all the 26 bones of the foot.

The ankle joint

The ankle joint proper – as opposed to the other joints contained within the ankle and foot – is between the top and sides of the first bone of the foot (the talus) and the enlargements (malleoli) of the lower ends of the tibia and fibula: the fibula articulates with the outside of the talus; and the tibia articulates with the top of the talus and its inner side. As a result, the talus is almost enclosed on three sides. This gives the joint an intrinsic stability, which is reinforced both by the range of ligaments at the front and back of the foot – there are more than 100 of them in the foot as a whole – the 'ankle strap' muscles that surround the joint and a number of tendons.

The joint itself allows only two movements: plantar flexion, which points the foot up, and dorsiflexion, which points it down. This may sound relatively trivial, but these actions are an essential part of walking.

The arches of the foot

The prime function of the ankle joint is to transmit to the ground the weight of the body and the forces exerted when walking or running. These forces are considerable, and the brunt of them is borne by the talus. However, the foot is constructed according to sound engineering principles that have been used by bridge builders for centuries.

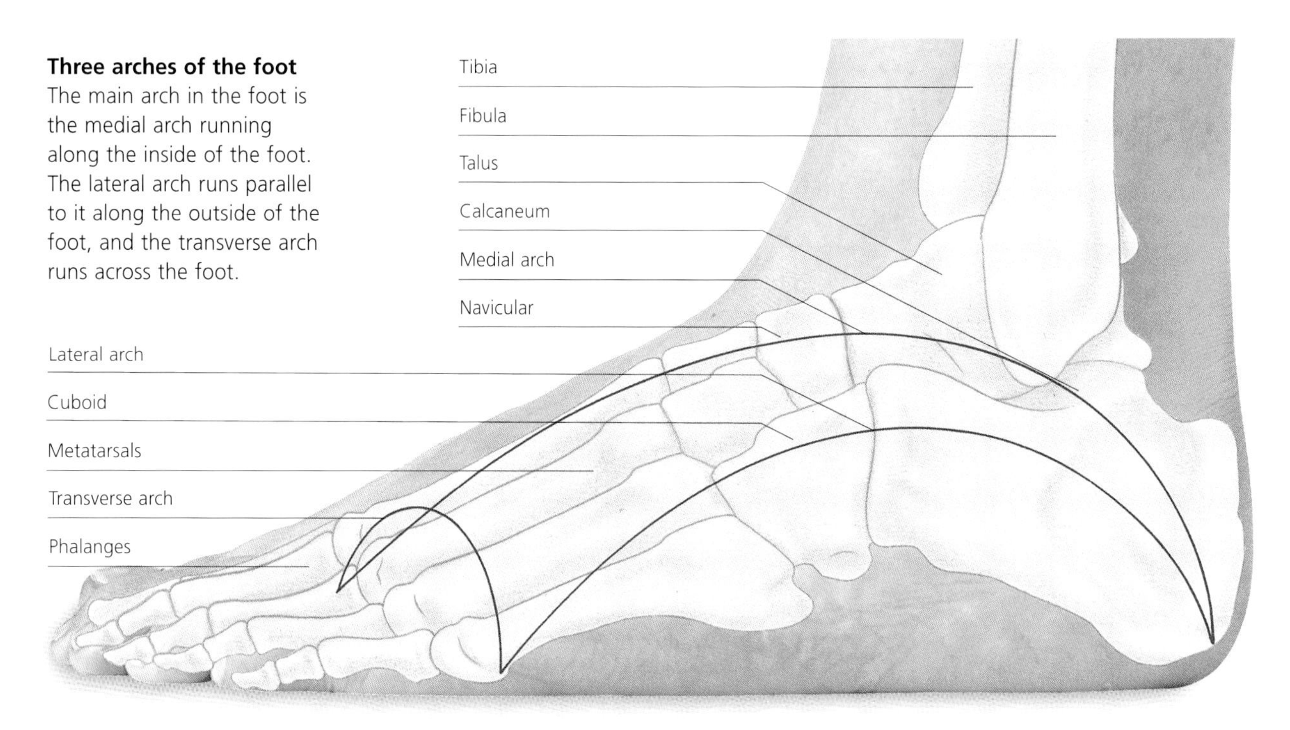

Three arches of the foot
The main arch in the foot is the medial arch running along the inside of the foot. The lateral arch runs parallel to it along the outside of the foot, and the transverse arch runs across the foot.

In this case the bridge is the medial arch of the foot, and the talus forms its keystone. It is a flexible bridge, though, that is raised and lowered as we walk. The shape of the bridge must be able to change so that we can walk comfortably on uneven surfaces, and a series of joints between the 26 different bones of the foot allows small movements that make this possible; it also distributes the forces that are transmitted throughout the foot.

On the inside of the foot, *tibialis anterior* supports the navicular bone at the top of the arch.

Tibialis posterior sweeps round underneath the arch to support the same bone from below (it also turns the foot in).

The talus and navicular bones are at the top of the medial arch. The spring ligament runs between them, under the foot, protecting the arch against the shock of a sudden jolt.

Victims of fashion

I leave platform shoes to my daughter these days, but I still wear high heels from time to time. However, wearing platform shoes puts a considerable strain on the muscles of the lower leg, which pulls the ankle joint out of position. High heels, on the other hand, shift the weight of the body forwards, which strains the knees and the muscles and ligaments of the arches; there is also an increased risk of bunions, corns and deformation of the toes. Ideally, you should stick to shoes with low, sensible heels, but if you must be fashionable, maintenance exercises can reduce the effects (see pages 130–31).

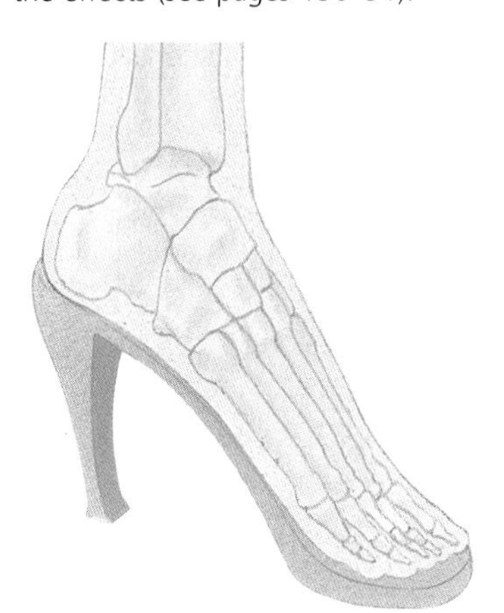

A suspension bridge

A subtle arrangement of muscles and ligaments controls the movement of the medial arch and brings it back into shape. The muscles shown act in a similar way to the cables of a suspension bridge. Small intrinsic muscles between the bones of the foot maintain and relax tension, according to circumstances, in order to preserve the arch's shape and strength.

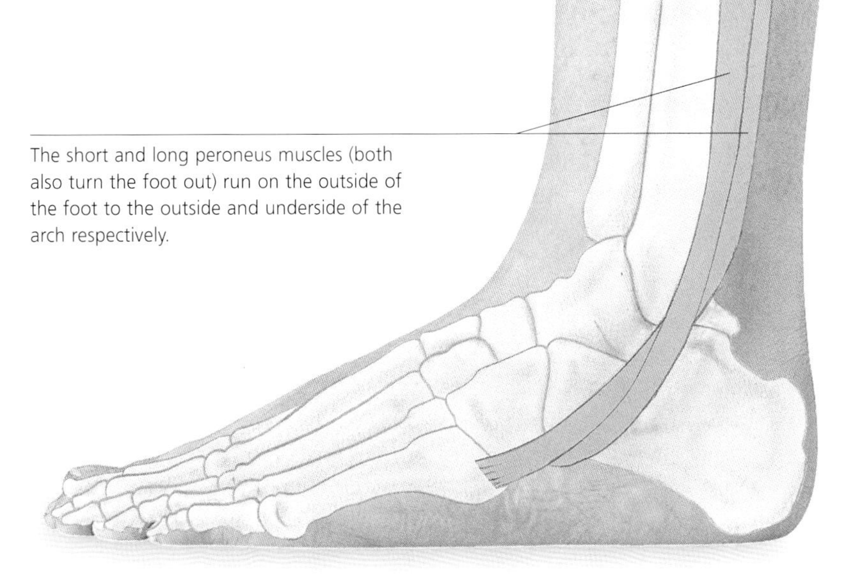

The short and long peroneus muscles (both also turn the foot out) run on the outside of the foot to the outside and underside of the arch respectively.

Ankle and foot complaints

Achilles rupture

The Achilles tendon (tendo calcaneus) links the calf muscle (*gastrocnemius*) to the heel bone (the calcaneum), lifting the latter up when the calf muscle contracts, either as part of taking a step, standing on tiptoe or stretching up.

Problems with the Achilles tendon are fairly common. At the less-serious end of the scale, tendinitis may result from friction (caused by a new pair of shoes, for example) or exercise (such as dancing or a long walk) taken after a period of inactivity with no warm-up routine.

In the middle of the scale, a partial tear or rupture may result either from excessive exercise or a minor blow – the position of the tendon makes it very susceptible to such injuries. In both these cases, rest, ice, compression and elevation are needed (see pages 74–75), with a programme of graded stretching exercises (see pages 110–11).

Unfortunately the tendon's poor blood supply slows healing, and after it has healed it is often slightly shorter than before – this is because most people sleep with their feet pointed in, so that the tendon is slack. The result is that the tendon feels tight and a little painful while walking, and may be prone to tear once more. Again, stretching exercises, with the tendon being gently stretched to its limit, are the best way of avoiding this problem.

A complete rupture of the tendon is normally caused by a sudden, hard blow to the ankle, or by a sudden movement when the tendon is taut: it feels as though you have been kicked. As a result, a rupture is not an uncommon injury on the football field, or when an occasional player attempts squash or tennis in middle age; women who wear high heels are particularly vulnerable, because the height of the heels means that the tendon is rarely stretched fully, and so becomes shorter. With a complete rupture, surgery may be necessary to join the torn ends together, and the lower limb must be immobilised in plaster of Paris. A full range of remedial exercises is then needed to stretch the tendon and restore full movement at the ankle joint.

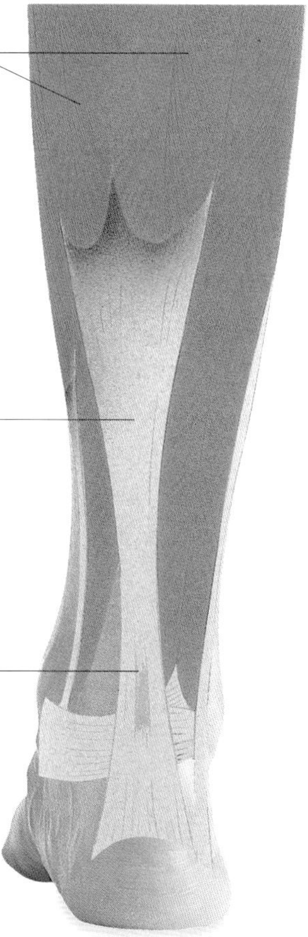

Gastrocnemius

Tendo calcaneus
(Achilles tendon)

A partial rupture of the tendon

Achilles heel
Gastrocnemius acts as a flexor at the ankle joint. A sudden movement of the joint can cause the tendon to be damaged.

AT A GLANCE: Achilles rupture
Cause: unusual and excessive exercise; taut calf muscles; sudden movement when the tendon is taut
Medical treatment: anti-inflammatory drugs; sometimes surgical suturing of the two ends and immobilisation in plaster of Paris
Physiotherapy: RICE; ultrasound treatment; stretching and balancing exercises
Self-help: RICE (see pages 74–75); exercises to stretch calf muscle (see page 110–11)
Avoidance: wear low-heeled shoes; keep up general fitness levels; warm-up routine and warm-down routine (see pages 114–19); stretching exercises (see page 130–31)
Prognosis: good, if condition is not ignored when chronic

Bunions

A bunion forms at the joint at the base of the big toe, and involves a thickening of the skin over the joint, as well as an enlargement of the bone itself; generally, there is also a mild bursitis (see page 45). Bunions, which can be very painful, are the result of excessive pressure or friction, normally as the result of wearing tight, ill-fitting shoes. Rest and a pair of new, well-fitting shoes can often reduce the size of a bunion. In the short term, pressure in the joint can be relieved by aspirating some of the fluid with a syringe. However, in serious cases, surgery may be necessary to remove the affected tissue.

AT A GLANCE: Bunions
Cause: excessive pressure, usually from tight shoes
Medical treatment: aspiration of fluid; surgery
Physiotherapy: not applicable
Self-help: exercises (see pages 110–11); change of footwear
Avoidance: wear shoes that fit properly; exercises (see pages 130–31)
Prognosis: good if footwear changed and condition not too far advanced

Fallen arches

The complex mechanism of the feet means that fallen arches, or 'flat feet', can result from an interplay between a large number of forces.

The medial arch, for example – the main arch of the three in the foot – can be affected by weakness in the muscles to the big toe that help hold the arch up. This, in turn, occurs when the feet are turned in or someone has 'knock knees' (a lack of external rotation at the hip). The result is that the arch drops: this can cause a deep, dragging pain along the foot, and may also affect the knee and hip joints, causing pain in the lower back.

If your transverse arch drops, however, it will feel as if there is a stone beneath your middle toes – the weight is being borne by bones not designed for the purpose, and which do not have any cushioning tissues.

In general, fallen arches are the result of defects in posture, though their effect can be worsened by ill-fitting footwear, and especially by high heels. So treatment is based on re-educating posture and walking habits and mobilising and strengthening the joints of the hip, knee, ankle and foot where necessary. While this is being done, pads may be placed in the shoes to raise the arch artificially, but it is vital that the muscles are also strengthened sufficiently so that they can once more hold the arch in place and the pads can be discarded.

AT A GLANCE: Fallen arches
Cause: lack of external rotation at the hips; weak ankles; short big toe; incorrect walking; knock knees; high heels
Medical treatment: rigid arch orthoses (pads)
Physiotherapy: postural training; mobilisation of hip, knee, ankle and foot, as appropriate; ankle and foot exercises; balancing exercises
Self-help: correct posture (see pages 20–27); wear flat shoes; exercises (see pages 110–11)
Avoidance: wear flat shoes; walk barefoot as much as possible; maintain correct posture (see pages 20–27)
Prognosis: good

Normal arches
This footprint shows the natural arches of the foot where weight is distributed evenly to the ground.

Fallen arches
Here the footprint shows almost the entire sole of the foot in contact with the ground. The foot is turned out slightly indicating poor posture.

High arches
This footprint shows the least contact between the foot and the ground. Here the foot is turned inwards from the mid-line; those affected will be 'pigeon-toed'.

SECTION THREE

SELF-HELP FOR ACHES AND PAINS

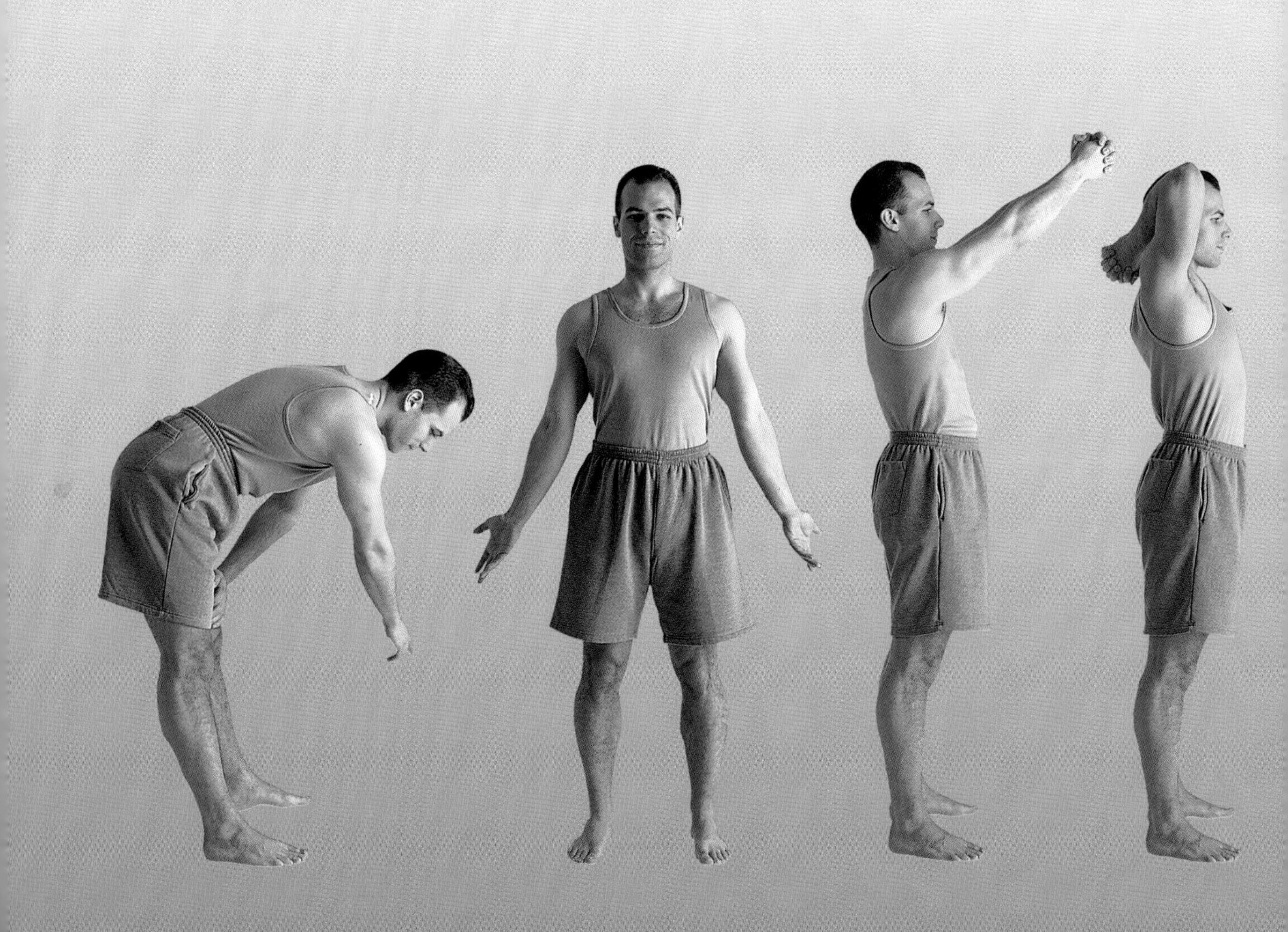

Whether you are suffering from one of the common complaints that I've just described or you have less distinct aches and pains, there is normally something that you can do to help yourself. And this section of the book tells you what it is. However, you should seek out professional advice if you are in any doubt about your condition and, of course, you should always be guided by the advice given by your doctor or physiotherapist.

First you'll find a description of home physiotherapy equipment and how to use it, and then I will introduce RICE – it's nothing to do with cooking, but an acronym that sums up how to treat some minor injuries. Next comes the core of this section: for each area of the body there's a diagnostic questionnaire that leads you from symptoms of musculo-skeletal injuries to their likely cause, and then directs you to short-term measures and remedial exercises, as well as suggesting when you should seek medical advice.

But it is important to remember that solving a problem in the short term does not mean that the problem will not return. Any injury weakens the tissues, and you should follow a maintenance exercise programme in order to reduce the chances of any recurrence. Follow the cross-references in this section to find the appropriate maintenance exercises to use in your case: you will find these in section four of this book.

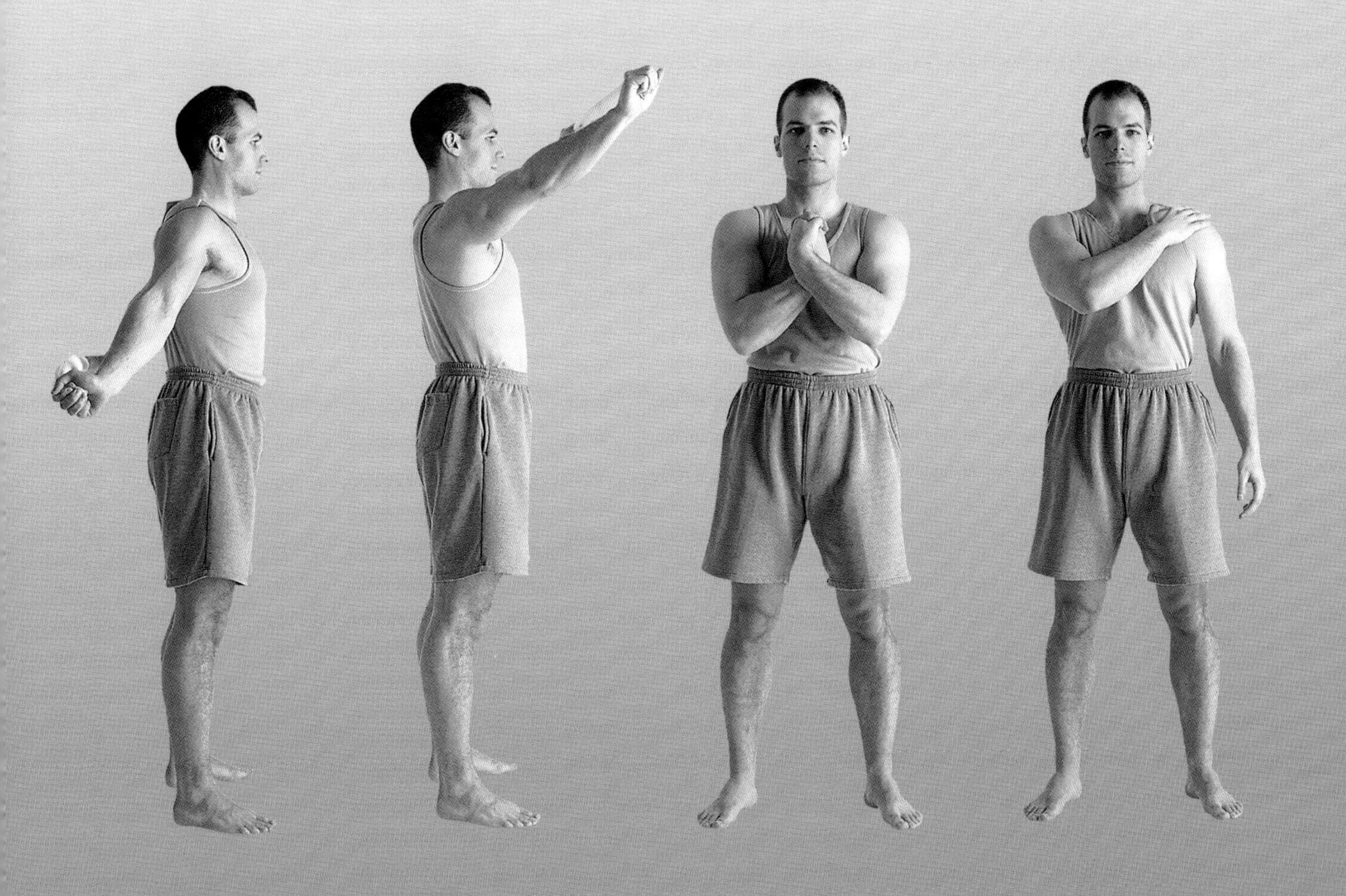

Equipment to ease the pain

The short-term treatment of musculo-skeletal injuries and strains often involves the use of creams, lotions, bandages and sprays, and it is worthwhile having a stock of them at home – though even if you don't you can often make do with a combination of the contents of your home first aid kit and your freezer.

In some cases, however, physiotherapy aids can play an important part in long-term treatment, and in prevention, too. Over the past few years some of them have become available to the general public, and while they are not essential they can be very useful – ask your local physiotherapist or pharmacist where you can buy them, or look in medical supplies stores.

Your home physiotherapy kit

It is well worth keeping a stock of the following items, especially if you take regular exercise. At a pinch, though, you can raid the freezer and use a bag of frozen peas as an ice pack (a freezer sleeve for cooling a wine bottle works well on children's limbs and adults' wrists); or take a hot bath and do some stretching exercises instead of using a heat lotion – always remembering to warm up properly beforehand and warm down afterwards (see pages 114–19). And, at night, you can always rest stiff, sore muscles on a warm hot-water bottle.

▲ **Safety watchpoint** Always follow the instructions given on any preparation or machine. It is a mistake to think that more does you good: in some cases, overuse can be counter-productive and, in extremes, dangerous.

ICE PACKS

These are used to reduce bruising and swelling. You can buy them at sports shops and pharmacists. Sprays are also available, but ice packs are more effective since the former only cool the area superficially and the effect does not last long. (See RICE, pages 74–75.)

HEAT LOTIONS AND PADS

These aids are used to ease stiff and sore muscles, and they can be bought at sports shops and pharmacists. (Do not use them when there is swelling or bruising, as heat dilates the blood vessels and so makes the problem worse.) Lotions are often the most effective, since the act of massaging them in kneads the muscle fibres and encourages them to relax.

BANDAGES

Bandages are used to support a vulnerable joint and to reduce any swelling. It is advisable to keep a range of different sizes at hand. (See step-by-step bandaging, page 75.)

SUPPORTS AND BELTS

These are useful when you know that a particular joint may be vulnerable, because they not only give a bit of extra support to the area but also make you more aware of how you move. However, using a support is no substitute for strengthening the muscles surrounding a joint and they should only be used occasionally – otherwise the muscles are encouraged to rely on the support and become weaker, exacerbating the problem.

CERVICAL COLLARS

These strips of foam are specially shaped to fit the neck and serve to support the cervical spine and limit movement; some pharmacists stock them. They help reduce muscle spasm and prevent any sudden movements in conditions such as acute neck pain (see pages 48–49). It is important that you buy a neck support that fits you properly and put it on correctly – check with your physiotherapist.

▲ **MEDICAL ALERT** Always consult a doctor if you develop acute neck pain, especially if it happens after an accident or fall or if there is any pain in your shoulder or down your arm.

Are you sitting comfortably?

As we have seen, correct posture is vital to the health of the musculo-skeletal system (see pages 20–23), and that principle applies just as much when you are sitting as when you are standing. In fact, it is often more important, because many of us spend much of our lives sitting at a desk or a computer, or driving a car, and need all the help we can get to maintain good posture while we are concentrating on something else. One answer is to buy one of the many different aids to sitting correctly – from simple lumbar rolls to custom-designed posture chairs. They all help to maintain the correct curvature of the spine so that the body's weight passes down the spine and is absorbed by the pelvis and thighs rather than the lower back.

An 'orthopaedic' back chair
These chairs can be adjusted in various ways so that the lower back is fully supported, the body's weight is distributed evenly down to the pelvis and thighs and the seat tilts forward at an angle of five degrees with the knees at right angles and the feet firmly planted on the ground. Such chairs are expensive, but well worth the money if you sit at a desk for long periods or suffer from back pain. However, it sometimes takes time to get used to the new, correct position and the unaccustomed re-distribution of weight to the knees.

The posture or 'Balans' chair
The Balans chair has no back, so it is more like a prayer stool than a conventional chair. Its shape places the spine in its correct alignment and reduces the compression on the lumbar spine, since the weight is being borne by the thighs and the knees. It takes time to get used to the rather odd position, but the chair is very effective – unless, however, you have knee problems.

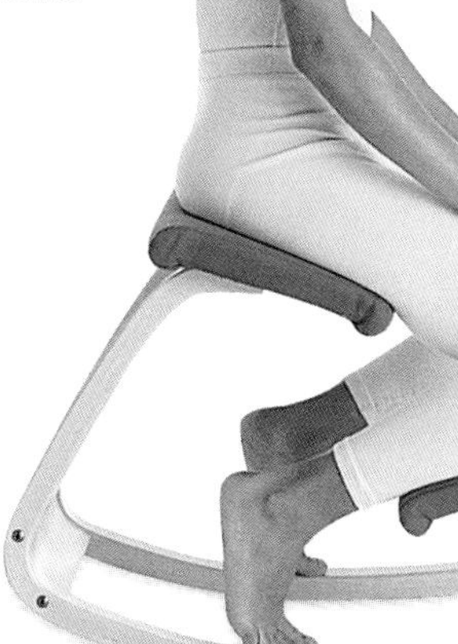

A lumbar roll
Placed at the base of a chair, this supports the lumbar spine. You can cover the roll with a pair of tights, and use them to tie it around your chair and keep it in position.

A chair wedge
Used on the seat of a chair – the thick end should be put at the back to adapt a horizontal seat into one with a forward angle of between five and ten degrees.

Relieving pain

Transcutaneous Electrical Nerve Stimulation (TENS) utilises low-voltage electricity to relieve pain. It is not a new principle: doctors in ancient Greece used to make their patients take baths with electric eels – I should think that just one treatment usually did the trick! But the modern-day TENS machine was developed once gate theory (see page 37) came to be generally accepted, and now you can buy one through a physiotherapist or by mail order. The electrical stimuli not only block the passage of pain sensations but also stimulate the production of endorphins, the body's natural painkillers (see page 38).

The advantage of a TENS machine is that you can reduce the sensation of pain as often as you want, for just a few minutes or as long as several hours – sometimes it can eliminate pain completely.

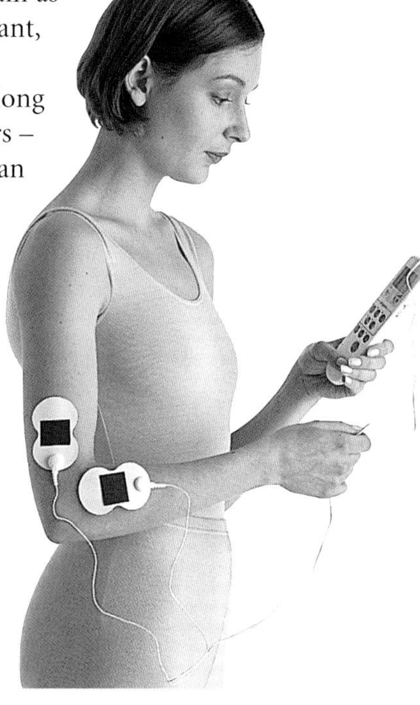

Using a TENS machine
It is simple to use a TENS machine and the procedure is completely safe if you follow the instructions. The size of a small personal stereo, it has either two or four pads. A jelly-like substance, which acts as a conductor for the current, is placed on the skin around the site of the pain and the pads are placed over it. (Some models have conductors built into the pads.) When you switch on, you will feel a tingling, rather like pins and needles, over the area, but it is not unpleasant. Adjust the intensity to suit yourself.

Ultrasound

Most people know that ultrasound machines are used to look at a baby in the womb, but physiotherapists use them, too, to treat a wide range of aches and pains. And now scaled-down ultrasound machines can be bought by the general public. Ultrasound – sound waves of a frequency so high that the human ear cannot detect them – has three main effects on the tissues of the body: these fall into the categories of mechanical, chemical and thermal.

The mechanical effect is really a very fast, mini-massage of the tissues, which helps them to relax, aids circulation and improves drainage, so reducing swelling. It can also speed up the disintegration of small pieces of bone and grit in the joints – a problem that is especially common in the knee joint.

As far as its chemical effect goes, ultrasound increases the permeability of membranes, so that salts and other products can be transported through them more easily, and also dilates the small blood vessels. This means that swelling reduces more quickly. Ultrasound also subdues the pain signals, probably by means of the gate control effect (see page 37).

Heat is produced by an ultrasound machine as a side-effect, but it is a useful one, because the heat can be directed precisely at a particular area or problem. Sprays or lotions have a more superficial effect. The heat relaxes the tissues and improves the circulation of blood.

Using an ultrasound machine
There is a wide range of ultrasound machines, and most of them have different instructions regarding intensity and length of treatment. All of them need a conducting substance to be applied to the skin, but if you run out of this, don't worry – olive oil will do.

▲ **MEDICAL ALERT** Do not use an ultrasound machine if you are pregnant or suffer from phlebitis or thrombosis; in cases of acute inflammation; if you suffer from haemophilia; over the heart or eyes, or over tumours, whether they are benign or malignant.

Relieving muscle tension

Over time, tension in the muscles can lead to tissue damage, strain on the joints and tension headaches. So it is best to deal with any muscle tension as quickly as you can. There is a wide variety of relaxants on the market – from aromatherapy oils to wooden massage rollers – and, of course, there's always the old standby of a hot bath. Try them, by all means, and choose the one that suits you best, though the effect may sometimes be more psychological than anything else. But perhaps the most effective method of all is massage – either by your partner or by means of a massage machine.

▲ **MEDICAL ALERT** Massage should not be used over an inflamed or septic area; over the abdomen of pregnant women; or on people who have circulatory problems.

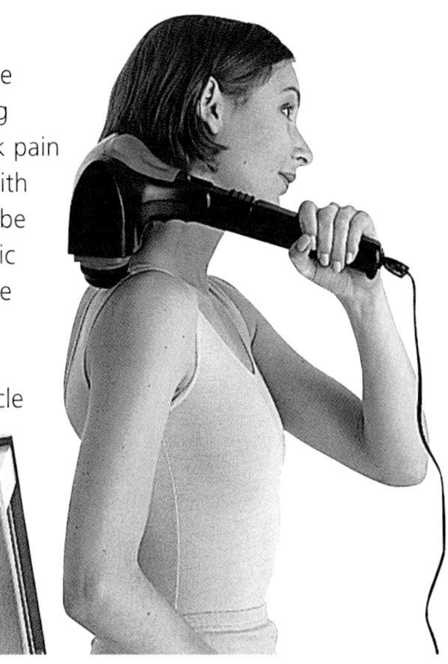

Massage machines
Many different types are available, from vibrating cushions that ease back pain to hand-held devices with various heads that can be used to massage specific areas of the body. These only give a superficial massage, but they are useful in reducing muscle spasm and tension, and inducing relaxation. They also help improve the circulation and reduce pain. Do not use a massage machine for more than 15 minutes at a time as many models have a powerful motor in rather a small case and tend to overheat after a while.

Wobble to fitness

A wobble board is simply a circular piece of wood mounted on a hemispherical wooden rocker, which either allows movement in just two directions or all directions, depending on the design. The aim is to stand on the board in a correct posture (see pages 20–21) and try to maintain your balance and keep the board level. It sounds easy, doesn't it? It isn't.

Using a wobble board helps strengthen the muscles of the leg, and the ankle strap muscles in particular. It puts the joint through its full range of small, accessory movements, and also uses all the muscles of the foot, helping to strengthen the arches. It improves balance and coordination, too, and helps you to re-learn the sense of proprioception – that is, the position of all your muscles and joints relative to the outside world – that can be lost temporarily but alarmingly when, for example, you have a chronically twisted ankle.

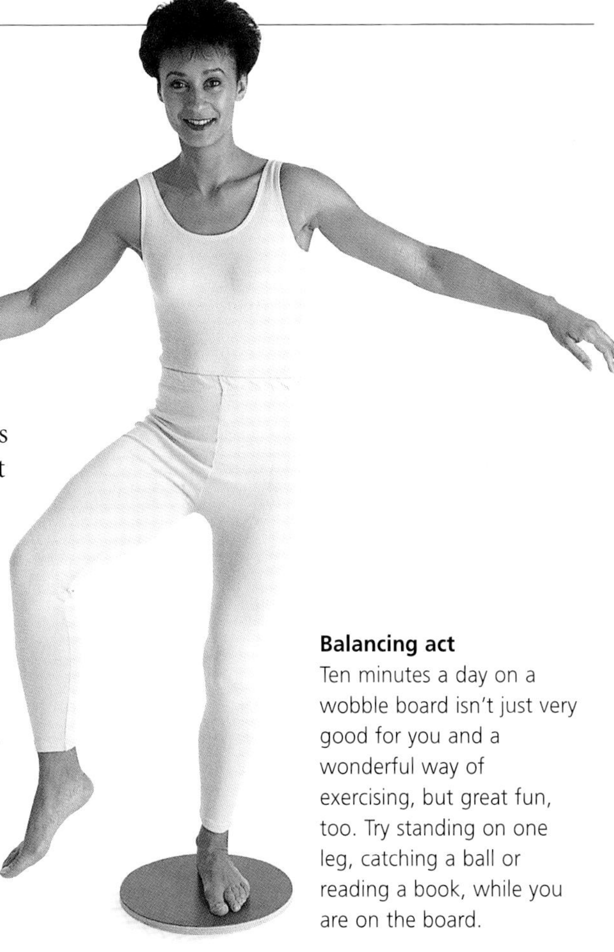

Balancing act
Ten minutes a day on a wobble board isn't just very good for you and a wonderful way of exercising, but great fun, too. Try standing on one leg, catching a ball or reading a book, while you are on the board.

Physiotherapy first aid

These two pages are not about first aid for any injuries that are serious or involve major internal or external bleeding: in such cases, call for an ambulance, consult your doctor or look the problem up in a first aid book, as appropriate. The measures given below are intended as the first line of defence when you have a minor injury: sprains, muscle strains, bangs and bruises, and minor joint problems. In many cases, you will have to consult a doctor or physiotherapist after you have taken these initial measures. The information can also be used to help your body heal after you have taken medical advice.

The aim of these measures is to stop bleeding inside the tissues. This will keep bruising to a minimum, lessen swelling and relax any muscles that are in spasm. Overall, they make it easier for the body's healing processes to get to work. The steps can be summed up by the acronym 'RICE': rest, ice, compression and elevation.

The problem-solver charts on the following pages will suggest when RICE is appropriate, when to use exercises, or when it would be advisable to consult your doctor.

REGAINING MOVEMENT

It is important that you start moving the injured muscle, tendon or joint after 24 hours of RICE (unless otherwise indicated by the problem-solver chart or by your doctor), in order to prevent scarring of the muscle tissue, shortening of a tendon, or loss of movement at a joint. Specific exercises for the different areas of the body are given in the pages that follow. To begin with, try gentle swinging and stretching exercises that do not involve weight-bearing – isometrics are particularly helpful when there is any pain (see below) – then start a course of exercises to strengthen the muscles surrounding the joint once there is a full range of movement.

Isometrics and isotonics

There are two types of muscular contraction: isometric and isotonic. In basic terms, an isotonic muscle contraction involves the movement of a joint, whereas an isometric contraction does not involve movement, and the muscle tightens without changing length; the abdominal, gluteal and pectoral muscle groups, for example, all tighten isometrically.

It may be painful to contract a muscle isotonically immediately after an injury, but isometric contractions – making a conscious effort to tighten a muscle without moving a joint – may be pain-free. Isometric exercises are useful in that they help maintain a muscle's strength, but they impede blood flow, so you should only attempt them for about ten minutes and take an hour's rest between each session. Incorporate both isometric and isotonic contractions in your exercise routine as soon as you can.

▲ **MEDICAL ALERT** Do not try isometric exercises if you have a heart condition or circulatory problems unless you have checked with your doctor first. Some isometric exercises are prescribed as part of the treatment for such conditions, but only under medical supervision.

Rest

Take the weight off any injured part of your body: sit or lie down if you have a leg injury; put an injured arm in a sling made from a scarf.

Ice

Wrap the area in an ice pack. Never put ice or an ice pack straight on to the skin as it may cause an ice burn. Wrap the pack in a tea towel or cloth beforehand. Leave the ice pack on for ten minutes and repeat the application at hourly intervals.

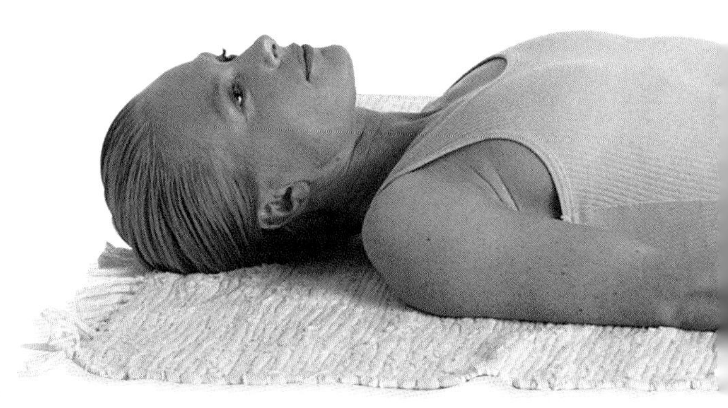

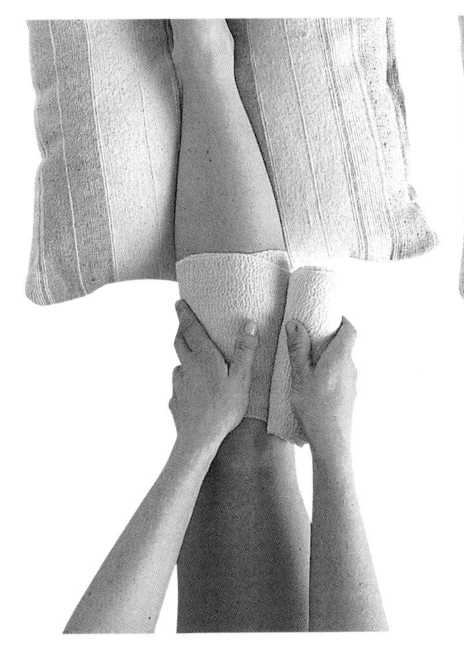

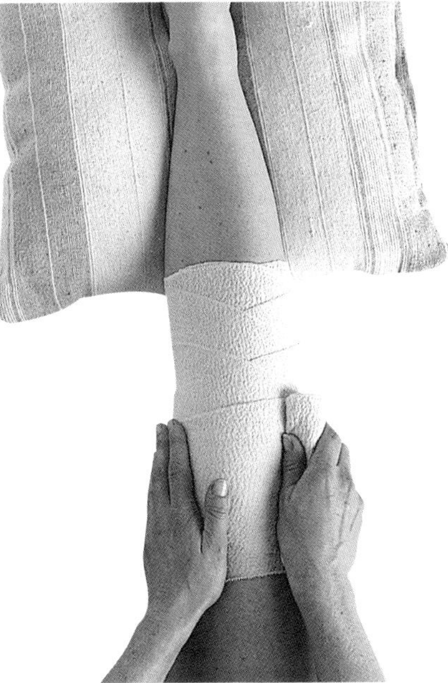

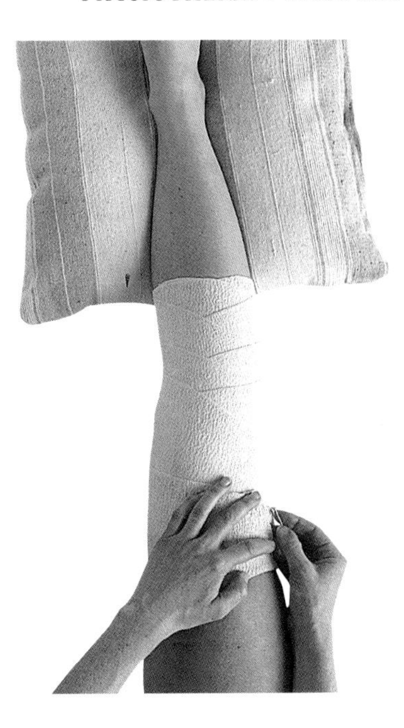

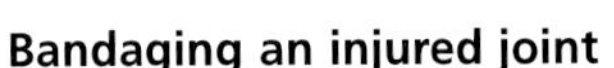

Bandaging an injured joint

1 Place your hands either side of the limb a few inches below the joint. Move the roll of the bandage round and under the limb, then over the other end of the bandage to fix it.

2 Continue making circles round the limb, starting each one about an inch higher than the previous, bringing the bandage back down as you go round, to create a criss-cross pattern.

3 Make sure the bandage is not too tight, or it may impede blood flow. It should be firm, though, and run well above and below the joint. Fasten the loose end with a large safety pin.

Compression

Bandage the area to reduce swelling and give support. However, it is important that you give support and compression without inhibiting the blood flow.

Elevation

Lift and support the injured part. If possible, the injury should be higher than the heart. This eases the pressure on the blood vessels and aids the drainage of fluids from the site.

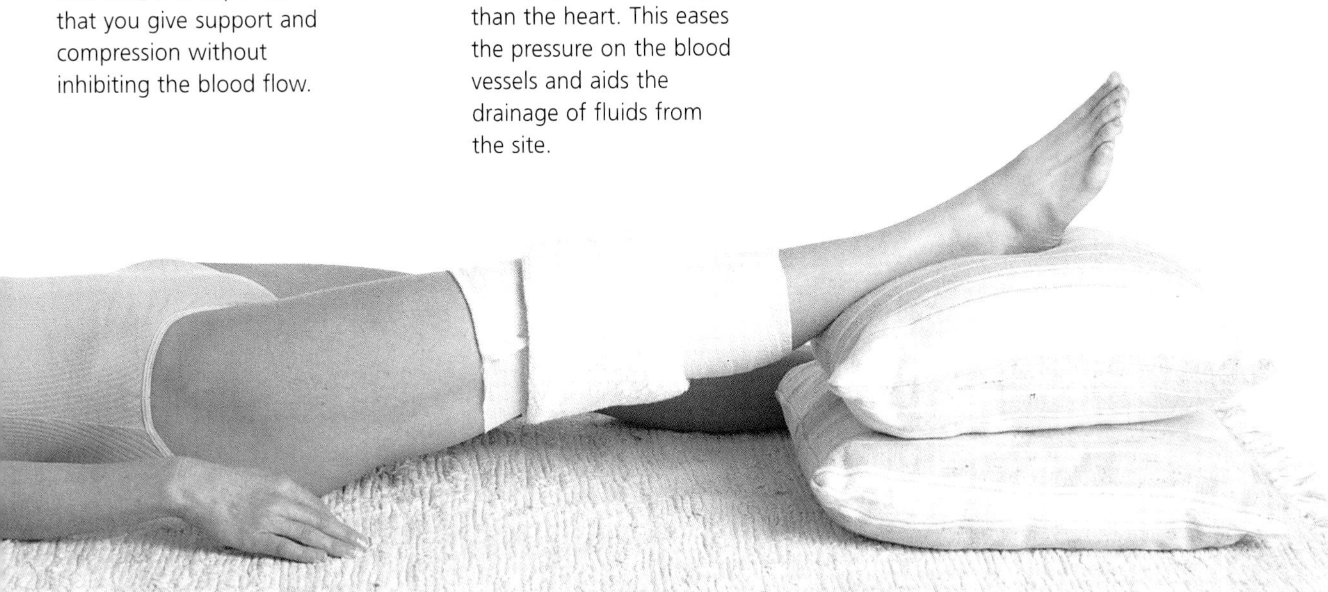

Head and neck problems

In most cases, neck pains – which are often, but not always, associated with headaches – are caused by a build-up of tension in the muscles of the neck and upper back.

The main muscle involved is *trapezius* (see pages 13 and 53), because it is the main support for the head when it is tilted forwards – when you are looking at a computer screen, for example, or absorbed in a hobby. Other muscles in the neck, beneath and alongside *trapezius*, also help maintain the position of the head.

There are two common causes of muscle tension in this area: emotional stress (see pages 32–33) and bad posture (see pages 20–27). The former might seem surprising – but think how we hunch our shoulders, not just against the rain or cold but in fear, or as a reaction to stress. An increase in muscular tension is an integral part of the body's natural 'fight or flight' response to perceived danger – and that, essentially, is what the body interprets stress to be.

The results of bad posture are more obvious: *trapezius* and the other muscles are constantly tight, and often the muscle fibres on different sides of the body have fallen out of balance, because they have been attempting to maintain a posture for which the body is not designed.

Whatever the cause, continued tension in the neck and back muscles results in pain, and often in headaches as a result of the unnatural pull on the bones of the skull. It also distorts the muscle fibres: if you have a habit of tilting your head to one side, the contracted fibres of the muscles on the side to which you tilt may lose the ability to slide over each other and thus tie themselves in knots; at the same time, the muscle fibres on the other side may become damaged by being overstretched – and this damage can itself exacerbate the problem.

Use the flowchart opposite to analyse the nature of your neck pain and follow the appropriate course of action. However, if you are in any doubt about the nature or cause of a neck problem, consult a doctor without delay.

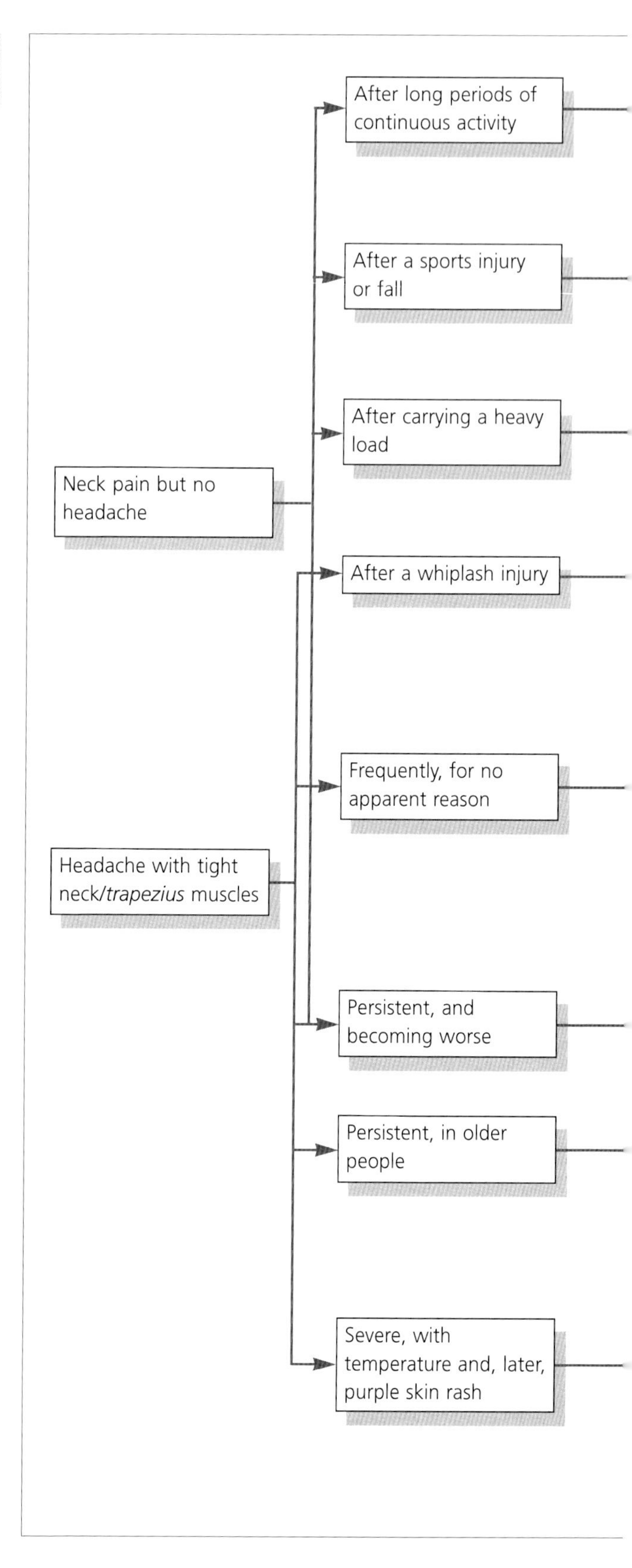

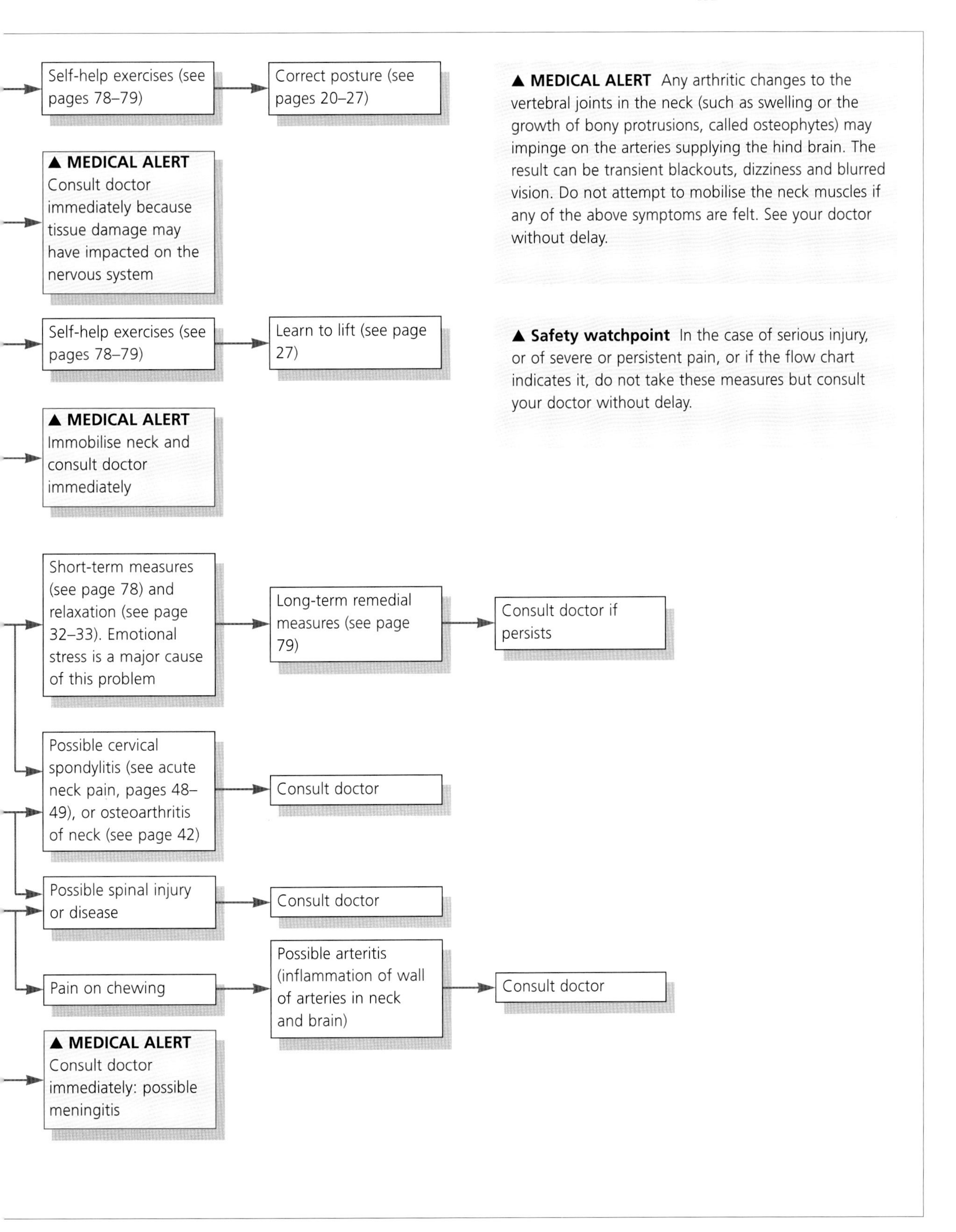

▲ **MEDICAL ALERT** Any arthritic changes to the vertebral joints in the neck (such as swelling or the growth of bony protrusions, called osteophytes) may impinge on the arteries supplying the hind brain. The result can be transient blackouts, dizziness and blurred vision. Do not attempt to mobilise the neck muscles if any of the above symptoms are felt. See your doctor without delay.

▲ **Safety watchpoint** In the case of serious injury, or of severe or persistent pain, or if the flow chart indicates it, do not take these measures but consult your doctor without delay.

Self-help head and neck exercises

A few, simple techniques can often be used to relieve headaches and neck pain in the short term.

SHORT-TERM MEASURES FOR HEADACHES

▼ Locate the acupressure points on your head and press (pinch the ear lobe) each one firmly for a count of five, using the ball of the thumb or the tips of your fingers. Build the pressure up gradually – but do not cause pain.

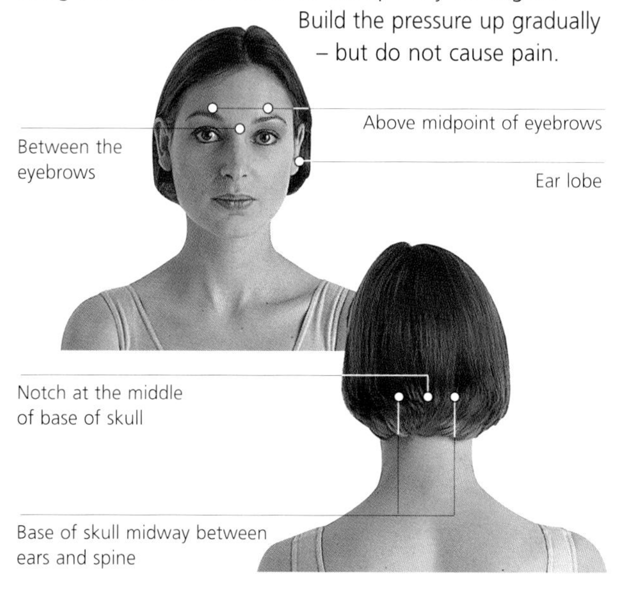

SHORT-TERM MEASURES FOR NECK PAIN

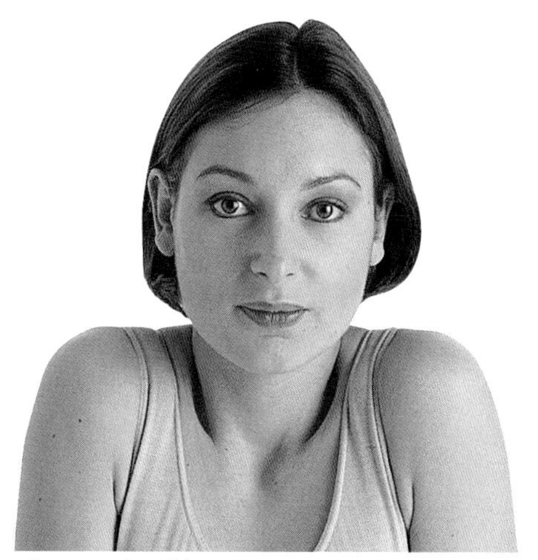

1 ▲ Push your shoulders forwards and up, then rotate them back and down, pushing the crown of your head towards the ceiling. Repeat three times.

2 Raise your shoulders, tightening them up towards your ears. Hold for a count of two, then let them flop back. Repeat three times.

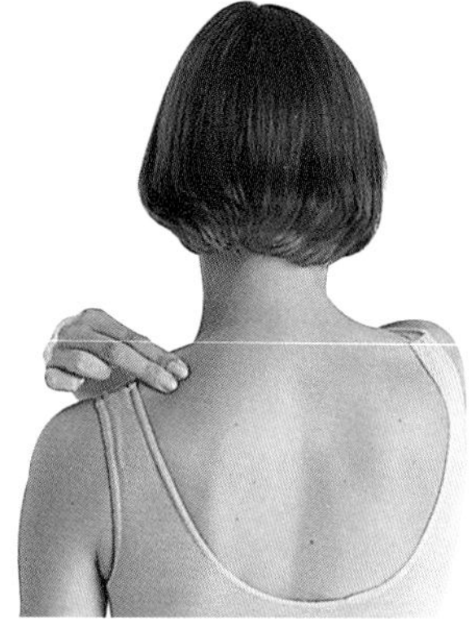

3 ◀ Relax your left arm, resting it against a cushion or your thigh. Pinch and roll *trapezius* between your finger and thumb along the line of its join to your left collar bone. Continue up the neck to the head and return. Repeat, using your left hand on your right shoulder.

4 ▶ Tilt your head back slightly, so that trapezius and the other neck muscles become shorter, and knead the muscles down the neck to the shoulders. Don't forget to massage the muscles next to the cervical vertebrae, those up to the external occipital protuberance (the central peg at the base of the skull) and the ones a few inches either side of it.

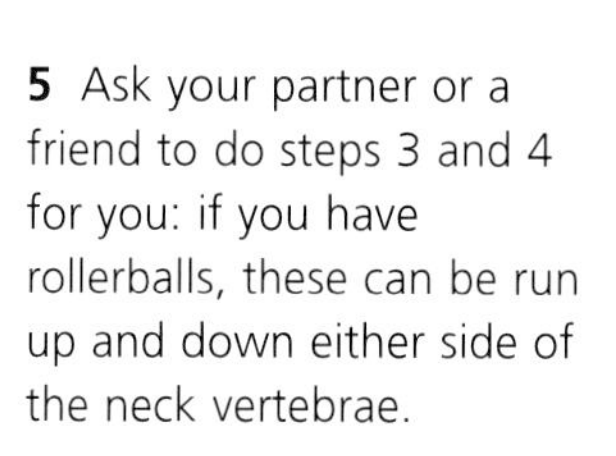

5 Ask your partner or a friend to do steps 3 and 4 for you: if you have rollerballs, these can be run up and down either side of the neck vertebrae.

6 To finish off, rub some muscle lotion into the muscles and, if you have one, attach an immobilising collar (see page 70) to your neck. This will give the muscles time to relax thoroughly and recover.

▲ **Safety watchpoint** Do not allow anybody unqualified to massage the area around the base of your neck and the base of your skull too powerfully or deeply. The procedure can be extremely dangerous in untutored hands.

LONG-TERM MEASURES FOR HEADACHES AND NECK PAIN

In the long term, you can relieve chronic headaches and neck pain and prevent them recurring by performing a few basic exercises designed to relieve muscle tension.

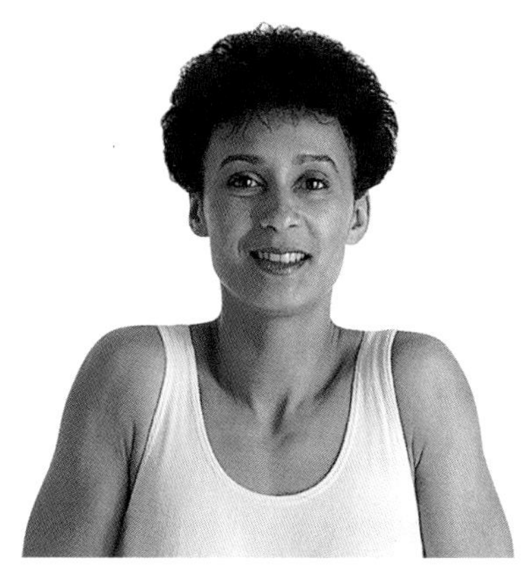

1 ▲ Raise both shoulders towards your ears. Hold and let them drop. Repeat three times.

2 Circle both shoulders forwards and upwards, then back and down. Repeat three times, then reverse.

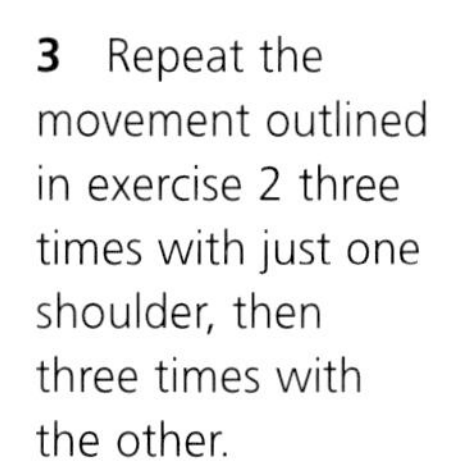

3 Repeat the movement outlined in exercise 2 three times with just one shoulder, then three times with the other.

4 ▶ Turn your head to look over your left shoulder and return. Repeat three times. Turn to look over your right shoulder three times.

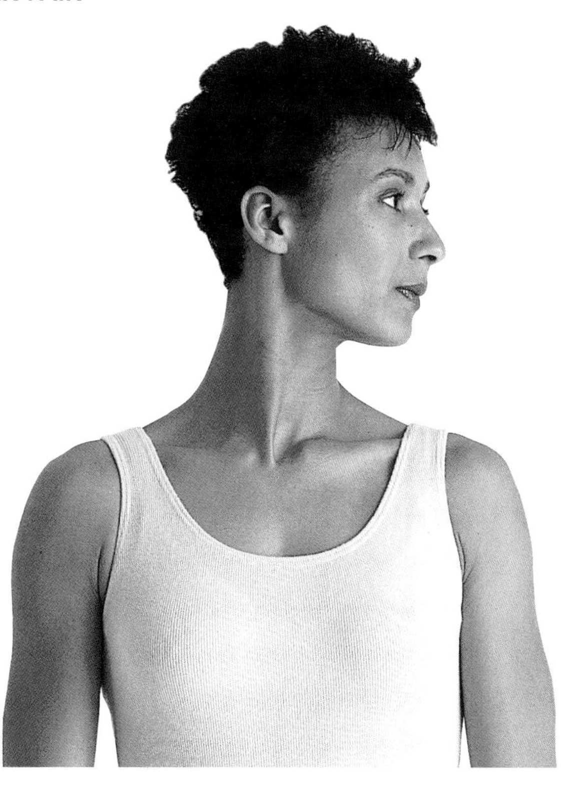

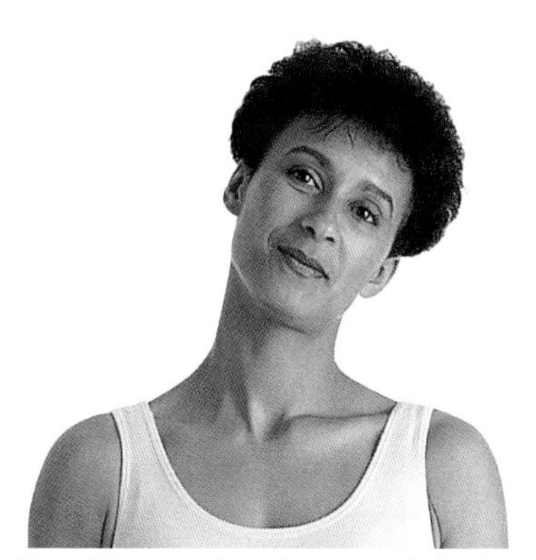

5 ▲ Tilt your head to your left shoulder, avoiding lifting your shoulder to your head, and return. Repeat three times, then repeat three times tilting to your right shoulder.

6 Put your chin on your chest and return. Repeat three times.

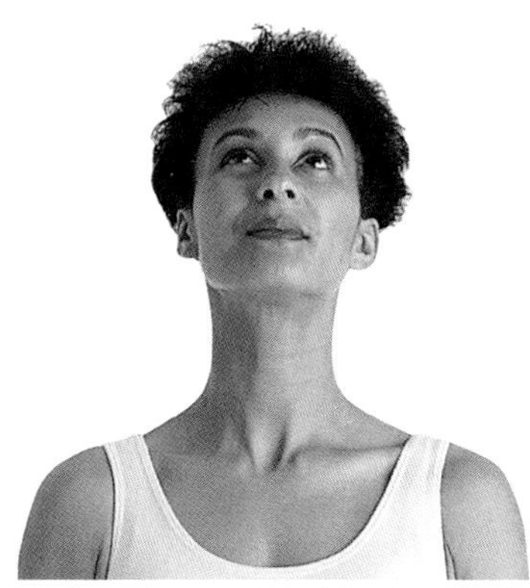

7 ▲ Push your head back to look at the ceiling and return. Repeat this three times.

8 Move your head clockwise in a 360 degree circle. Repeat three times, then move your head round anti-clockwise three times.

9 If necessary, rub muscle lotion into your muscles and attach an immobilising collar.

▲ **Safety watchpoint** It's important that you push your body only to the point of discomfort and not beyond it. If you feel light-headed, stop. Most people naturally become slightly light-headed after exercising neck muscles, but this feeling is a sign that you are beginning to overdo things.

▲ **Safety watchpoint** These exercises are only intended for the treatment of minor strains and tensions. If your problem is more serious, or you are receiving medical treatment for an injury or condition, make sure that you consult your doctor or physiotherapist before starting them.

Back problems

More working days are lost as a result of back problems than for any other reason. This is hardly surprising, when you consider what a complex structure the spine is and the strains that are put on it. The spinal column is still better suited to walking on all fours, as most other vertebrates do, rather than walking upright.

In general terms, back problems may be caused by bad posture (see pages 20–27), old age, disease, pregnancy (the hormones of pregnancy make the ligaments slacker, so that the whole structure becomes less stable) or excessive strain – which may be caused by carrying a heavy weight incorrectly, for example, or twisting the body rapidly and without sufficient control.

The result can be any one of a variety of problems, or a combination of them. One of the short muscles linking the vertebrae may be pulled for example, or a ligament strained. Then a sudden strain may cause a disc to prolapse – to protrude beyond its fibrous, enclosing ring (see slipped disc, pages 50–51). Spinal discs may degenerate, too, either through lack of use or as a result of ageing, and lose their water content. The facet joints may be jammed together as a result of this thinning of the discs, and the resulting inflammation can press on the roots of spinal nerves. Osteoarthritis (see page 42), the onset of which can be delayed by exercise, can also lead to the growth of osteophytes – bony protrusions – into the central canal of the spine, narrowing it (a 'stenosis') to the extent that the bone starts to press on the spinal cord.

Most of these problems can be avoided, in the main, if regular exercise is taken, or they can be treated with a fair expectation of success. However, this is not the case in ankylosing spondylitis, a condition in which calcium is laid down in the ligaments, and the joints become inflamed, causing them to lock up and become rigid. This disorder runs in families, is fairly rare and normally only affects young adult men. Usually it attacks the sacro-iliac joint and causes pain and stiffness in the lower back, especially in the mornings.

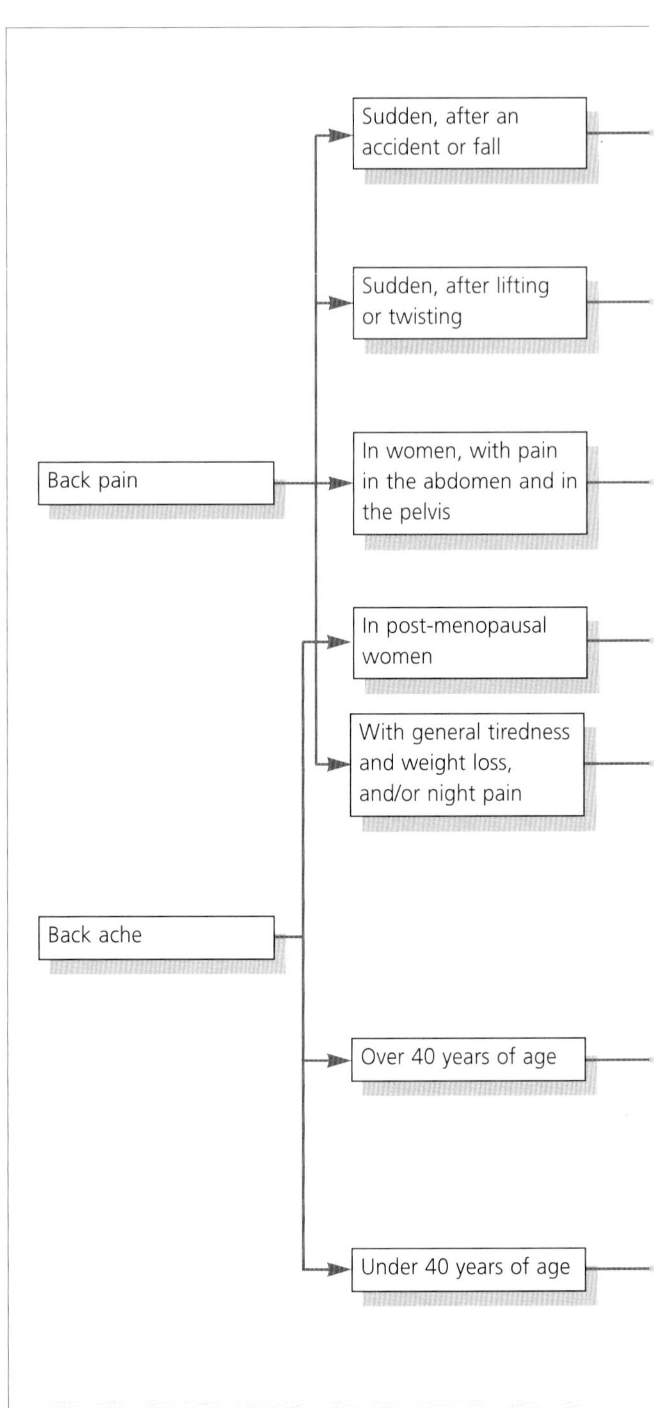

▲ **Safety watchpoint** In the case of serious injury, or of severe or persistent pain, or if the flow chart indicates it, do not take these measures but consult your doctor without delay. Also consult your doctor immediately if pains, numbness or pins and needles become worse.

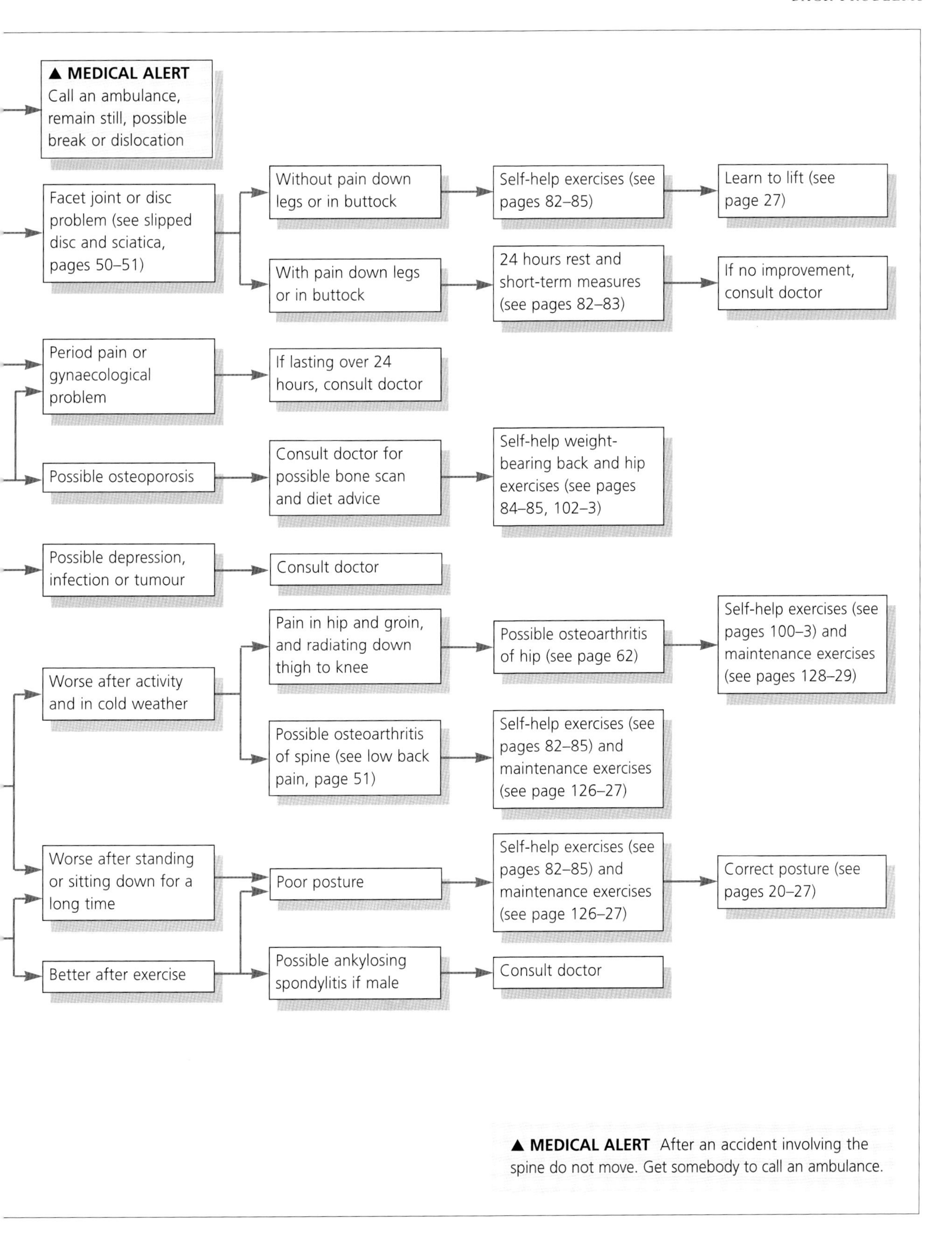
▲ MEDICAL ALERT
Call an ambulance, remain still, possible break or dislocation
Facet joint or disc problem (see slipped disc and sciatica, pages 50–51)
Without pain down legs or in buttock
Self-help exercises (see pages 82–85)
Learn to lift (see page 27)
With pain down legs or in buttock
24 hours rest and short-term measures (see pages 82–83)
If no improvement, consult doctor
Period pain or gynaecological problem
If lasting over 24 hours, consult doctor
Possible osteoporosis
Consult doctor for possible bone scan and diet advice
Self-help weight-bearing back and hip exercises (see pages 84–85, 102–3)
Possible depression, infection or tumour
Consult doctor
Worse after activity and in cold weather
Pain in hip and groin, and radiating down thigh to knee
Possible osteoarthritis of hip (see page 62)
Self-help exercises (see pages 100–3) and maintenance exercises (see pages 128–29)
Possible osteoarthritis of spine (see low back pain, page 51)
Self-help exercises (see pages 82–85) and maintenance exercises (see page 126–27)
Worse after standing or sitting down for a long time
Poor posture
Self-help exercises (see pages 82–85) and maintenance exercises (see page 126–27)
Correct posture (see pages 20–27)
Better after exercise
Possible ankylosing spondylitis if male
Consult doctor
▲ MEDICAL ALERT After an accident involving the spine do not move. Get somebody to call an ambulance.

Self-help back exercises

SHORT-TERM MEASURES

These exercises are designed to help relieve acute back pain in the short term. Try to repeat each one six times morning and evening, though make sure that you do not strain. Increase to ten repetitions as you feel more comfortable. First, lie down on an exercise mat or a bed with a firm mattress. Make sure that your body is straight.

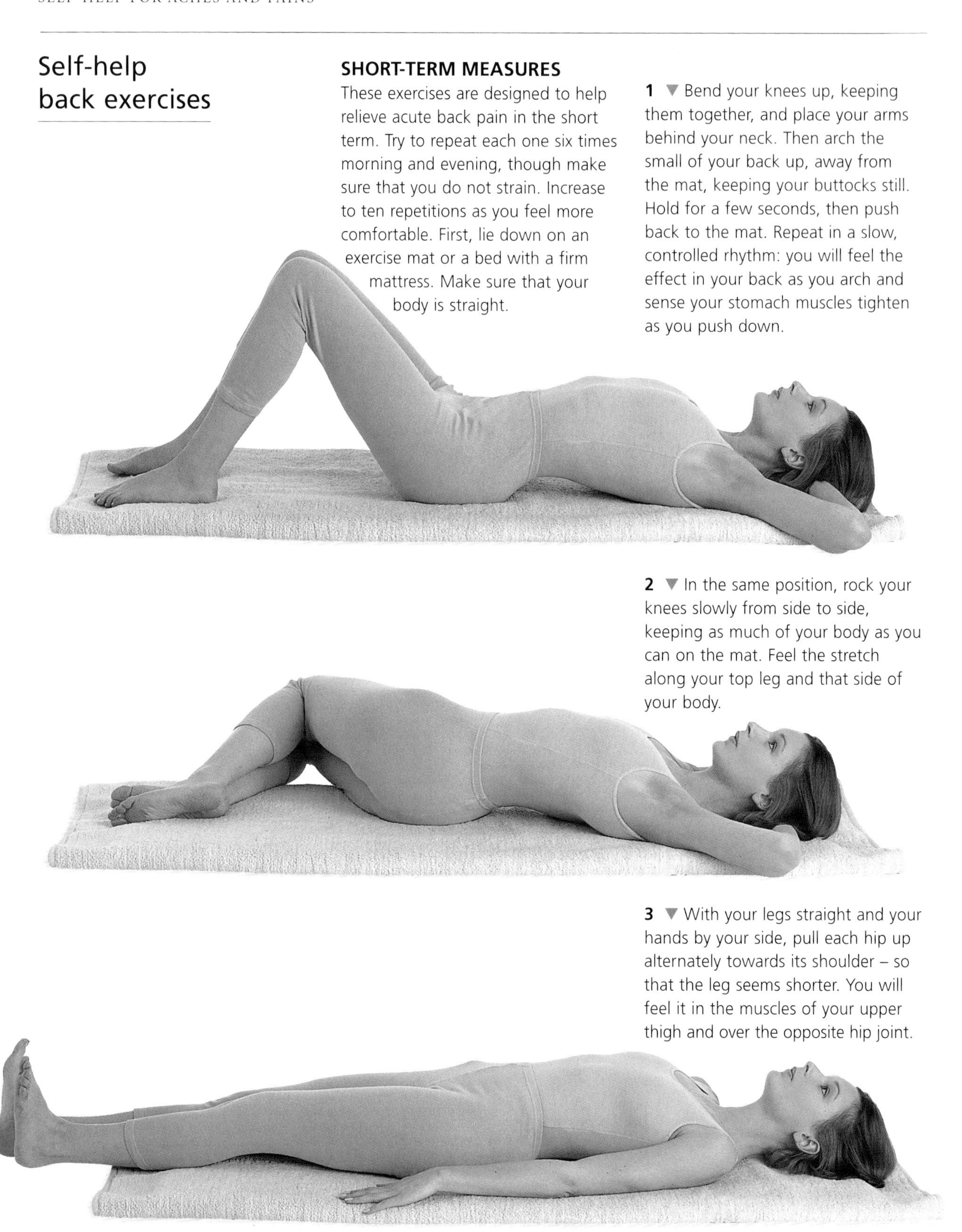

1 ▼ Bend your knees up, keeping them together, and place your arms behind your neck. Then arch the small of your back up, away from the mat, keeping your buttocks still. Hold for a few seconds, then push back to the mat. Repeat in a slow, controlled rhythm: you will feel the effect in your back as you arch and sense your stomach muscles tighten as you push down.

2 ▼ In the same position, rock your knees slowly from side to side, keeping as much of your body as you can on the mat. Feel the stretch along your top leg and that side of your body.

3 ▼ With your legs straight and your hands by your side, pull each hip up alternately towards its shoulder – so that the leg seems shorter. You will feel it in the muscles of your upper thigh and over the opposite hip joint.

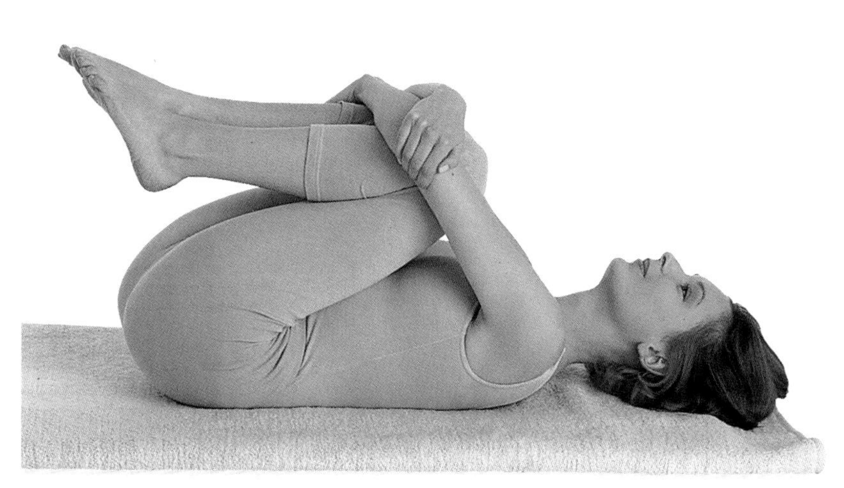

4 ◀ Bend your knees and hug them into your chest, feeling the stretch over your lower spine. Relax fully between repetitions.

5 Finish your routine by repeating exercise 1.

▲ **Safety watchpoint** Make sure that you do not strain at any stage or you might make matters worse. If any exercise increases the severity or extent of the pain – if it starts to shoot down your leg, for example – stop immediately and lie flat. If in any doubt, consult your doctor.

LONG-TERM MEASURES

Once the immediate problem of acute back pain has been dealt with, it is vital that you follow a long-term exercise programme in order to prevent any relapse and relieve nagging, minor pains. Make the exercises below and the weight-bearing ones overleaf part of your daily routine, morning and night – they will only take a few minutes.

1 ▼ Lie down with a lumbar roll supporting the small of your back – a cushion or rolled-up towel will do; reduce the height of the roll until you feel comfortable. Relax in this position for ten minutes each day. Over time, gradually increase the height of the roll (up to the height of about four cushions) and keep the position for up to 20 minutes.

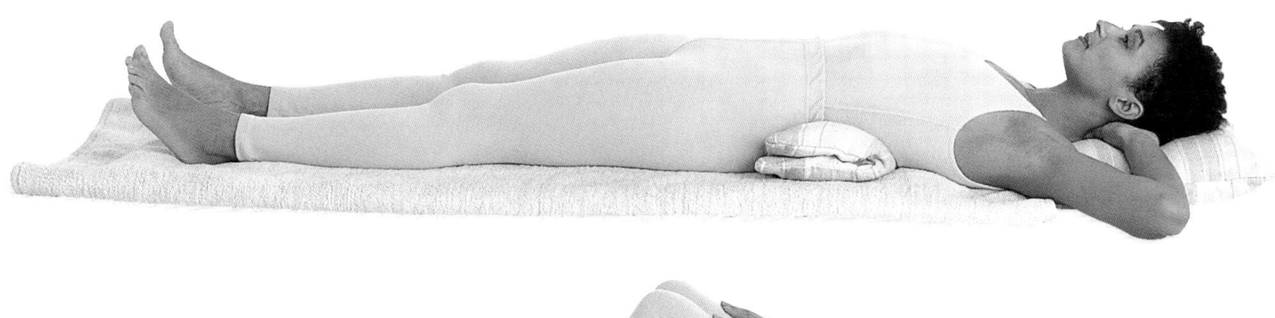

2 ▶ Bend your knees and try to touch them with your hands, lifting your head and shoulders off the mat. Make sure you do not strain your neck – your abdominal muscles should do the work. Hold for a count of five, increasing to ten over time, then lower slowly.

LONG-TERM MEASURES (continued)

3 ▶ Stand up with your feet shoulders' width apart. Without bending forwards or backwards, slide one arm down your side towards your knee, feeling the stretch down the opposite side. Then do the same with your other arm. Repeat this exercise six times.

4 ▶ Repeat, stretching first one hand and then the other as far up to the ceiling as you can, without bending forwards or backwards or moving your feet. Repeat six times.

5 ▼ Put your hands on your hips and twist to look behind you while keeping your hips and legs still; then twist to look back over the other shoulder. Repeat six times and feel the stretch in your spine and rib cage.

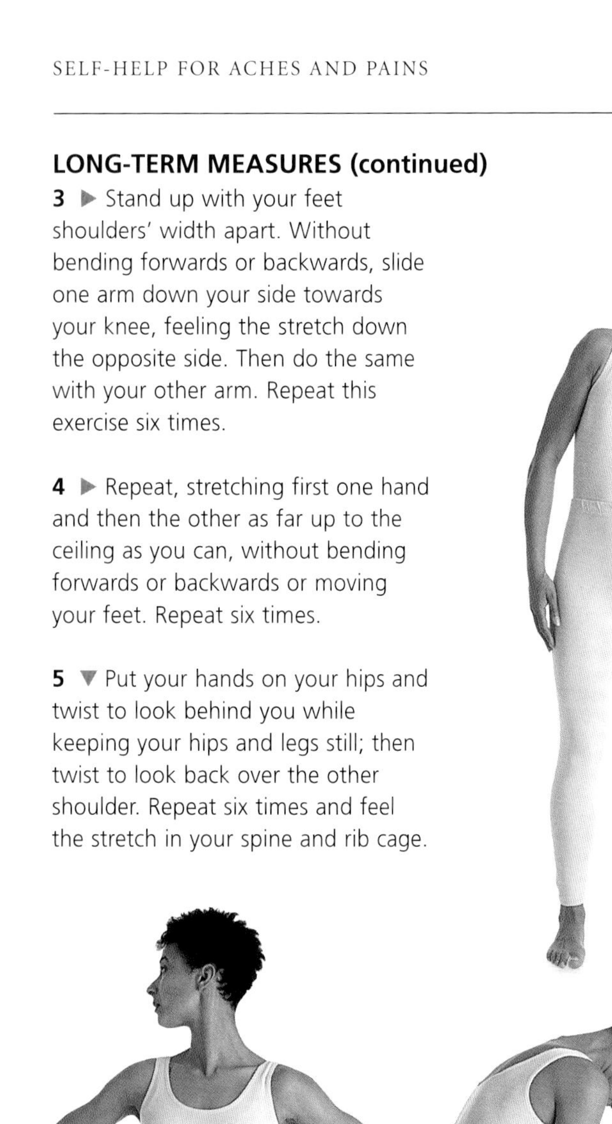

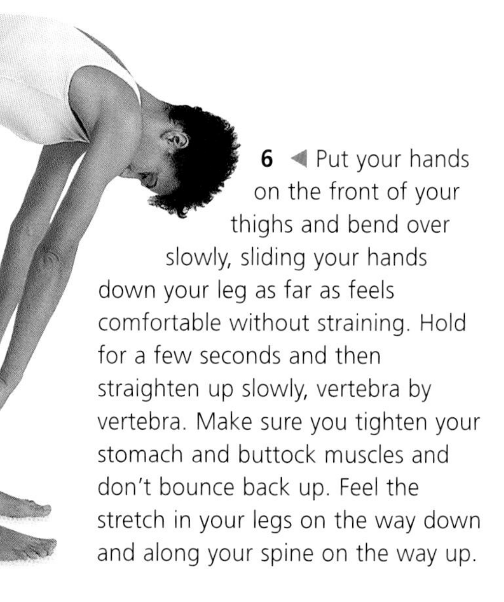

6 ◀ Put your hands on the front of your thighs and bend over slowly, sliding your hands down your leg as far as feels comfortable without straining. Hold for a few seconds and then straighten up slowly, vertebra by vertebra. Make sure you tighten your stomach and buttock muscles and don't bounce back up. Feel the stretch in your legs on the way down and along your spine on the way up.

7 ▶ Put your hands on your hips and arch your back, pushing your shoulder blades together and looking up at the ceiling – don't put your neck too far back or you may strain it. Feel the stretch across your chest and the tightness between your shoulder blades.

8 Repeat exercises 6 and 7 alternately three times, then finish off with exercise 6 again.

9 ▶ Rotate your hips for one minute as if you were moving a hula hoop or dancing – some music may help.

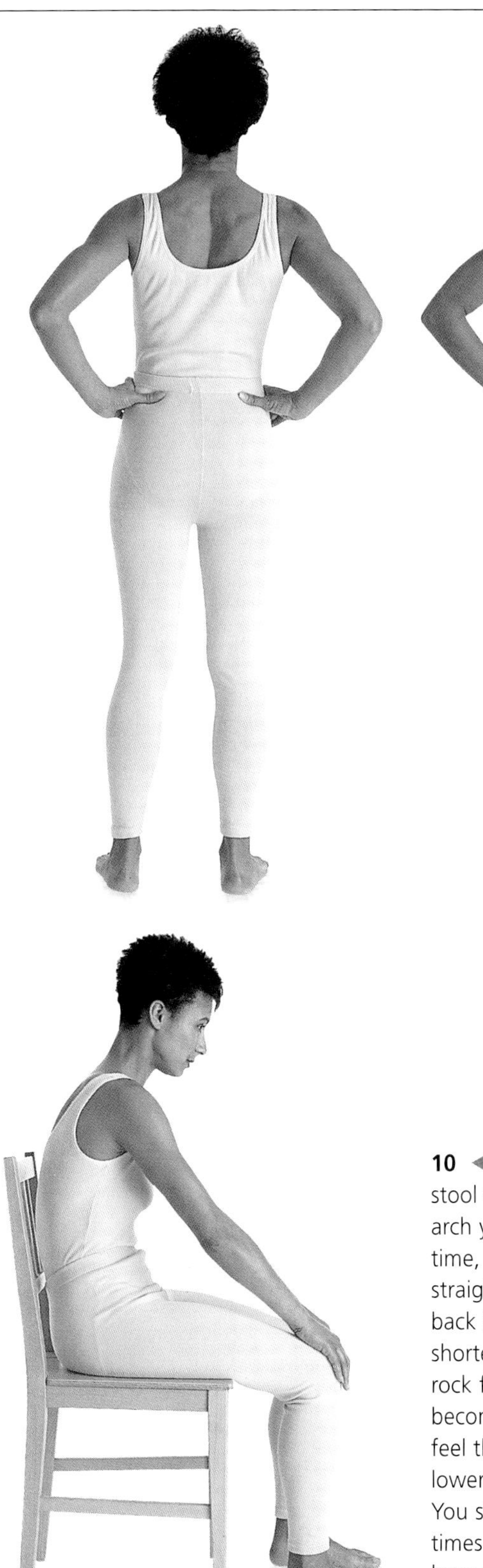

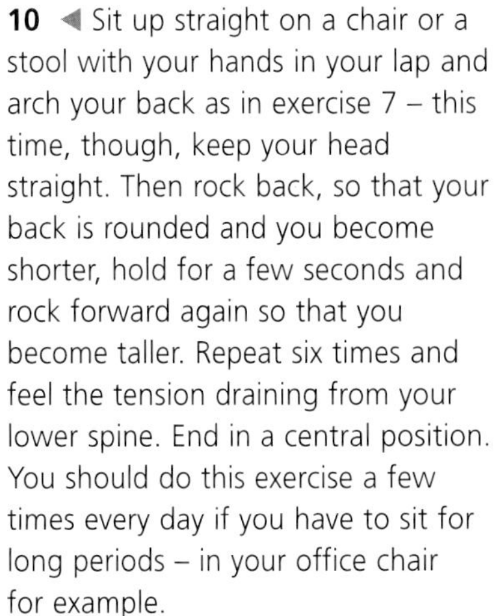

10 ◀ Sit up straight on a chair or a stool with your hands in your lap and arch your back as in exercise 7 – this time, though, keep your head straight. Then rock back, so that your back is rounded and you become shorter, hold for a few seconds and rock forward again so that you become taller. Repeat six times and feel the tension draining from your lower spine. End in a central position. You should do this exercise a few times every day if you have to sit for long periods – in your office chair for example.

Shoulder problems

The shoulder allows the greatest range of movements of any joint in the body. This is largely due to the complex array of muscles that constantly adjust the alignment of the bones. There are two types of muscles in the shoulder: phasic muscles (see page 23) that move the shoulder blade and maintain posture, and small rotator cuff muscles that move the arm (see page 54).

Most shoulder-joint problems stem from the fact that the muscles that move the humerus are short compared to the length of the bone. Even the largest, *deltoid*, only inserts half way down the humerus. In order to work efficiently, therefore, the muscles need to operate at their best possible angle of pull. To achieve this, the head of the humerus must manoeuvre around the socket of the shoulder joint. If these accessory movements are lost for any reason, the muscles cannot work efficiently and tendons will be strained and become inflamed.

Poor posture – especially hunched and rounded shoulders – affects the muscles of the shoulder joint. *Trapezius*, a postural muscle, will be overstretched and the small muscles will be at the wrong angles to move the head of the humerus around its socket, resulting in tendinitis or more rarely a frozen shoulder (see pages 54–55).

The same conditions can result from weak muscles, especially if they are called on to perform some strenuous task, such as lifting a heavy weight, or activities that involve sudden jerks. Repetitive movements that strain the muscles, such as painting a ceiling, pruning high bushes or swimming front crawl, can have the same effect.

Osteoarthritis (see page 42) of the shoulder is uncommon as it is a non-weight-bearing joint. However, it can occur, especially if the shoulder joint has been used excessively over a long period of time, as with fast bowling in cricket.

Sometimes, pain in the shoulder arises not in the joint itself but in the neck. If a nerve is pinched where it leaves the spinal column, the pain can be felt in the shoulder and sometimes radiating down the arm (see pages 40–41).

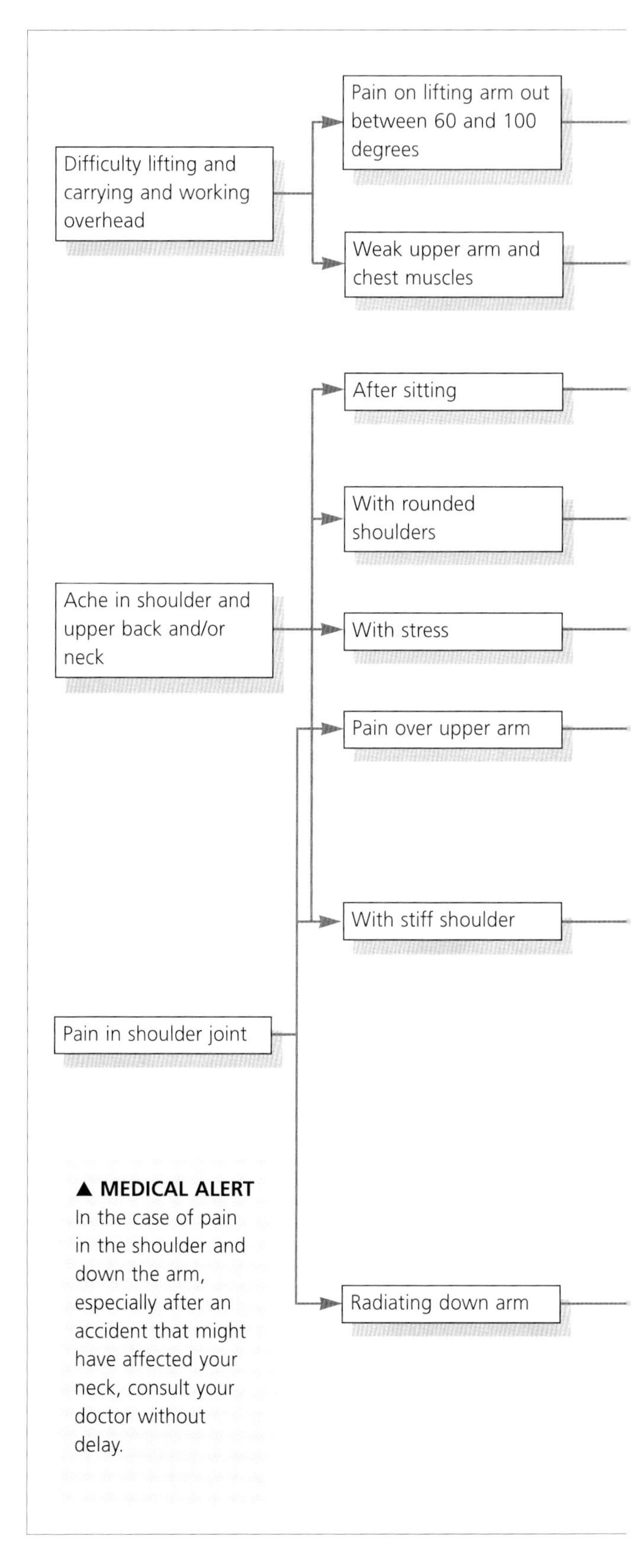

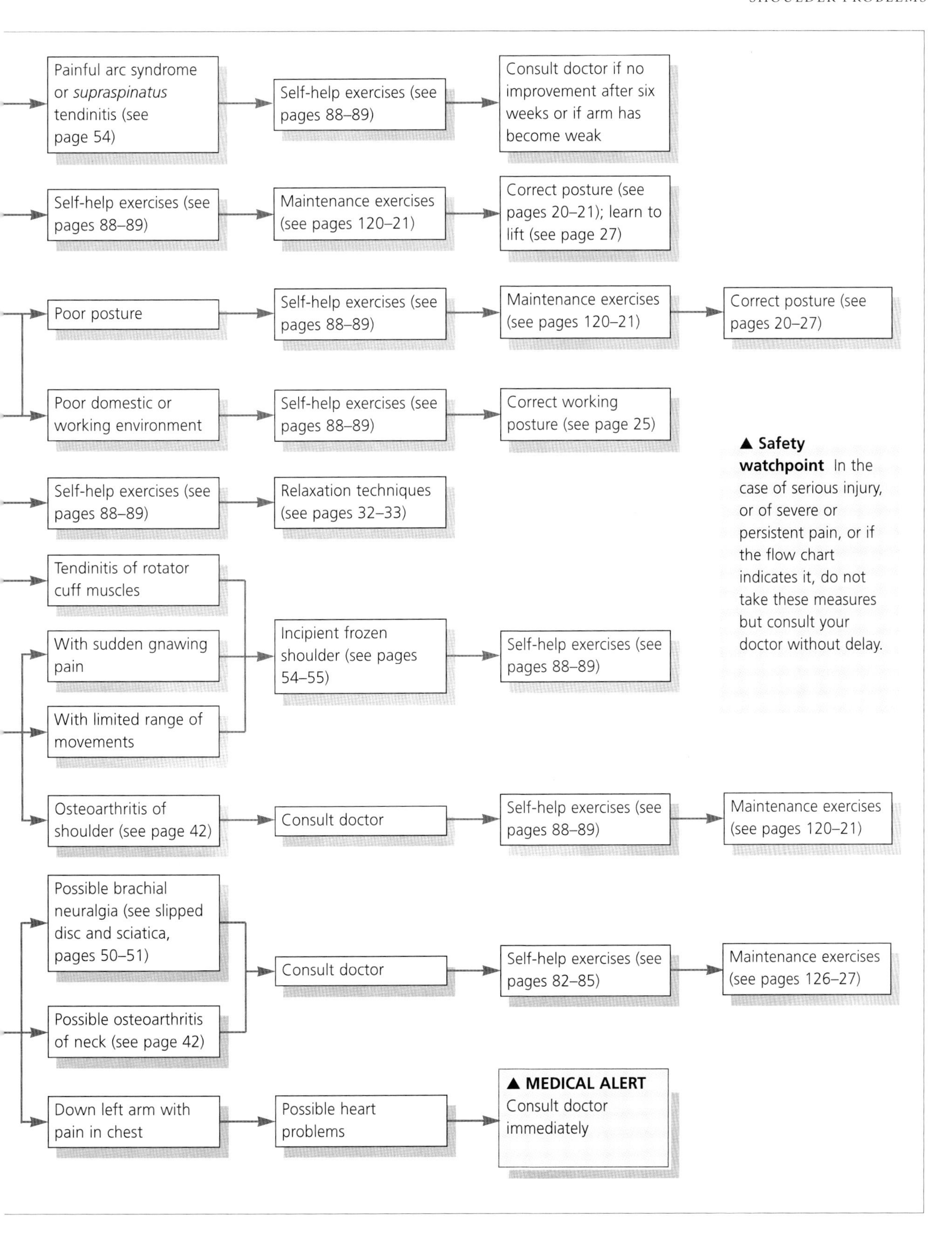

▲ **Safety watchpoint** In the case of serious injury, or of severe or persistent pain, or if the flow chart indicates it, do not take these measures but consult your doctor without delay.

Self-help shoulder exercises

SHORT-TERM MEASURES

These exercises are designed to provide prompt treatment for conditions that affect the shoulder, such as frozen shoulder, *supraspinatus* tendinitis and problems of the rotator cuff muscles in general. Use them morning and evening, but make sure that you do not overdo things.

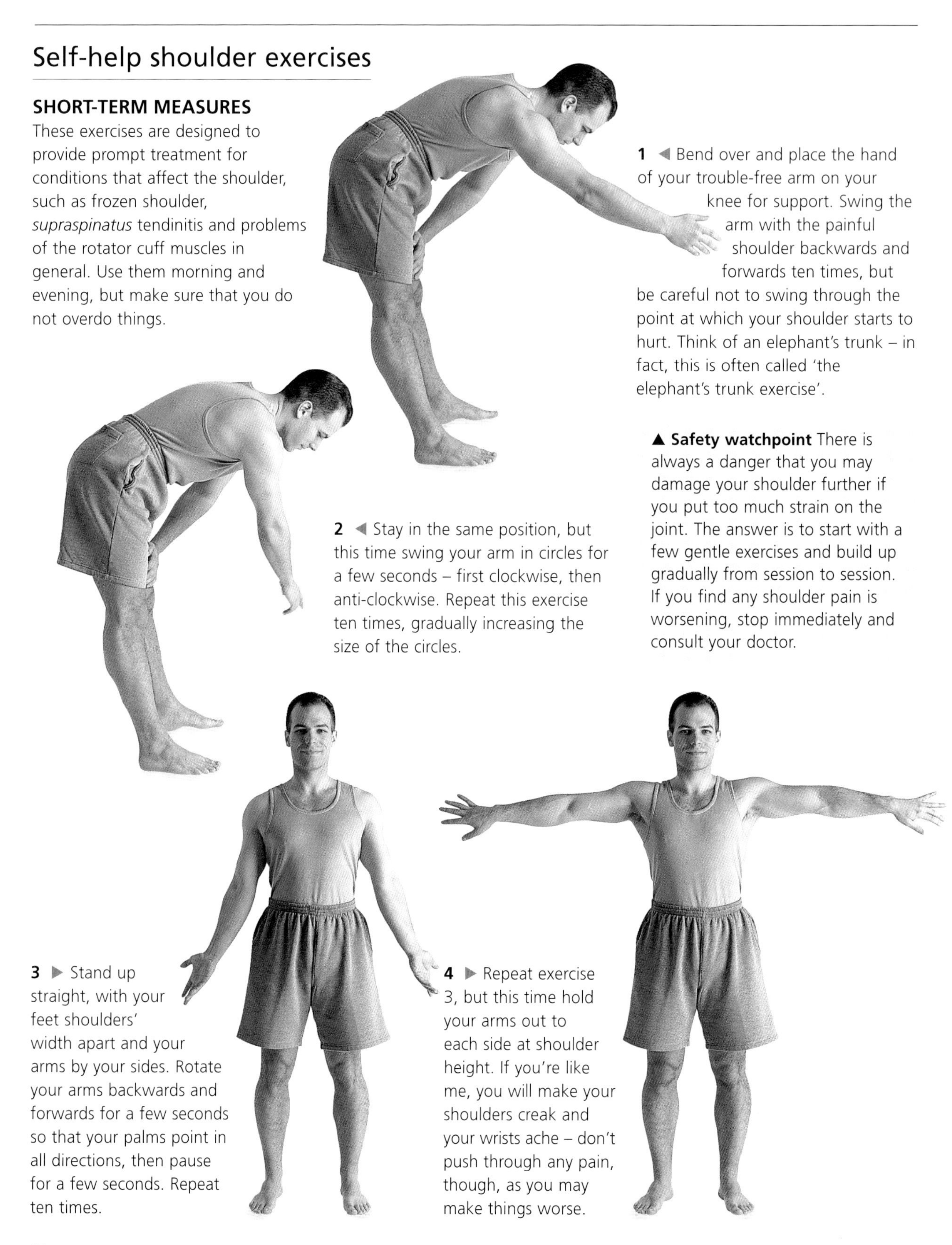

1 ◀ Bend over and place the hand of your trouble-free arm on your knee for support. Swing the arm with the painful shoulder backwards and forwards ten times, but be careful not to swing through the point at which your shoulder starts to hurt. Think of an elephant's trunk – in fact, this is often called 'the elephant's trunk exercise'.

2 ◀ Stay in the same position, but this time swing your arm in circles for a few seconds – first clockwise, then anti-clockwise. Repeat this exercise ten times, gradually increasing the size of the circles.

▲ **Safety watchpoint** There is always a danger that you may damage your shoulder further if you put too much strain on the joint. The answer is to start with a few gentle exercises and build up gradually from session to session. If you find any shoulder pain is worsening, stop immediately and consult your doctor.

3 ▶ Stand up straight, with your feet shoulders' width apart and your arms by your sides. Rotate your arms backwards and forwards for a few seconds so that your palms point in all directions, then pause for a few seconds. Repeat ten times.

4 ▶ Repeat exercise 3, but this time hold your arms out to each side at shoulder height. If you're like me, you will make your shoulders creak and your wrists ache – don't push through any pain, though, as you may make things worse.

LONG-TERM MEASURES

Unless you take long-term measures to strengthen the muscles and ligaments that support the shoulder joint, there is a risk that your shoulder problem will recur – especially if an acute condition has led to damage in the joint. Follow this programme morning and night to maximise the chances of a full recovery.

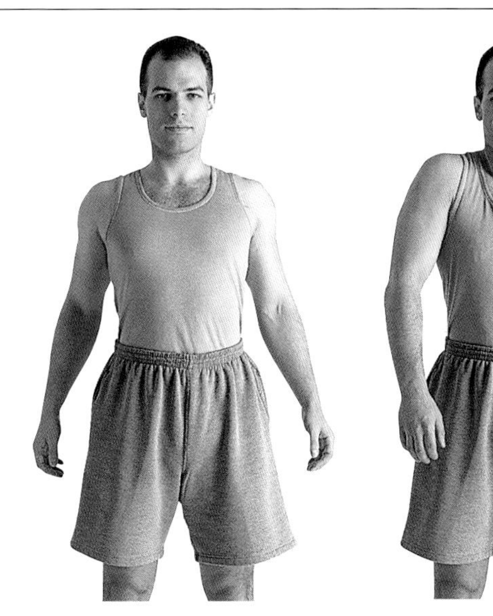

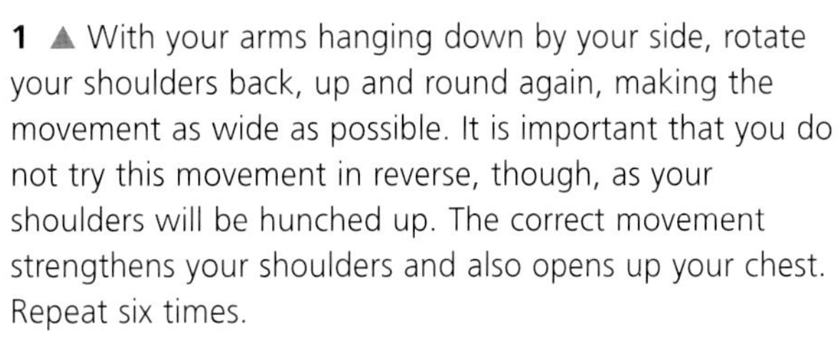

1 ▲ With your arms hanging down by your side, rotate your shoulders back, up and round again, making the movement as wide as possible. It is important that you do not try this movement in reverse, though, as your shoulders will be hunched up. The correct movement strengthens your shoulders and also opens up your chest. Repeat six times.

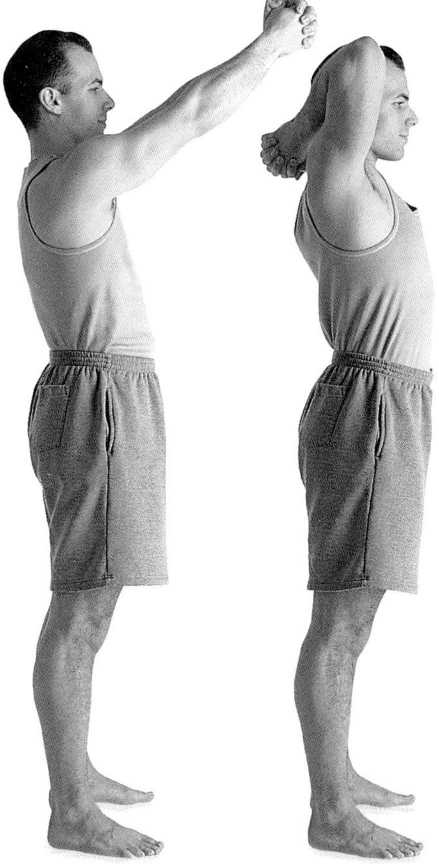

2 ▲ Hold your hands up high in front of you, clasp them together and then lift them above your head. Push them as far back as you can without straining, hold the position for a few seconds and then lower your hands so they rest behind your neck and relax. Repeat six times – you should feel the stretch in your chest.

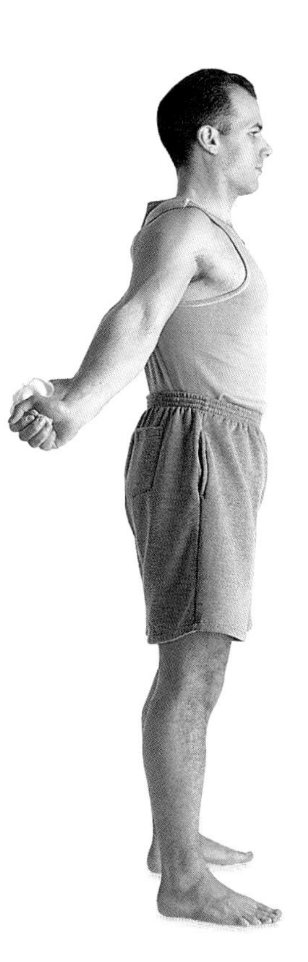

3 ◀ With your hands wide apart, grasp the two ends of a pole (a broom handle would do) or a rolled-up towel behind your back. Swing the object up, over your head and down in front of you. Reverse the motion, then repeat six times. You should feel the stretch down your back and in your shoulder and chest muscles. Reduce the distance between your hands as you get better at the exercise.

Elbow problems

Technically, we could all claim to be 'double-jointed' as far as the elbow is concerned, because the elbow joint is really two joints in one: a hinge joint between the humerus and the ulna; and a pivot joint where the head of the radius rotates around the ulna (see pages 52–53).

The hinge joint is a very tight joint, with many nerves and blood vessels within the capsule. Any damage that results in inflammation and swelling of the capsule – such as a fracture or dislocation – needs to be seen rapidly by a doctor. The excess fluid must be drained off before it compresses the vessels or nerves, causing permanent damage.

Other elbow problems, such as tennis elbow, are normally caused by unaccustomed repetitive movements of the forearm muscles – the wrist flexors and extensors. Each of these two muscle groups shares a common tendon attached to a small point of origin on the humerus. The tendon can easily become wrenched or torn and can even be pulled off the bone. Fluid will seep from the torn tissues, resulting in swelling and pain – a condition known as tendinitis. The point of origin and any movement of the muscles will be exquisitely painful.

In tennis elbow (see page 55) it is the tendon of the wrist extensors that is damaged. This is often due to repetitive domestic or occupational tasks (in tennis, it is the result of frequent backhand shots). With age, the tendons become less resilient, so that actions that were previously tolerated – digging, polishing or window cleaning, for example – can cause tears. Another cause is shaking hands firmly: people who have to shake hands frequently never grasp your hand firmly – they are warned not to.

The ulnar nerve, which supplies the forearm and the hand, passes in a shallow groove across the inner protrusion at the base of the humerus, otherwise known as the funny bone. If this point is knocked it will feel tender and there may be tingling down the forearm. Chair-bound people should not sit with their elbows pressing down onto the arms of their chairs for extended periods or they may damage the nerve permanently.

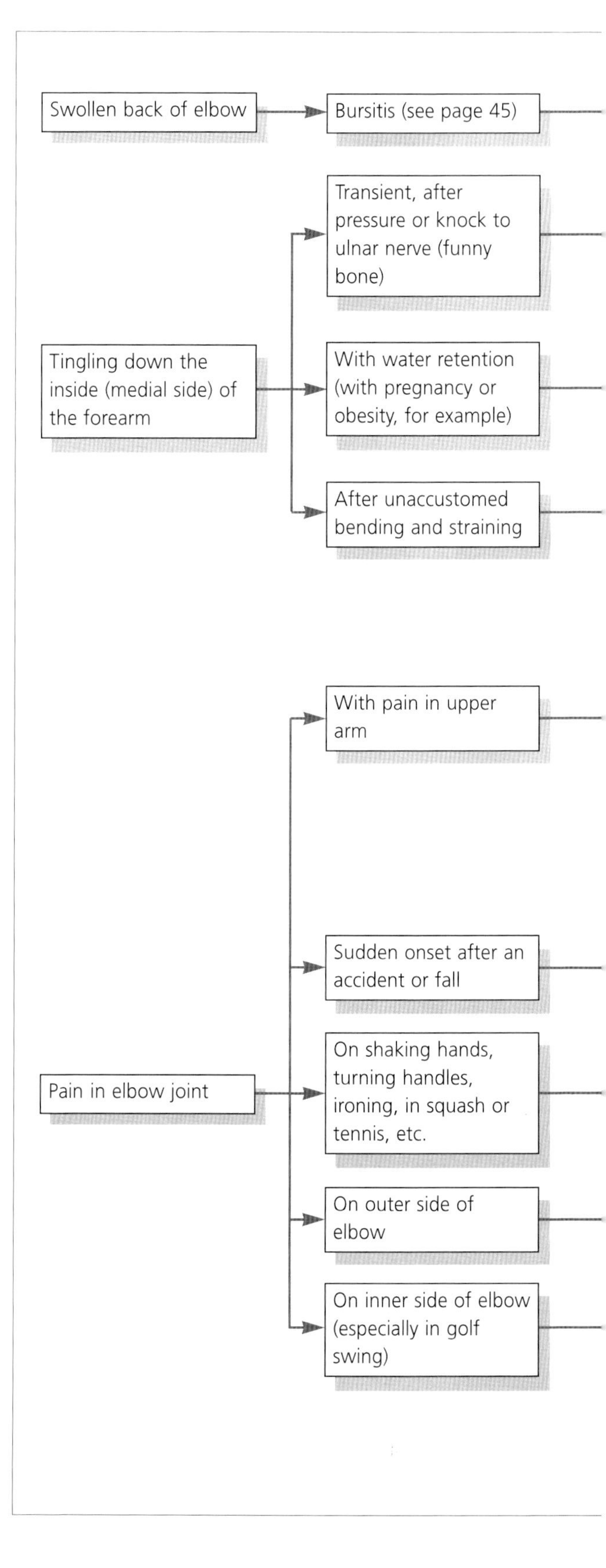

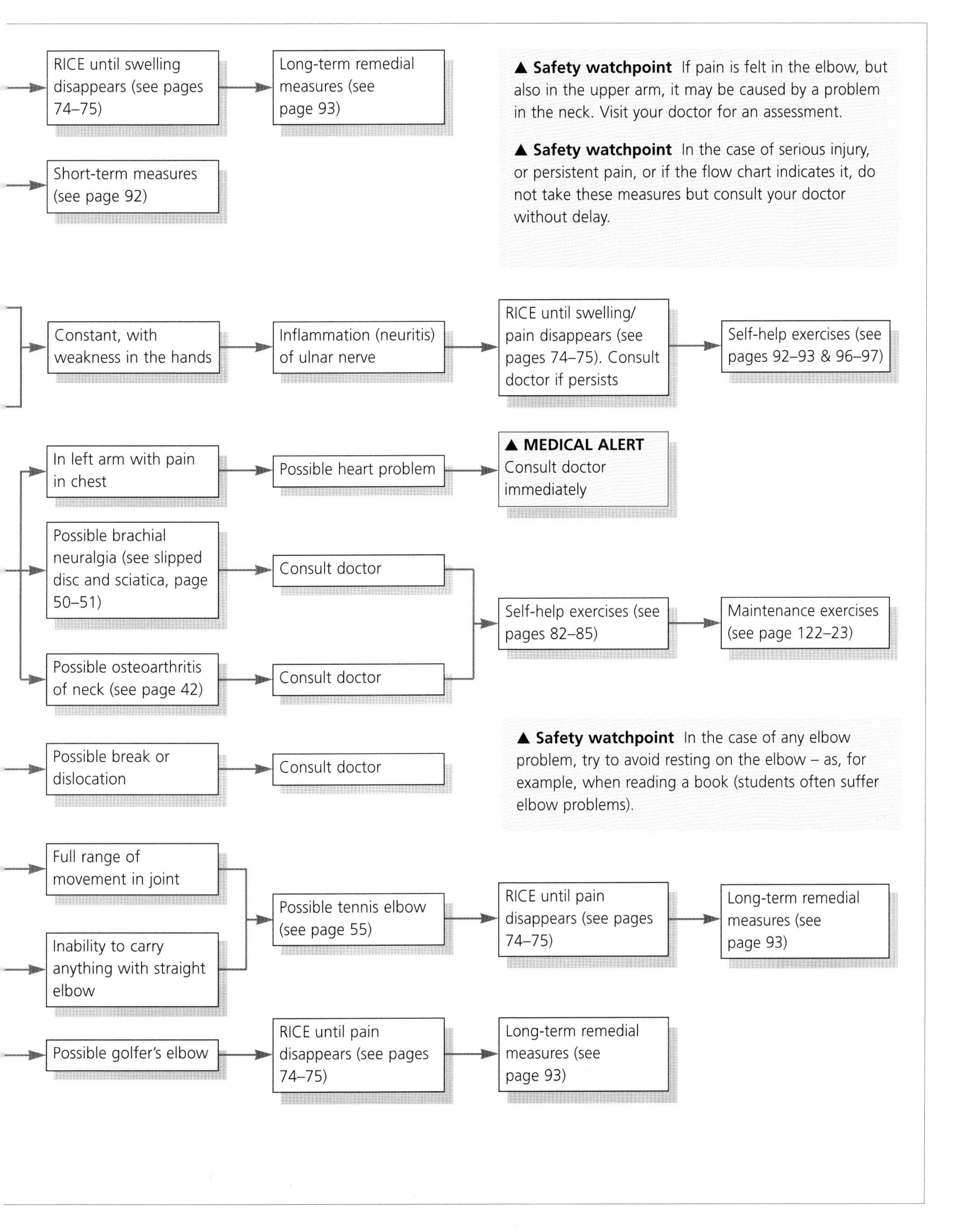

▲ **Safety watchpoint** If pain is felt in the elbow, but also in the upper arm, it may be caused by a problem in the neck. Visit your doctor for an assessment.

▲ **Safety watchpoint** In the case of serious injury, or persistent pain, or if the flow chart indicates it, do not take these measures but consult your doctor without delay.

▲ **Safety watchpoint** In the case of any elbow problem, try to avoid resting on the elbow – as, for example, when reading a book (students often suffer elbow problems).

Self-help elbow exercises

SHORT-TERM MEASURES

These exercises are designed to treat problems affecting the elbows and forearms, such as tennis elbow, sprains and pulled muscles. They increase mobility across the elbow joints and strengthen muscles and ligaments. Use them morning and evening, but don't do too many repetitions at first.

1 ▶ Stretch your arms out in front of your body, and cross one over the other at the wrist so that the thumb-edge of your hands is closest to the ground. Lace your fingers together, drop your hands down towards your stomach and then move them up so that they come to rest under your chin – make sure that your fingers are laced. Hold for a count of three, then reverse the movement. Repeat the complete exercise up to six times, swopping the crossover of your arms on alternate goes – you should feel the pull on the top of your forearms.

2 ▶ Kneel on all fours with your fingers pointing towards your knees and your palms on the ground. Rock gently backwards and forwards up to six times, making sure that your hands stay on the ground.

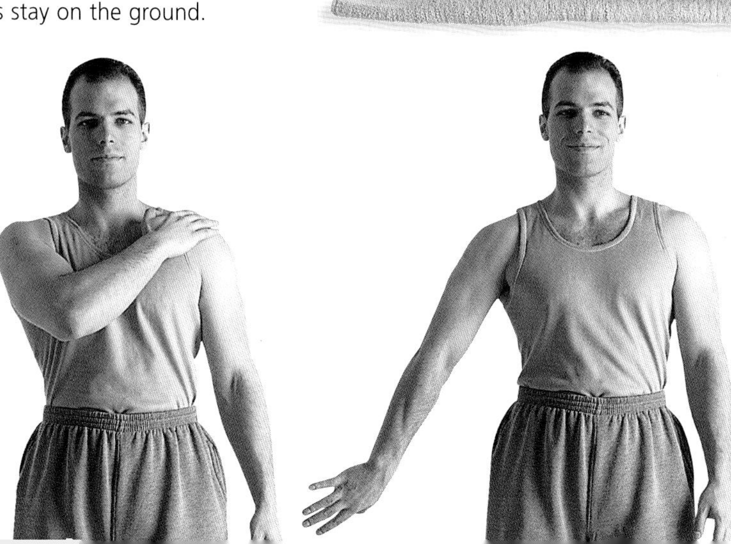

3 ◀ Touch the point of your shoulder with your opposite hand, then straighten and lower your arm, turning your hand so that the palm faces upwards while you do so. Repeat up to six times, to help increase mobility at the elbow.

LONG-TERM MEASURES

Once the initial pain and discomfort of an injury that affects the elbow has been relieved, it is vital that you continue with an exercise programme to try to make sure that the problem does not recur. These exercises are designed to strengthen the tissues and increase both mobility and flexibility.

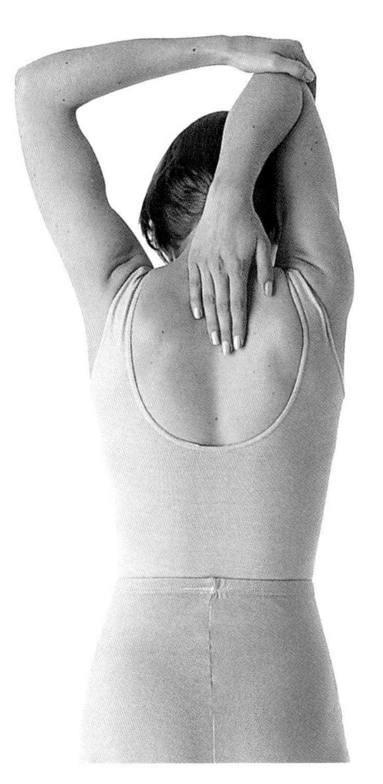

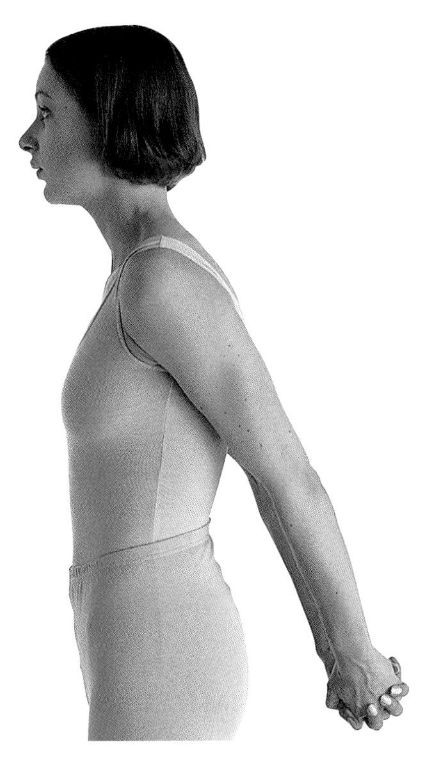

1 ▶ Place one hand behind the back of your neck with the fingers pointing down the spine. Then use your other hand to push the elbow down gently so that your fingers are moved down the spine a little. Don't force, just ease slightly when you begin to feel resistance. Hold for a count of five and then release. Repeat six times, changing hands between each go, and feel the stretch in your elbow and shoulder.

2 ▲ Clasp your hands behind your back. Keeping your elbows straight, raise your hands as high as possible without causing pain. Hold for a few seconds, then lower. Repeat six times – this frees up the elbow joint.

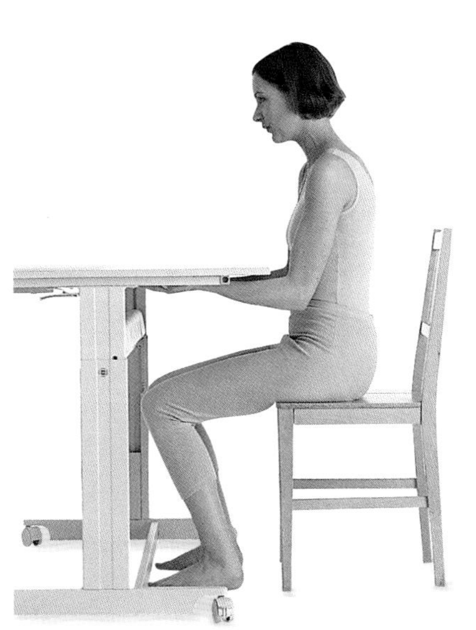

3 ▲ Sit at a heavy table or desk with your elbows bent and your palms on its underside. Now try to lift the table, without moving the rest of your body. Hold for a few seconds, then relax before trying again – up to six times. This is an isometric exercise that strengthens the muscles that work across the elbow joint.

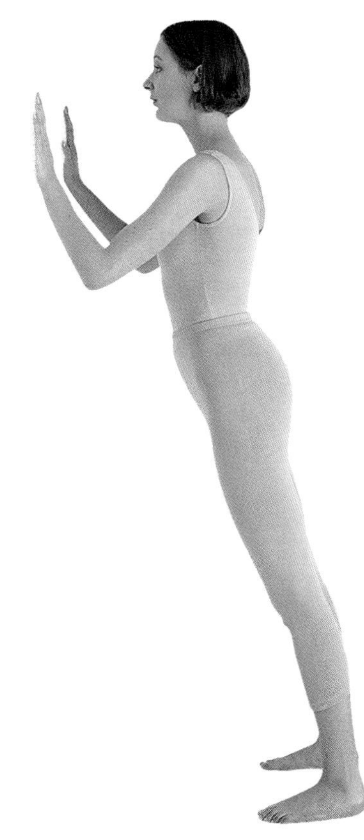

4 ◀ Stand at arm's length from a wall and place your hands on it shoulder's width apart at shoulder height. Bend your elbows until your face touches the wall. Stop for a moment and then push back up. Repeat six times.

▲ **Safety watchpoint** Never try to get up to the maximum number of repetitions on the first occasion that you try these exercises, nor should you push through any pain. It is important that you build up slowly, over a number of sessions, otherwise you may damage the tissues. If you feel that any pain is becoming worse, or spreading to a new area, stop doing the exercise and consult your doctor or physiotherapist.

Wrist and hand problems

The human hand is unique in the animal kingdom for its dexterity. The ability of the wrist to turn in and out, and of the thumb to oppose the fingers, makes the hand extraordinarily versatile. Normally, the wrist and hand can cope with constant, repetitive movements, such as those demanded by computers and other machines, but unaccustomed ones can cause the joint and surrounding soft tissues to suffer. The result can be tenosynovitis, in which both the tendons and their synovial sheaths become inflamed, the condition being known as RSI or AFT (see pages 58–59).

This inflammation of the tendons in the hand and fingers can compress the median nerve as it runs through the narrow channel in the wrist called the carpal tunnel. Initially, this only causes pins and needles, but eventually the muscles waste and sensation is lost in the hand. Carpal tunnel syndrome (see page 59) is also caused by rheumatoid arthritis and can occur during pregnancy.

Rheumatoid arthritis and gout also affect the hands. Acute gout affects the thumb and wrist, which become hot, red and painful. Gout is easily diagnosed by a blood test for high levels of uric acid. Rheumatoid arthritis affects all the joints of the hand and can cause considerable deformation.

The bones of the hands and wrists are susceptible to fractures – we instinctively put our hands out to break a fall. The wrist above the thumb is often fractured – a Colles fracture – by a fall on an outstretched hand, particularly when children are involved. The scaphoid bone at the base of the thumb may also be broken. This bone has a poor blood supply, so heals slowly and with difficulty, and if the problem is not treated there can be considerable pain in the deep tissues.

Pain in the wrist and hand can also be due to damage to ligaments and nerves. Often this results from continuous pressure on the heel of the hand, as when bicycling or making bread. Osteoarthritis often affects the wrist and hand in old age after a lifetime of heavy use; the base of the thumb is the most common site, especially in women.

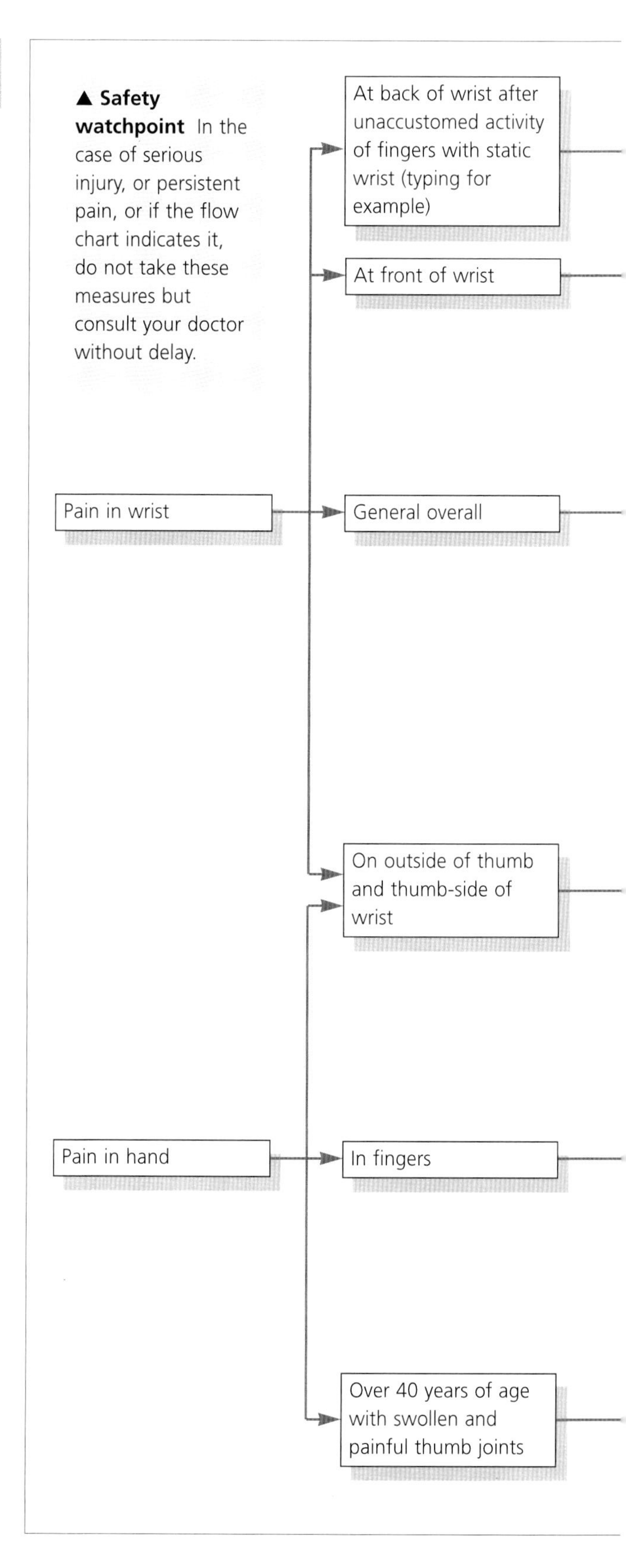

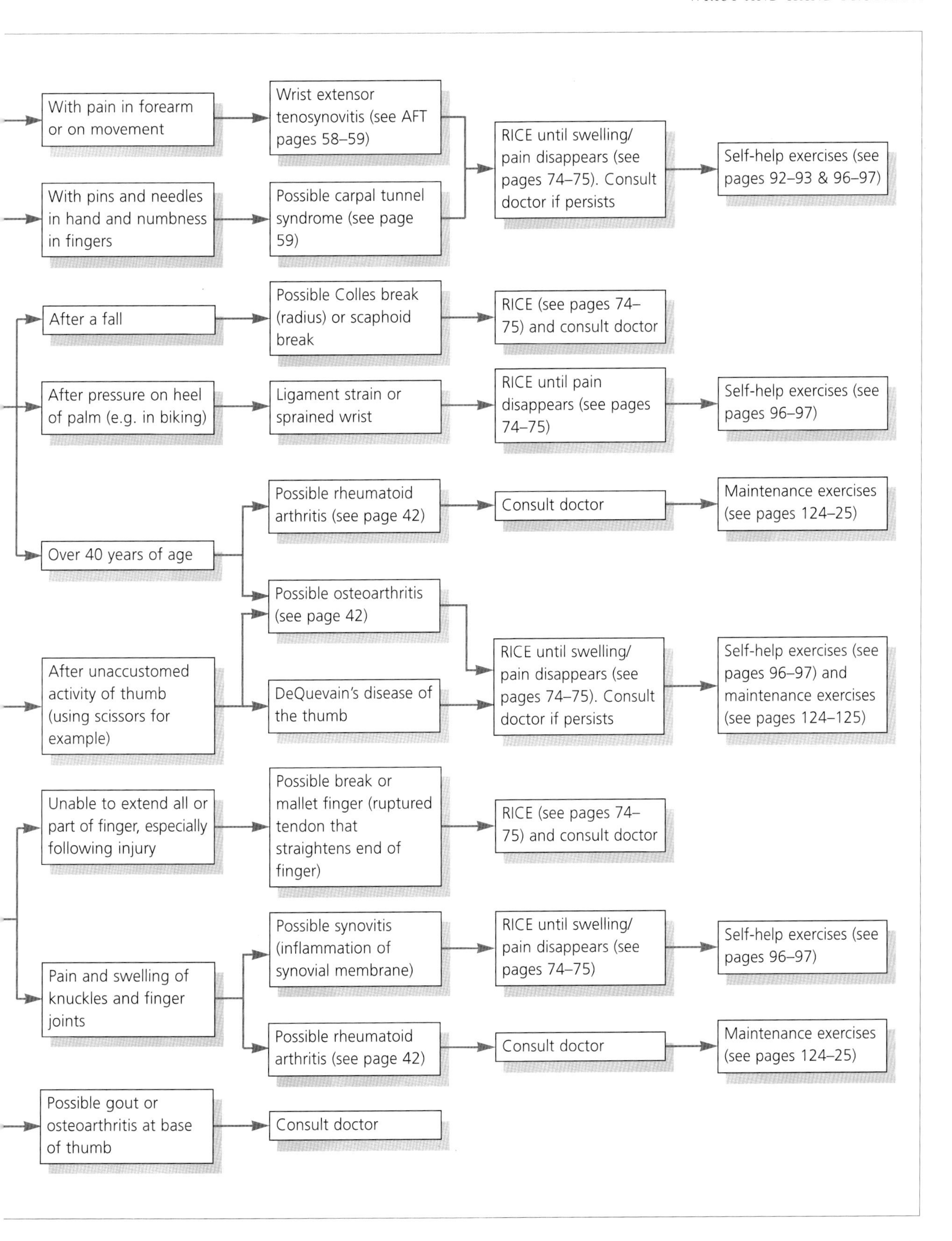
With pain in forearm or on movement
Wrist extensor tenosynovitis (see AFT pages 58–59)
With pins and needles in hand and numbness in fingers
Possible carpal tunnel syndrome (see page 59)
RICE until swelling/ pain disappears (see pages 74–75). Consult doctor if persists
Self-help exercises (see pages 92–93 & 96–97)
After a fall
Possible Colles break (radius) or scaphoid break
RICE (see pages 74–75) and consult doctor
After pressure on heel of palm (e.g. in biking)
Ligament strain or sprained wrist
RICE until pain disappears (see pages 74–75)
Self-help exercises (see pages 96–97)
Over 40 years of age
Possible rheumatoid arthritis (see page 42)
Consult doctor
Maintenance exercises (see pages 124–25)
Possible osteoarthritis (see page 42)
After unaccustomed activity of thumb (using scissors for example)
DeQuevain's disease of the thumb
RICE until swelling/ pain disappears (see pages 74–75). Consult doctor if persists
Self-help exercises (see pages 96–97) and maintenance exercises (see pages 124–125)
Unable to extend all or part of finger, especially following injury
Possible break or mallet finger (ruptured tendon that straightens end of finger)
RICE (see pages 74–75) and consult doctor
Pain and swelling of knuckles and finger joints
Possible synovitis (inflammation of synovial membrane)
RICE until swelling/ pain disappears (see pages 74–75)
Self-help exercises (see pages 96–97)
Possible rheumatoid arthritis (see page 42)
Consult doctor
Maintenance exercises (see pages 124–25)
Possible gout or osteoarthritis at base of thumb
Consult doctor

Self-help wrist and hand exercises

Injuries that affect the hands and wrist, such as RSI and carpal tunnel syndrome, can have a major impact, simply because we use our hands so much. This constant use means that long-term remedial measures are rarely necessary, but use these short-term ones twice a day.

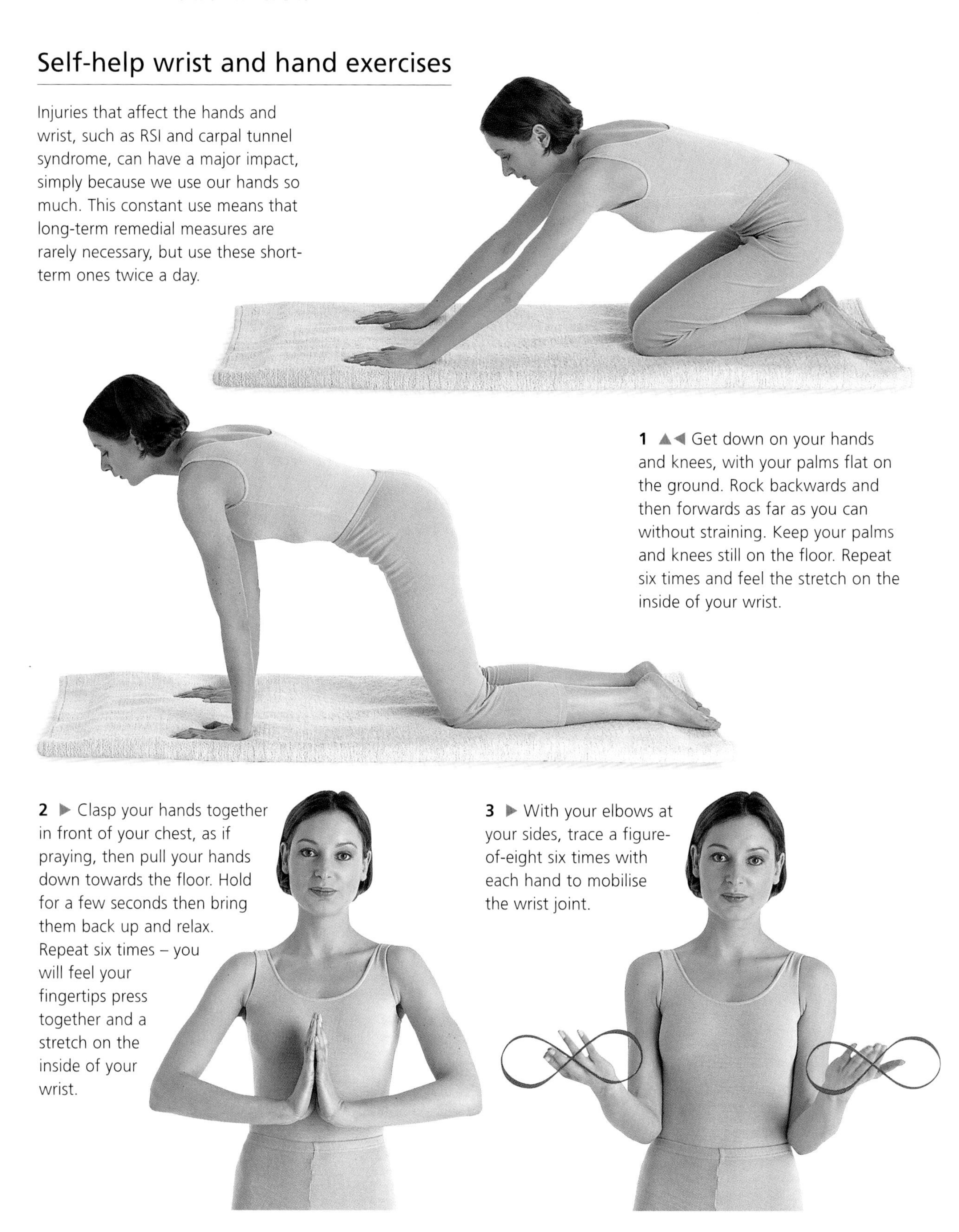

1 ▲◀ Get down on your hands and knees, with your palms flat on the ground. Rock backwards and then forwards as far as you can without straining. Keep your palms and knees still on the floor. Repeat six times and feel the stretch on the inside of your wrist.

2 ▶ Clasp your hands together in front of your chest, as if praying, then pull your hands down towards the floor. Hold for a few seconds then bring them back up and relax. Repeat six times – you will feel your fingertips press together and a stretch on the inside of your wrist.

3 ▶ With your elbows at your sides, trace a figure-of-eight six times with each hand to mobilise the wrist joint.

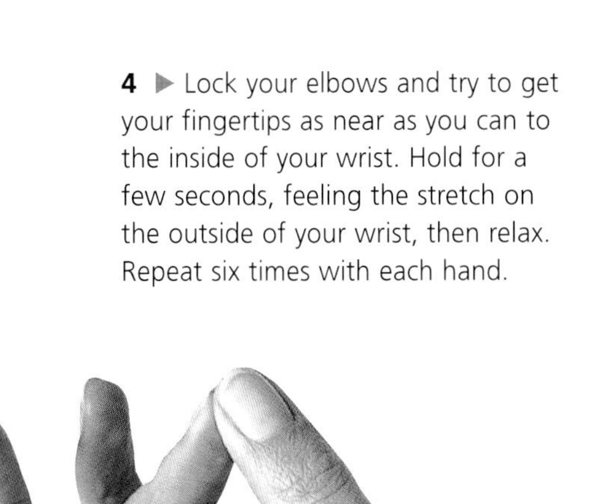

4 ▶ Lock your elbows and try to get your fingertips as near as you can to the inside of your wrist. Hold for a few seconds, feeling the stretch on the outside of your wrist, then relax. Repeat six times with each hand.

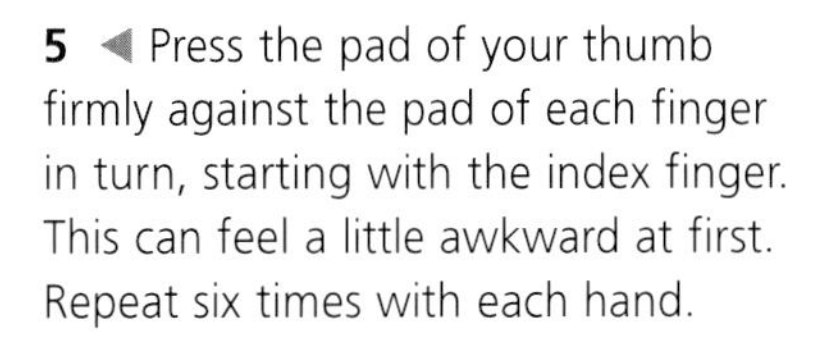

5 ◀ Press the pad of your thumb firmly against the pad of each finger in turn, starting with the index finger. This can feel a little awkward at first. Repeat six times with each hand.

6 ▶ Hold a towel or cloth in both hands and wring it as hard as you can. Repeat six times, bringing alternate hands forwards and backwards. This exercise improves pronation, supination and grip.

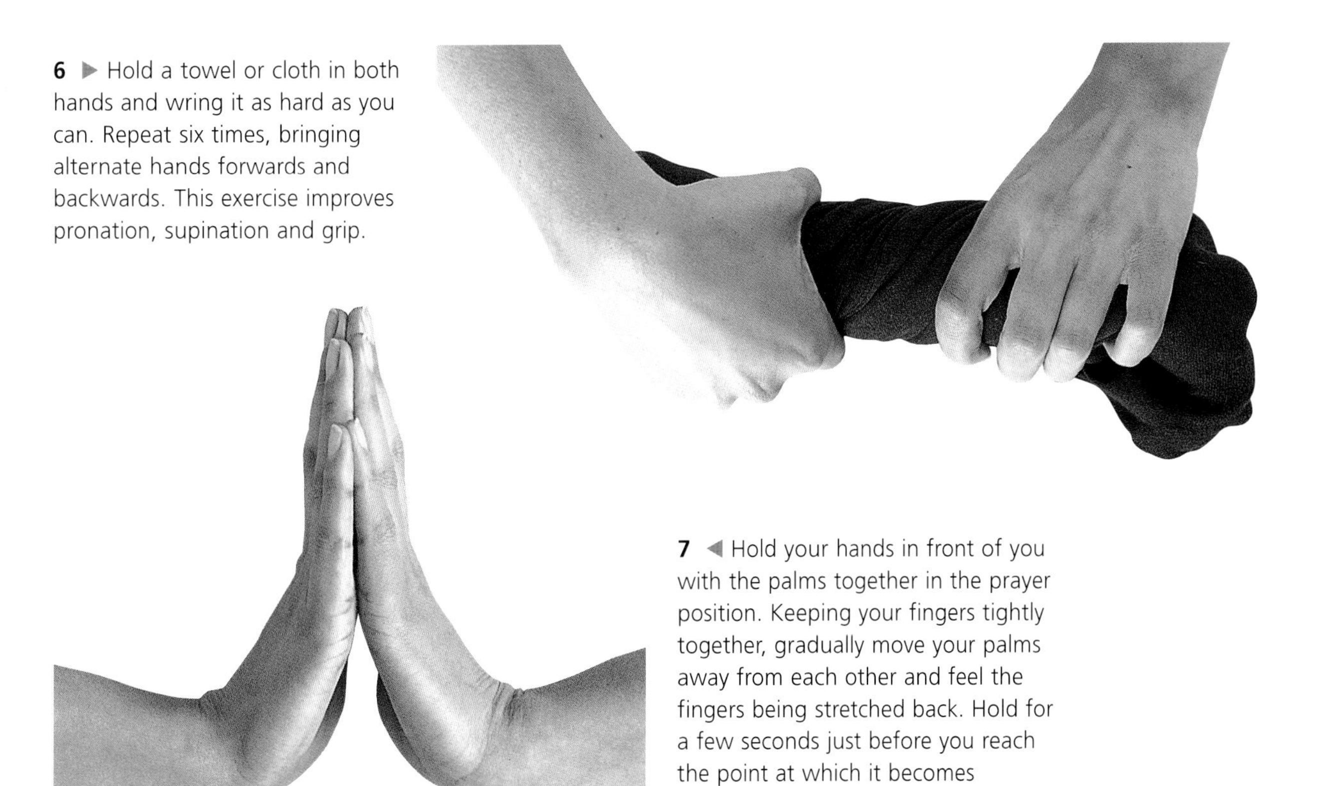

7 ◀ Hold your hands in front of you with the palms together in the prayer position. Keeping your fingers tightly together, gradually move your palms away from each other and feel the fingers being stretched back. Hold for a few seconds just before you reach the point at which it becomes painful, then relax. Repeat six times.

Hip problems

The hip is a rugged and stable joint, as it needs to bear the weight of the upper body and the stresses of moving about. Stability is given by the deep cup-shaped socket of the hip bone, strong surrounding ligaments and a tough joint capsule. What the hip gains in stability, however, it loses in having none of the small accessory movements common to most other joints, even though there is a wide range of gross movement.

Unfortunately, the hip is also one of the most vulnerable of joints, and is particularly susceptible to the effects of wear and tear. It is one of the most common sites for early arthritis, and some degree of osteoarthritis of the hip (see page 62) is almost inevitable in later years. In fact, hip replacement is one of the most common surgical operations performed in Western societies.

In part, the hip's vulnerability is due to the fact that its ligaments and bones receive sufficient blood, and so nutrients, only when there is all-round movement. A lack of nutrients causes the capsule and ligaments to thicken and dry out, producing stiffness and a loss of mobility – a vicious circle. Unfortunately, in the West the main use to which our hips are put is in walking, this action being a monotonous flexion and slight extension, with little variation or stretch. The lack of sideways movement affects the lubrication of the joint, which will quickly show the signs of wear and tear. By contrast, in the East, where people sit cross-legged for long periods, there is little osteoarthritis of the hip.

The muscles that surround the hip joint are also affected by failure to stretch them regularly through their full range. They become much more susceptible to painful sprains and tears. The hip is also vulnerable to fractures. The weakest part of the joint is the neck of the femur, particularly if old age or osteoporosis have made the bone brittle.

Pain in the hip joint may sometimes be referred from the lower back (see page 50). True hip pain is not made worse by bending, coughing or sneezing and, unlike referred pain, it may radiate down the front of the thigh to stop just above the knee cap.

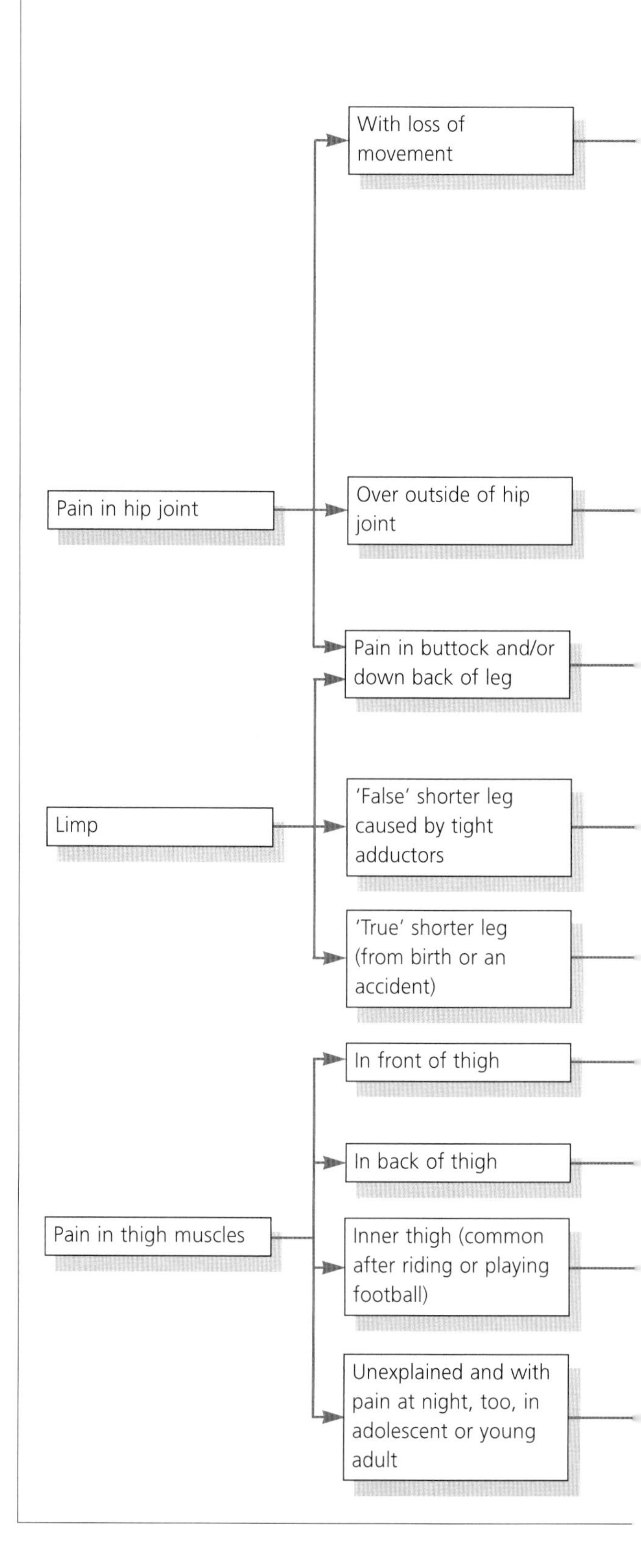

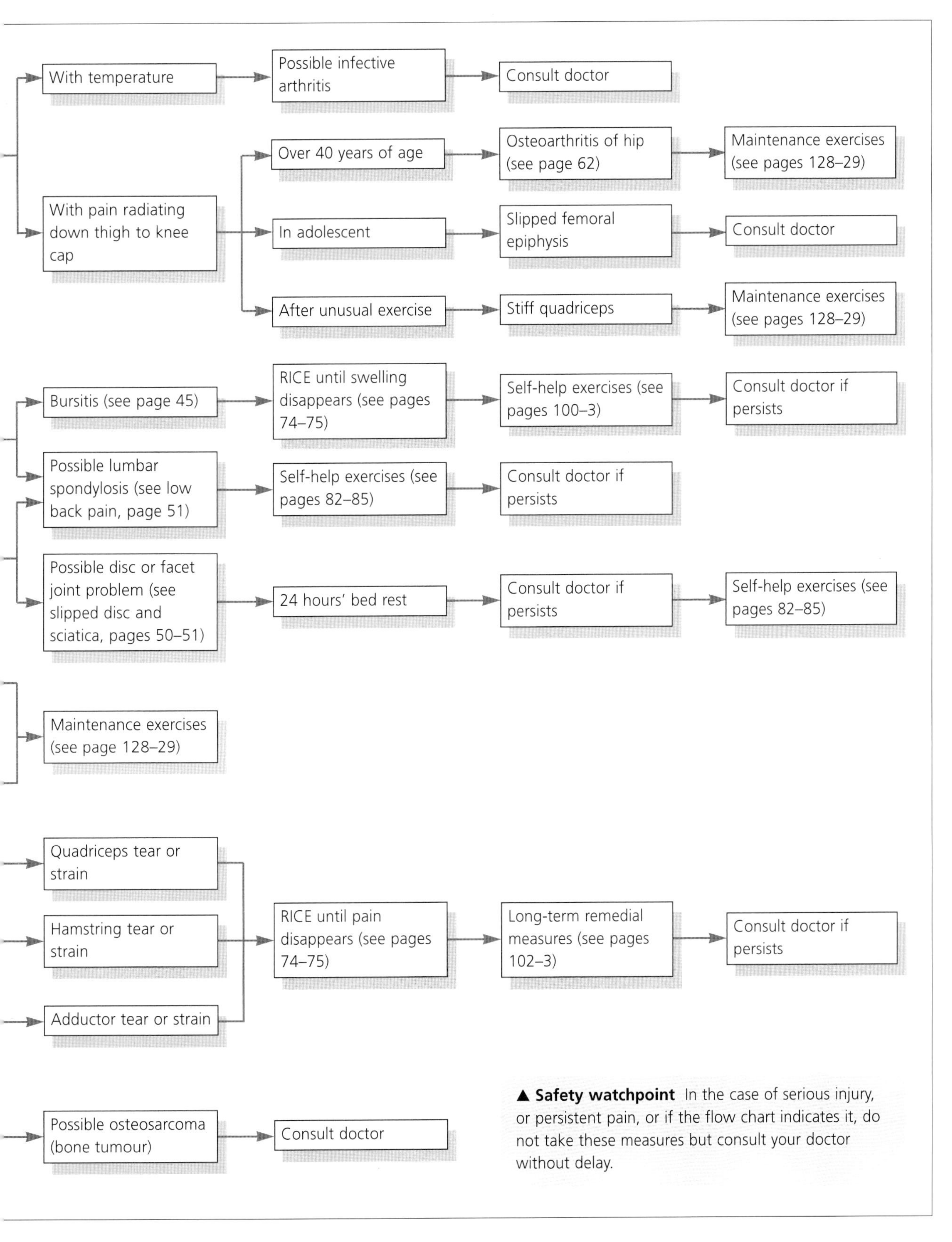

▲ **Safety watchpoint** In the case of serious injury, or persistent pain, or if the flow chart indicates it, do not take these measures but consult your doctor without delay.

Self-help hip exercises

SHORT-TERM EXERCISES

The majority of hip problems, which usually involve stiffness and pain, are caused by osteoarthritis. Its symptoms can be relieved and the condition improved by an exercise programme, but this is a long process. The routines on this page are really non-weight-bearing 'starter exercises', designed to free up hip joints and strengthen the muscles that work them before a more demanding long-term programme can be undertaken.

▲ **Safety watchpoint** As always, make sure that you do not strain when doing these exercises: if pain increases or spreads – in particular down your leg – stop immediately and consult your doctor. If the pain moves down into the leg it is probably a sign that your back is the root cause of the problem. Be especially careful not to strain your lower back when exercising your hips.

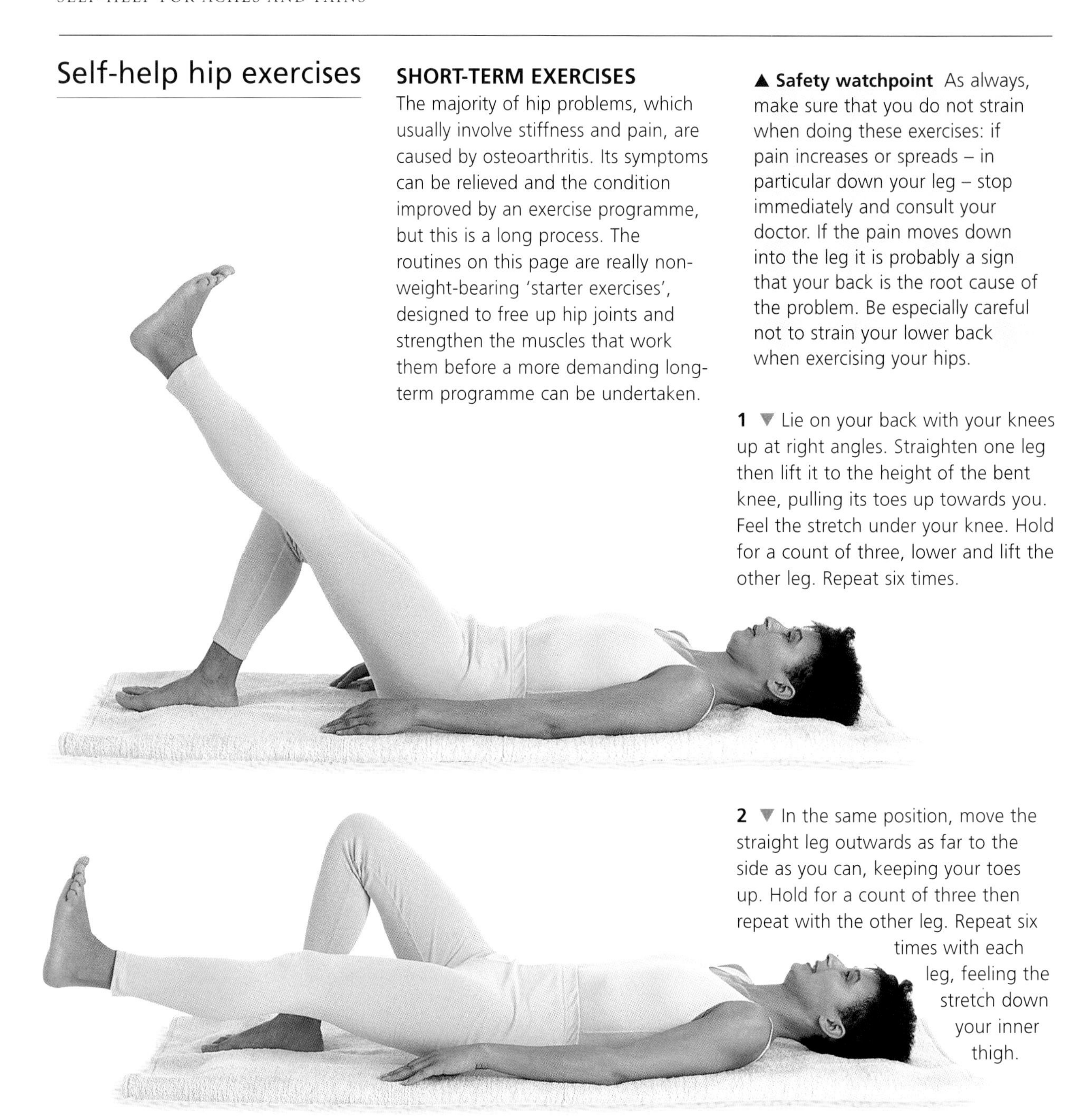

1 ▼ Lie on your back with your knees up at right angles. Straighten one leg then lift it to the height of the bent knee, pulling its toes up towards you. Feel the stretch under your knee. Hold for a count of three, lower and lift the other leg. Repeat six times.

2 ▼ In the same position, move the straight leg outwards as far to the side as you can, keeping your toes up. Hold for a count of three then repeat with the other leg. Repeat six times with each leg, feeling the stretch down your inner thigh.

3 ▶ Lie flat with both legs straight out in front of you on the mat. Turn both feet in towards each other by rolling the whole leg, then turn them out – keep your knees straight. Repeat six times. This exercise rotates the head of the femur in the hip, freeing up movement.

4 ▼ Lying on your back with your knees bent up, squeeze your knees together for a count of three, then let them drop down to either side. Repeat six times – the muscles of the inner thigh are worked as you squeeze and stretched as the knees drop.

5 ▶ Lie on your side with your lower leg bent, then raise your top leg – keeping your toes pulled up – and lower it. Repeat six times, then turn over and do the same with the other leg. You should feel a stretch in your inner thigh as the leg goes up and an ache in the hip joint as the muscles are worked.

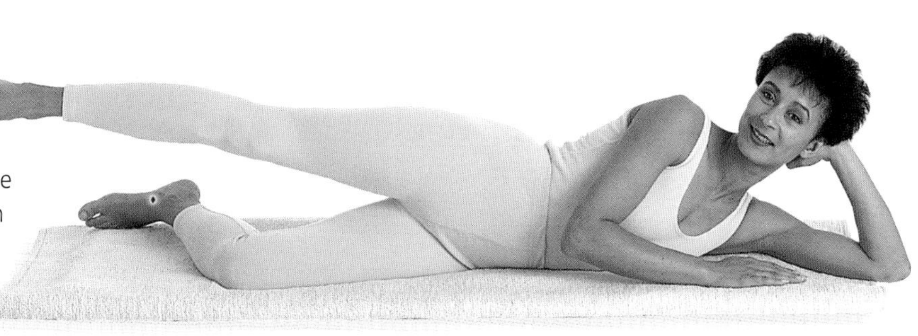

6 ▶ Lie on your side, but this time bend the top leg forward so that you can move the lower one. Lift and lower it six times, then turn over and repeat with the other leg. You will only be able to move the leg a little, but the ability to make this movement is one of the first to be affected by hip problems.

7 Lie on your stomach, then clench your buttocks tightly for a count of three and relax. Repeat six times.

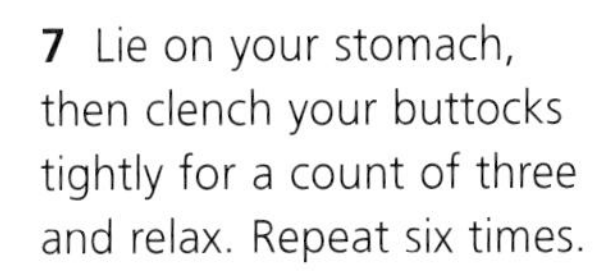

8 ▶ Lying on your stomach, raise one leg, without twisting or moving your lower back. Hold for a count of three and lower. Do the same with the other leg and repeat six times.

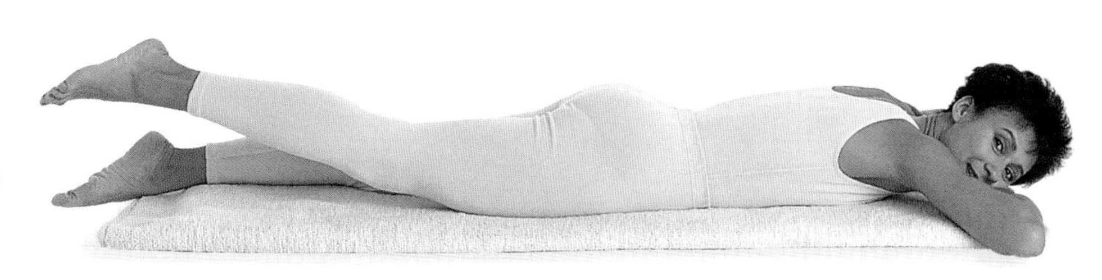

LONG-TERM MEASURES

When you are able to carry out the 'starter exercises' on the previous two pages with ease, and without any discomfort, it is time to move on to these weight-bearing exercises. Use the short-term exercises as a warm-up before trying them. Most people only move their hip joints in one plane (when walking) so this routine is designed to increase all-round mobility and strength.

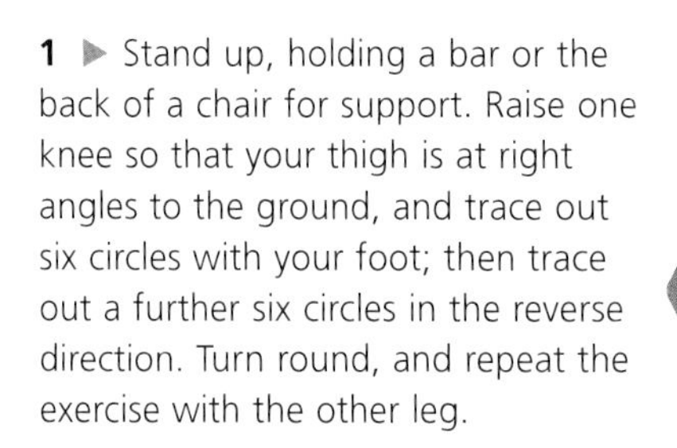

1 ▶ Stand up, holding a bar or the back of a chair for support. Raise one knee so that your thigh is at right angles to the ground, and trace out six circles with your foot; then trace out a further six circles in the reverse direction. Turn round, and repeat the exercise with the other leg.

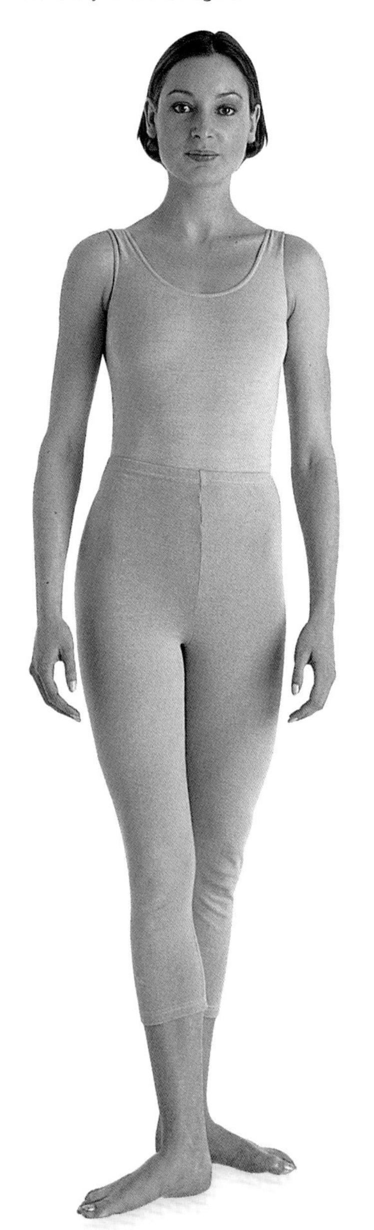

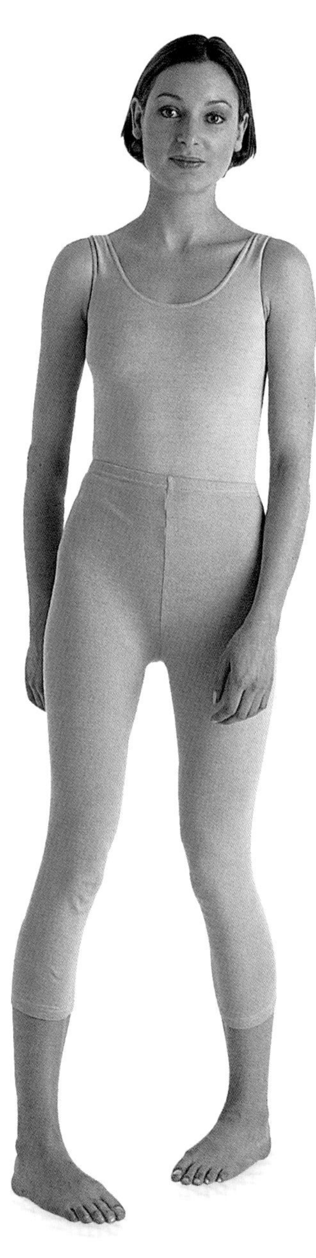

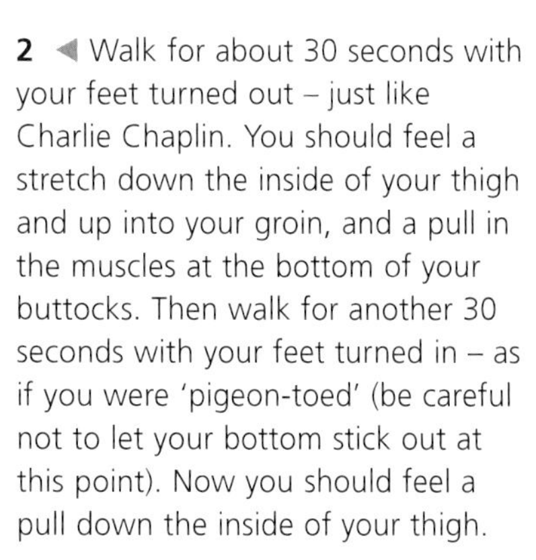

2 ◀ Walk for about 30 seconds with your feet turned out – just like Charlie Chaplin. You should feel a stretch down the inside of your thigh and up into your groin, and a pull in the muscles at the bottom of your buttocks. Then walk for another 30 seconds with your feet turned in – as if you were 'pigeon-toed' (be careful not to let your bottom stick out at this point). Now you should feel a pull down the inside of your thigh.

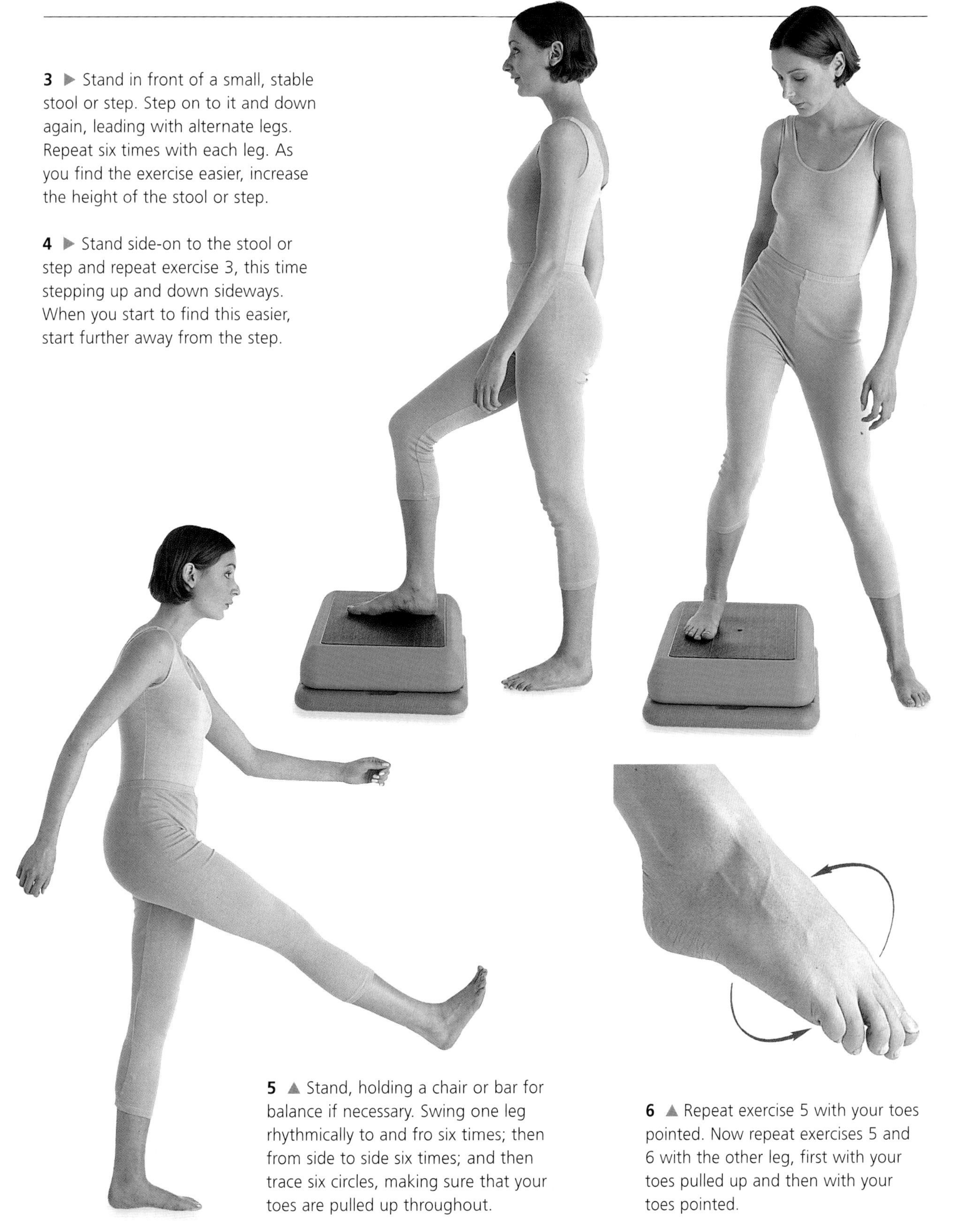

3 ▶ Stand in front of a small, stable stool or step. Step on to it and down again, leading with alternate legs. Repeat six times with each leg. As you find the exercise easier, increase the height of the stool or step.

4 ▶ Stand side-on to the stool or step and repeat exercise 3, this time stepping up and down sideways. When you start to find this easier, start further away from the step.

5 ▲ Stand, holding a chair or bar for balance if necessary. Swing one leg rhythmically to and fro six times; then from side to side six times; and then trace six circles, making sure that your toes are pulled up throughout.

6 ▲ Repeat exercise 5 with your toes pointed. Now repeat exercises 5 and 6 with the other leg, first with your toes pulled up and then with your toes pointed.

Knee problems

For any normally active person, the knee is a hard-working joint. Even when standing still, it has to transmit the weight of the body to the feet and ground and help keep the body upright.

The knee is a weight-bearing, simple hinge joint, with a limited but vital ability to rotate slightly (see pages 60–61). The rotational movements are made possible by pads of cartilage in the knee – the menisci – which separate the two articulating bones. The importance of rotation is that it allows the knee to 'lock' by pulling backwards and moving slightly inwards, so the weight of the body is transmitted straight through the joint and the thigh muscles are not under strain. People often 'lock' one or both knees while standing or leaning for any length of time.

The knee is a tight joint without much natural give. Failure to exercise it fully will further tighten it and squash surfaces together, eventually causing inflammation of the joint, cartilage and ligaments. As a weight-bearing joint, the knee is a common site of osteoarthritis, especially in the over 40s. If severe, the knee can be hot and painful.

The knee is particularly vulnerable to injury, especially during sports such as football. A sudden twist can tear a meniscus or a ligament and cause pain and swelling. Or a meniscus may be dislodged and obstruct the hinge mechanism, making the knee incapable of fully straightening or bending.

A swollen knee, as in housemaid's knee, may be the result of kneeling for too long or of bending the knee too frequently, which causes fluid to build up in the bursa just below the kneecap (patella). The inner surface of the patella itself may become abraded through friction with the underlying bone, causing pain and swelling.

The tendon that joins the patella to the tibia may become irritated or torn due to activities such as gymnastics or dancing. If the area is swollen, especially in young athletes, a doctor will need to check for Osgood Schlatter's disease (an injury of the growing point of the patellar tendon). Activity may have to be stopped or restricted for a while.

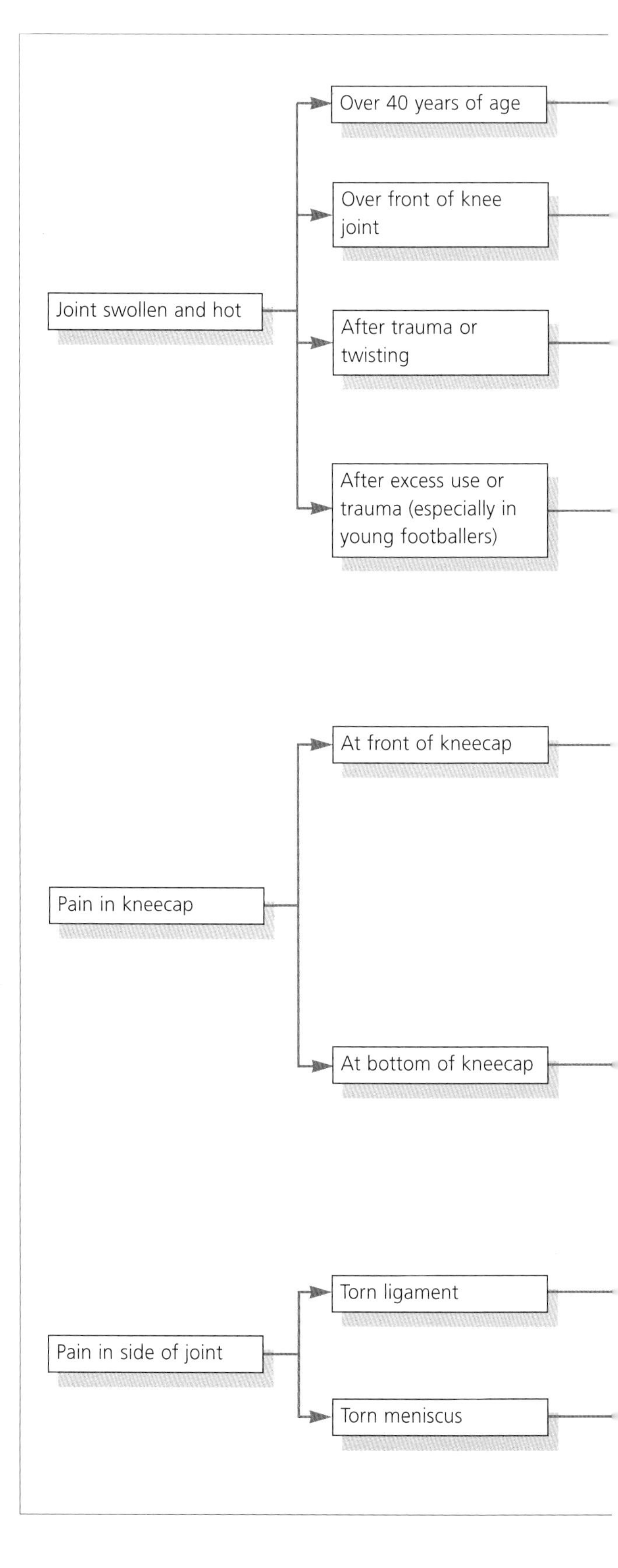

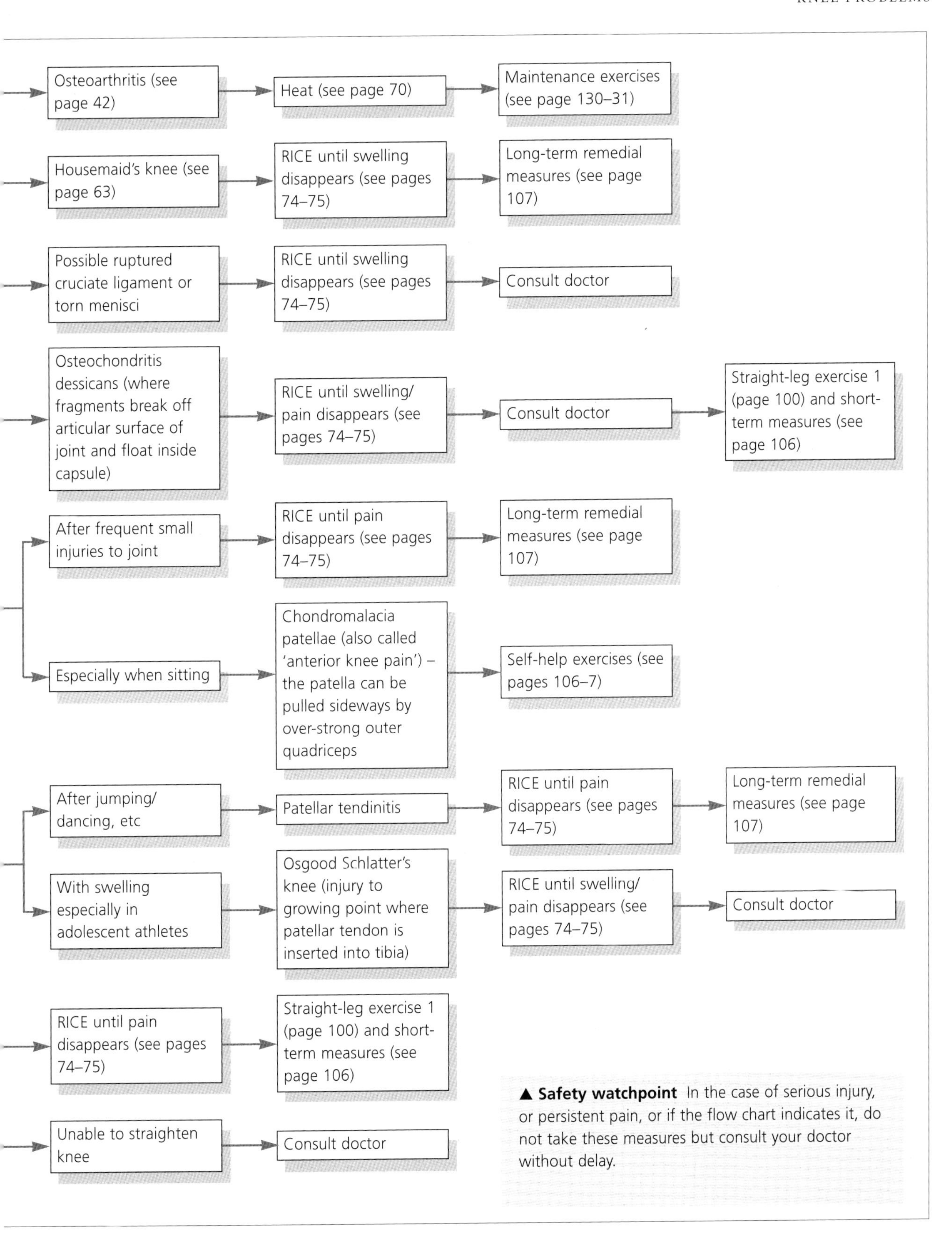

▲ **Safety watchpoint** In the case of serious injury, or persistent pain, or if the flow chart indicates it, do not take these measures but consult your doctor without delay.

Self-help knee exercises

SHORT-TERM MEASURES

The knee is notoriously vulnerable, especially when people have knee injuries from their youth that were not properly treated. The first line of attack when treating knee problems is not just to mobilise the joint itself but to strengthen the muscle groups that work over it.

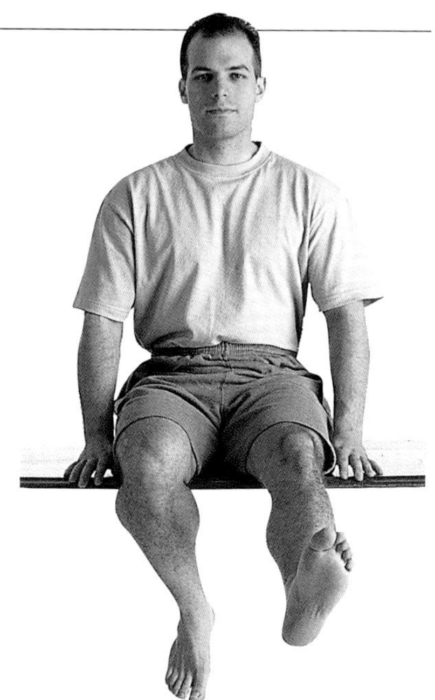

1 ▶ Sit on a table with your feet off the ground. Swing your legs backwards and forwards from the knee, six times each. Then repeat, but lock your knees when your leg is horizontal and hold for a count of three before releasing. Repeat six times, keeping your toes pulled up at all times. Finish off the exercise with a few loose swings.

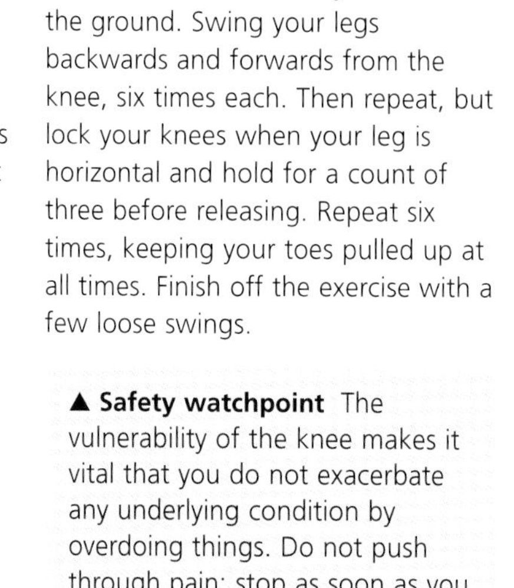

▲ **Safety watchpoint** The vulnerability of the knee makes it vital that you do not exacerbate any underlying condition by overdoing things. Do not push through pain: stop as soon as you feel any discomfort and consult your doctor or physiotherapist.

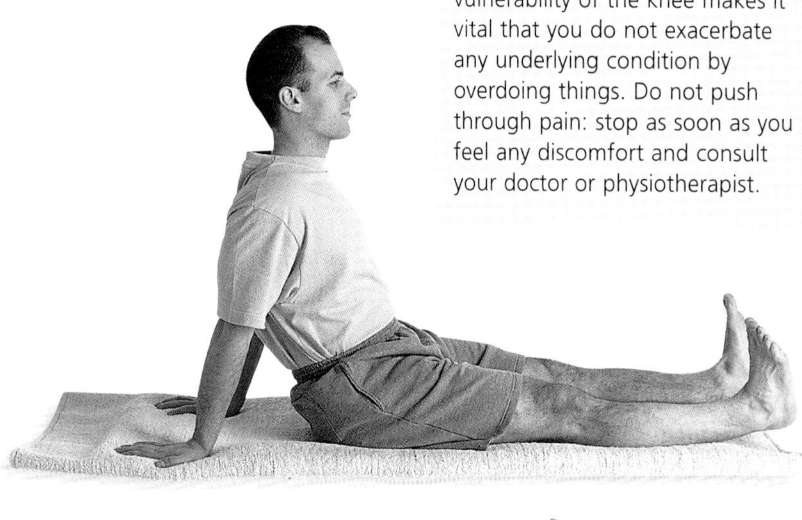

2 ◀ On a mat, sit up tall with your legs straight out in front of you, supporting yourself with the palms of your hands behind you. Pull your toes up and push the backs of your knees hard into the floor, so that your heels come slightly off the ground. Repeat six times, feeling your quadriceps muscles tighten.

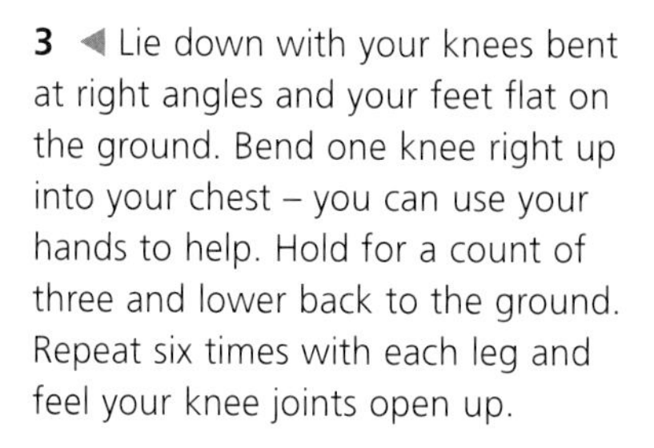

3 ◀ Lie down with your knees bent at right angles and your feet flat on the ground. Bend one knee right up into your chest – you can use your hands to help. Hold for a count of three and lower back to the ground. Repeat six times with each leg and feel your knee joints open up.

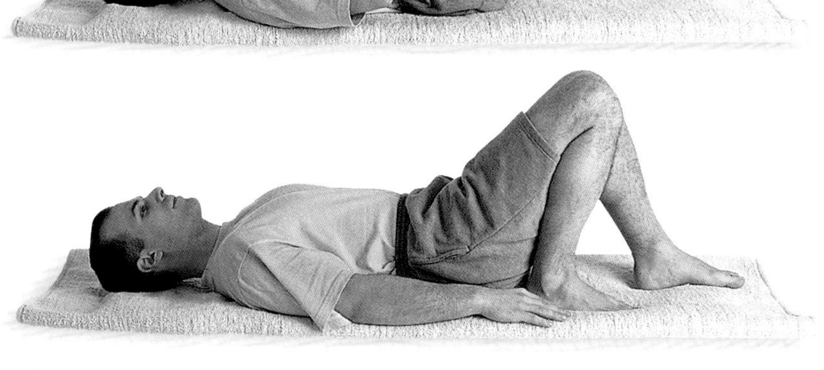

4 ◀ In the same starting position, slide the heel of one foot along the floor until it is as close to your buttocks as possible. You can use your hand to help, but be careful to keep your back straight. Hold for a count of three, and slide back. Repeat six times with each leg.

LONG-TERM MEASURES

The knee joint is designed to allow a range of fine, small movements, and it is these that are often lost first when the joint is affected by an injury or disorder. These exercises help restore fine movements and so increase the mobility of the joint, as well as strengthening it. Run through the short-term measures before you start this routine.

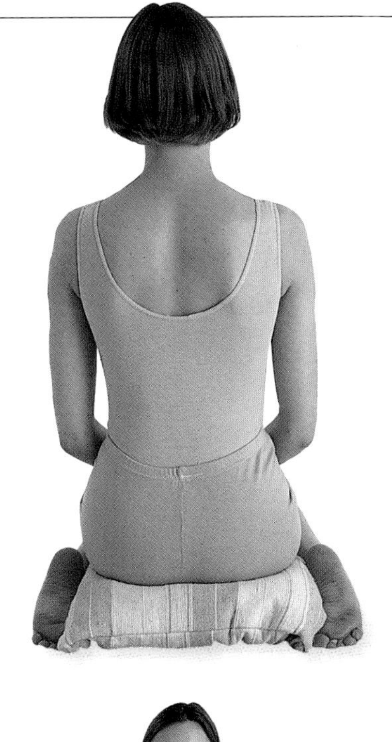

1 ◀ Sit on the floor with your knees bent and shoulders' width apart, and your feet tight up against the sides of your buttocks or under them if you can manage. You may need to put a cushion between your legs to begin with. Rest in this position for three minutes, then kneel up for 30 seconds before repeating the exercise once more. You should feel the stretch in your knee joints.

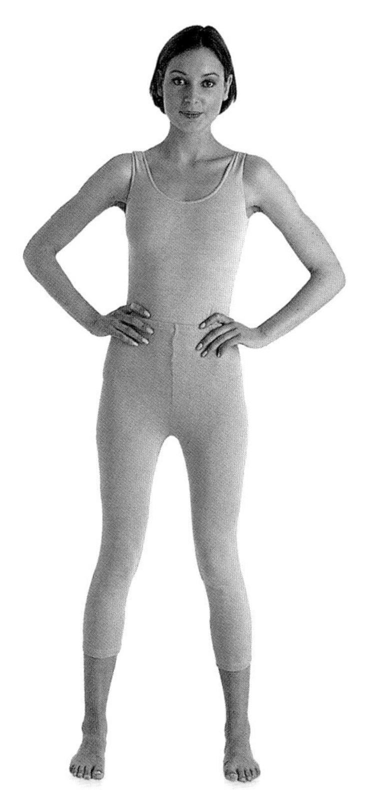

2 ▲ Stand with your feet shoulders' width apart and firmly planted on the ground. Put your hands on your hips and first turn your knees in towards each other – this is only a small movement – then out, away from each other. Repeat six times.

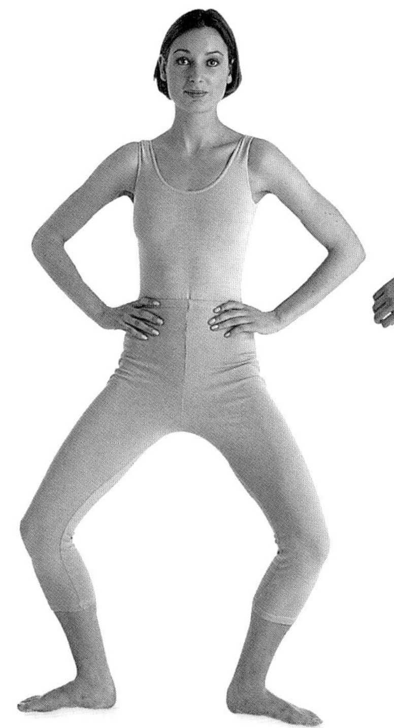

3 ▲ Take up the same position, but point your toes out. Keeping your back straight and your bottom tucked in, bend at the knees and lower (as if you were doing a plié in ballet). Repeat six times – you will probably feel an ache in your thighs.

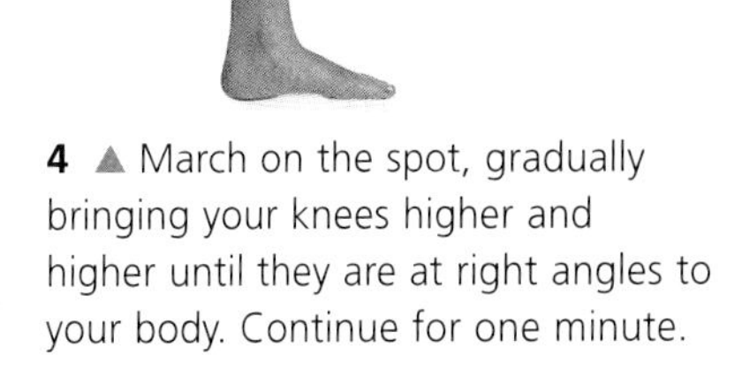

4 ▲ March on the spot, gradually bringing your knees higher and higher until they are at right angles to your body. Continue for one minute.

5 Repeat exercise 1 from the short-term measures as a warm-down.

Ankle and foot problems

The feet and ankles form the base on which our bodies are precariously poised. They have the job of maintaining balance and of cushioning the rest of the body against the jolts and shocks of running and walking (see pages 64–65).

The ankle is a simple hinge joint, but the foot is a complex bundle of 26 bones, forming three arches, with a correspondingly complicated array of muscles, tendons and ligaments to articulate them. All these need to be in good condition to cope with the daily pounding they receive, and to coordinate precisely in order to maintain balance.

Many of the problems that arise in the feet and ankles stem from two avoidable causes: insufficient exercise and badly fitting or ill-designed shoes. Weak ankles and dropped foot arches are the result. I wear high heels, but I also walk barefoot a lot and I use a wobble board (see page 73) at home to help prevent problems arising.

The area of pain in the foot normally indicates which arch of the foot is weak. Pain on the inner side or the front of the foot (or both) suggests a fallen medial arch, or flat feet – especially if the inner surfaces of the heels of your shoes are worn. Flat feet can also throw out your posture, leading to low back pain. Pain under the base of the toes may mean a fallen transverse arch, though if the pain is mainly under the big toe, it could be caused by a bunion. Pain on the outside of the foot may mean a fallen lateral arch, but is more likely to be from a chronic ankle problem.

A flat medial arch also increases the chance of twisting the ankle, as the ligaments that help to prevent the ankle rolling in are weakened. Once an ankle has twisted it is vulnerable unless care is taken to strengthen the muscles.

The two main calf muscles, *gastrocnemius* and *soleus*, can tear, especially if an unexpected, awkward movement causes the heel to drop. You will feel a sudden pain, which increases if you try to stand on tiptoe. The tendon of *gastrocnemius* (the Achilles tendon) is particularly vulnerable to blows, over-use or friction (see page 66).

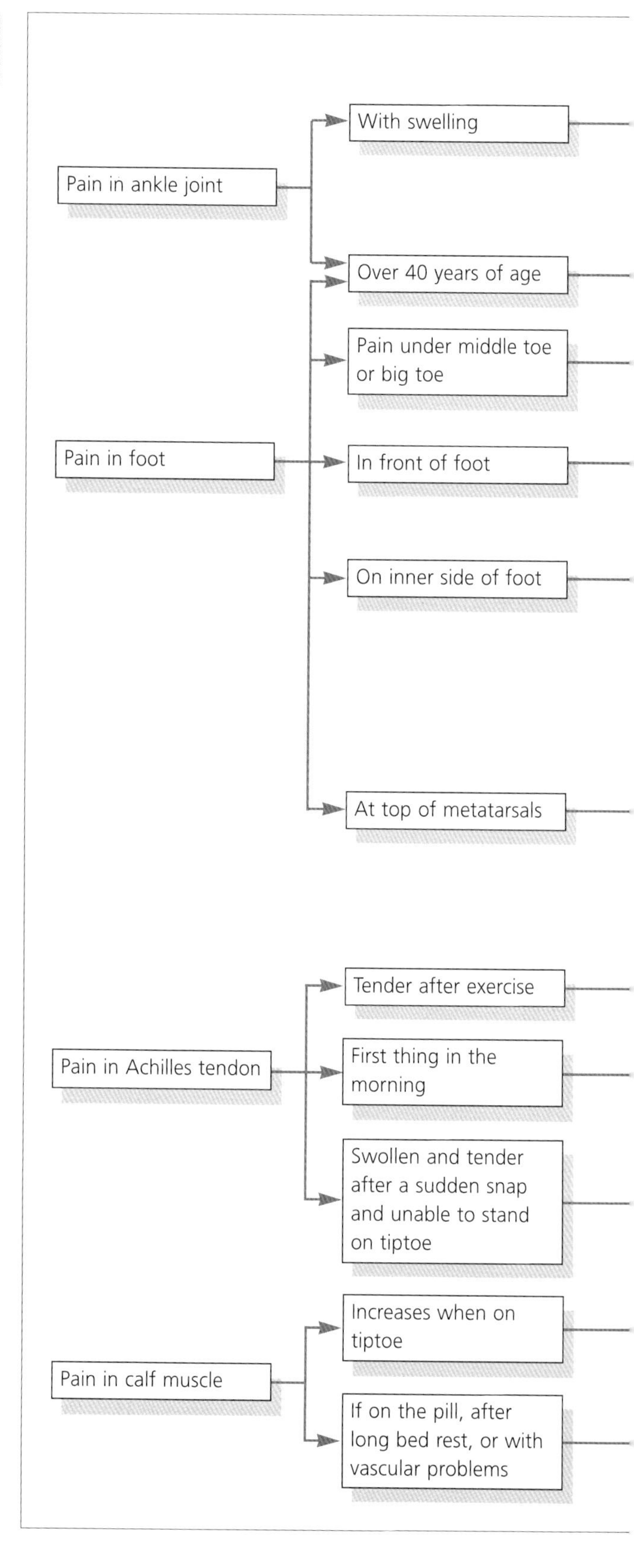

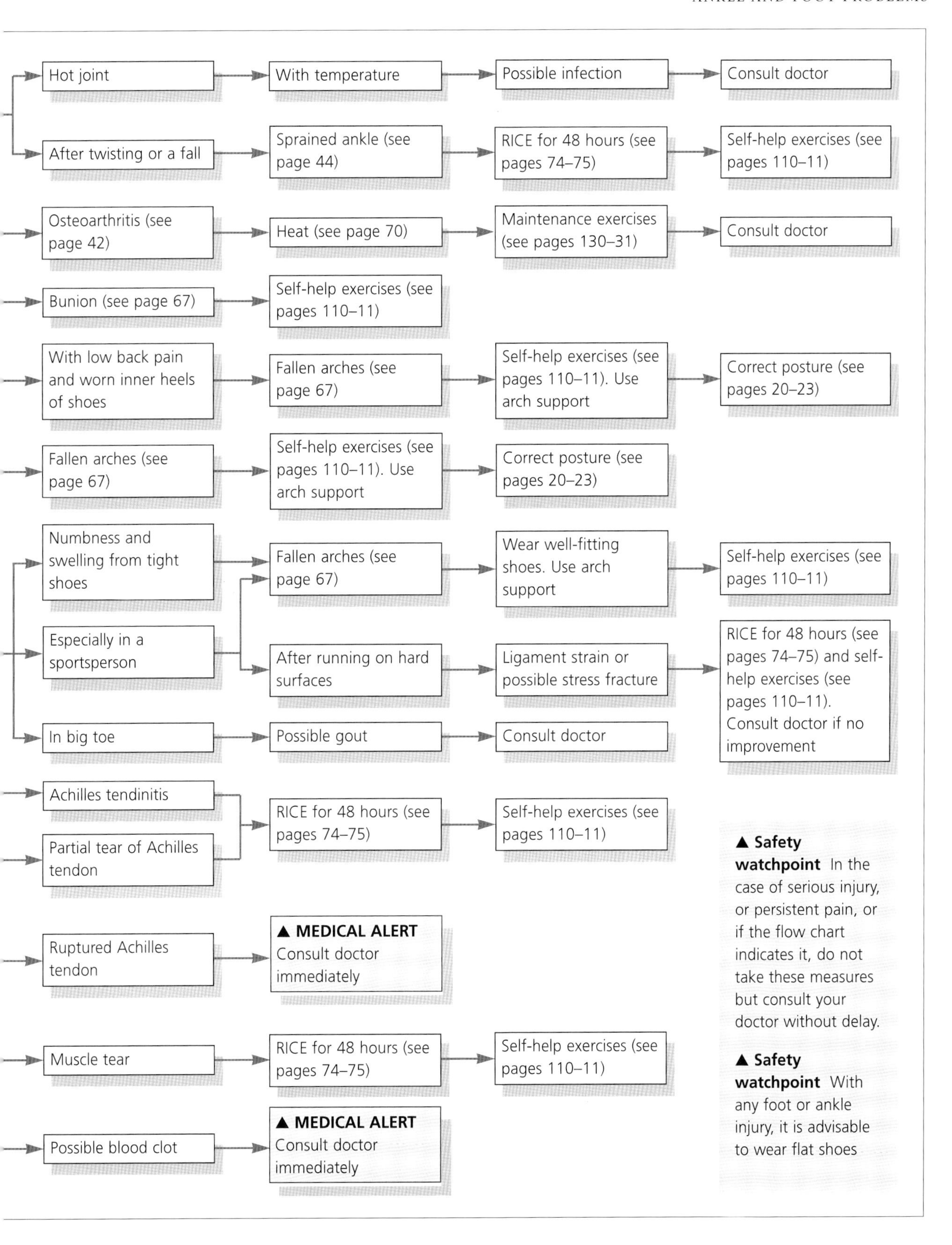

▲ **Safety watchpoint** In the case of serious injury, or persistent pain, or if the flow chart indicates it, do not take these measures but consult your doctor without delay.

▲ **Safety watchpoint** With any foot or ankle injury, it is advisable to wear flat shoes

Self-help ankle and foot exercises

Many of the problems affecting the ankle and foot are caused by ill-fitting shoes – high heels in particular. These exercises help restore strength and mobility, but it also helps to walk in barefoot whenever practical. Doing so not only strengthens the ankle but also improves balance and coordination.

▲ **Safety watchpoint** As with all exercise treatments, it is vital that you do not push yourself too far, too quickly, or there is a risk that you will make your condition worse. If the pain increases or spreads, stop immediately and consult your doctor or physiotherapist.

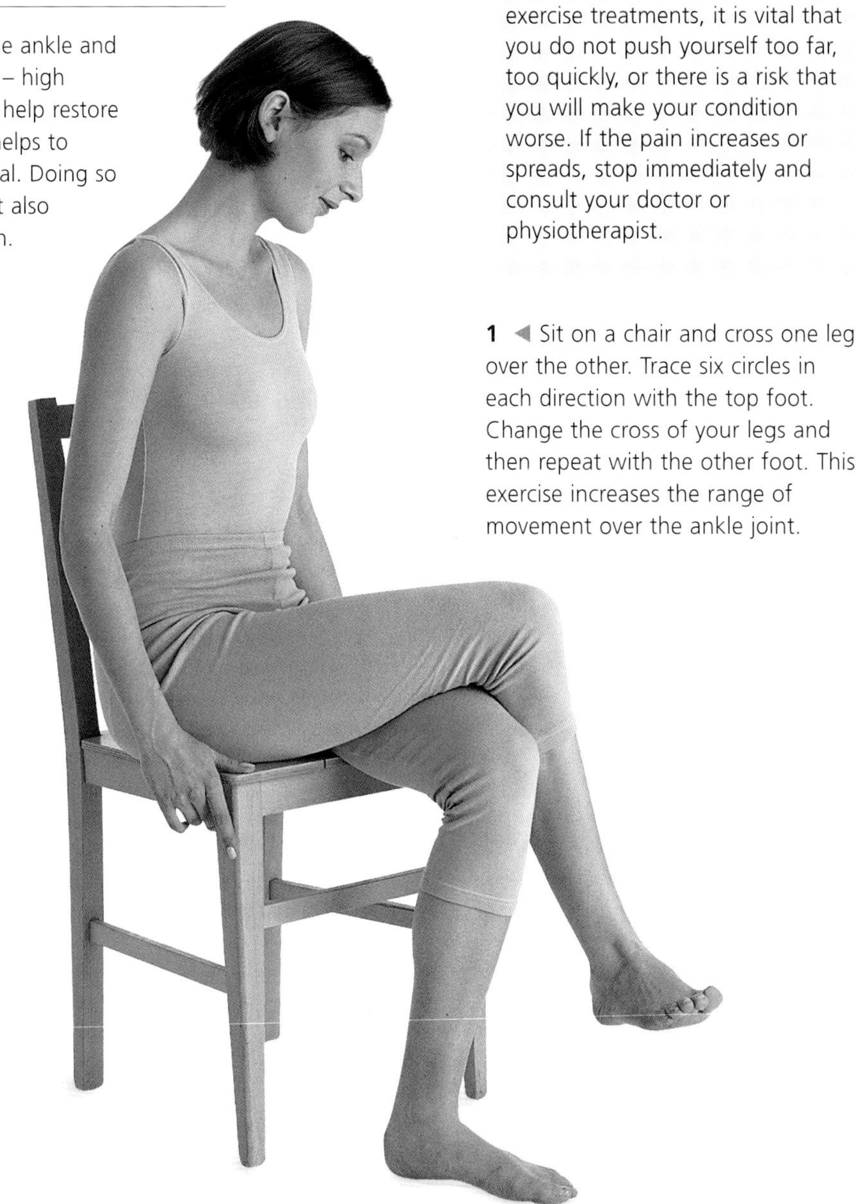

1 ◀ Sit on a chair and cross one leg over the other. Trace six circles in each direction with the top foot. Change the cross of your legs and then repeat with the other foot. This exercise increases the range of movement over the ankle joint.

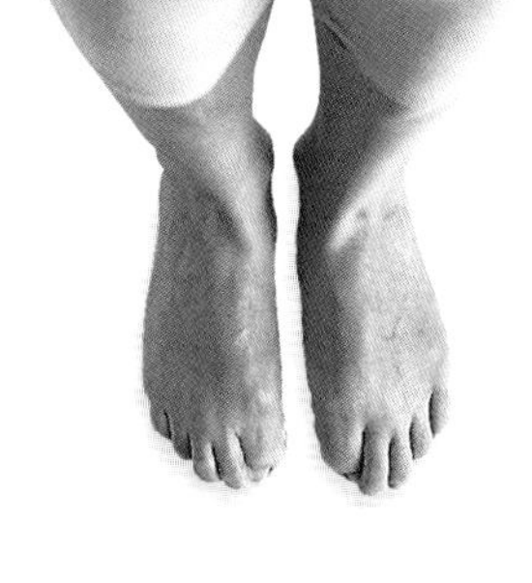

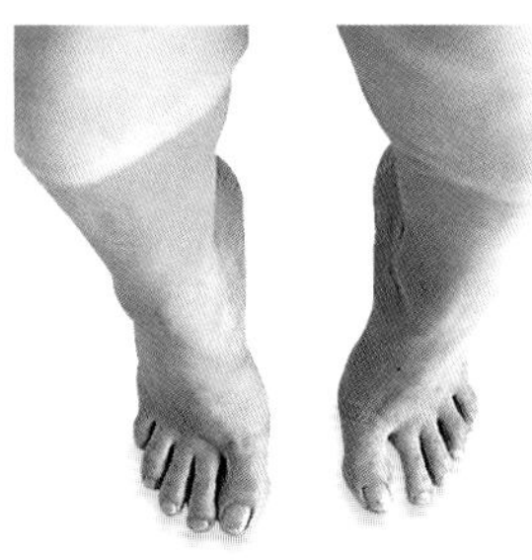

2 ▲ Sit on a chair with your feet on the floor and try to curl your toes under your foot (top). Hold for a count of three, then relax and try to splay your toes out (above). Repeat six times. This exercise pulls up the arches of the foot and helps prevent bunions.

3 ▶ Sit on a chair with your feet flat on the floor and your knees at right angles. Pull your toes up as far as possible, keeping your feet on the floor. Hold for a count of three, then relax. Repeat six times and feel the pull across the front of your feet.

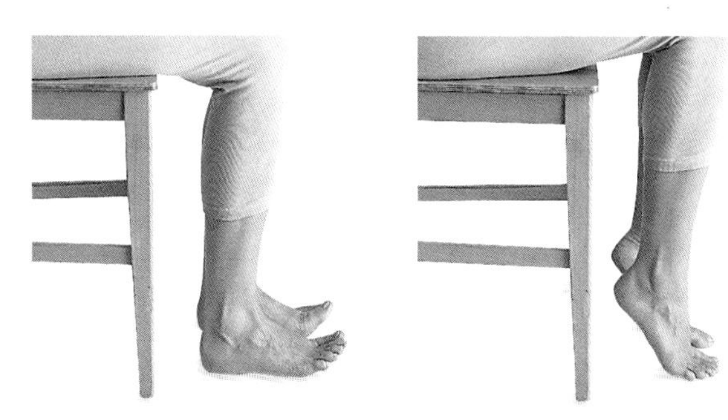

4 ◀ Now lift your heels up as far as possible, keeping your toes on the floor. Hold for a count of three, then relax. Repeat six times and feel the stretch over the front of your ankle.

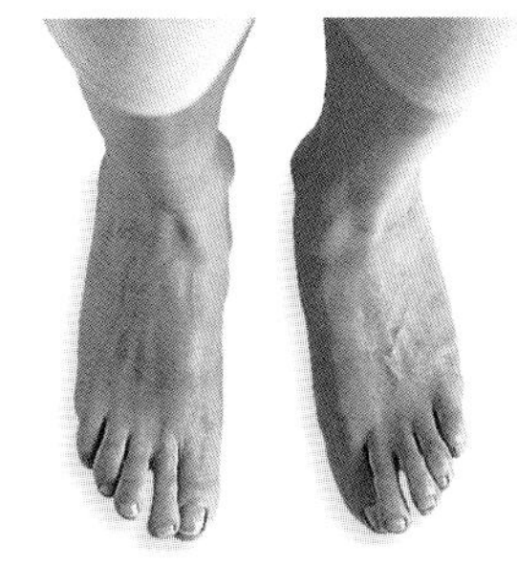

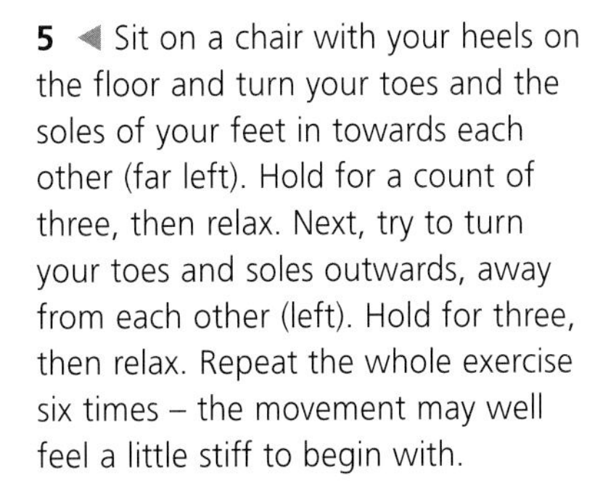

5 ◄ Sit on a chair with your heels on the floor and turn your toes and the soles of your feet in towards each other (far left). Hold for a count of three, then relax. Next, try to turn your toes and soles outwards, away from each other (left). Hold for three, then relax. Repeat the whole exercise six times – the movement may well feel a little stiff to begin with.

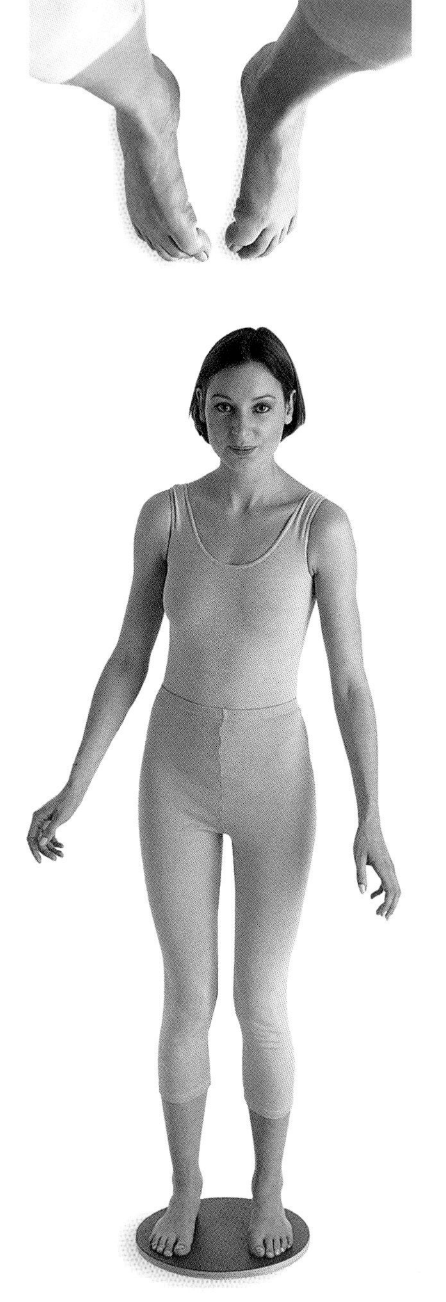

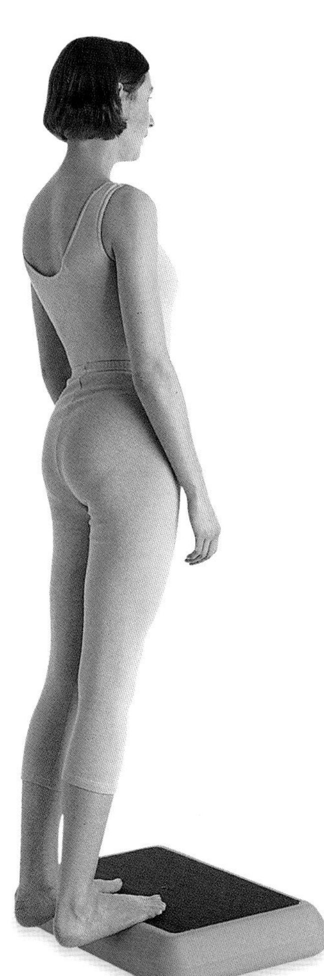

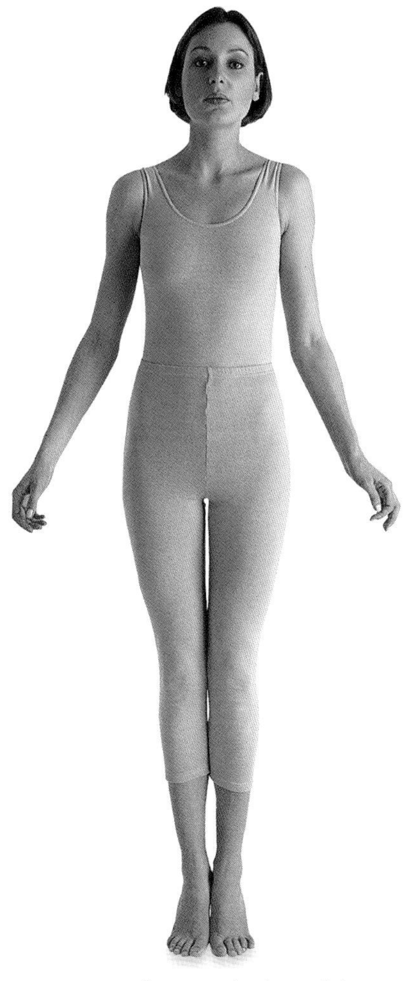

6 ▲ Stand on a wobble board with your feet shoulders' width apart for as long as you can – you should aim to build up to five minutes. As you start to find this easier, begin with your feet closer together; next try standing on one leg, then the other.

7 ▲ Stand on a step with your heels off its edge. Then lower your body so that your heels are lower than the step (you may need to hold onto something for balance). Hold for a count of three, then relax. Repeat six times. This exercise helps to stretch the Achilles tendons, and you are likely to feel them ache.

8 ▲ Keeping your body straight, raise up to stand on tiptoe, making sure that your ankles are touching at all times (you may need to hold onto something for balance). Hold for a count of three, then relax; repeat six times. This exercise sounds easy, but is surprisingly difficult when done properly.

SECTION FOUR

KEEPING UP THE GOOD WORK

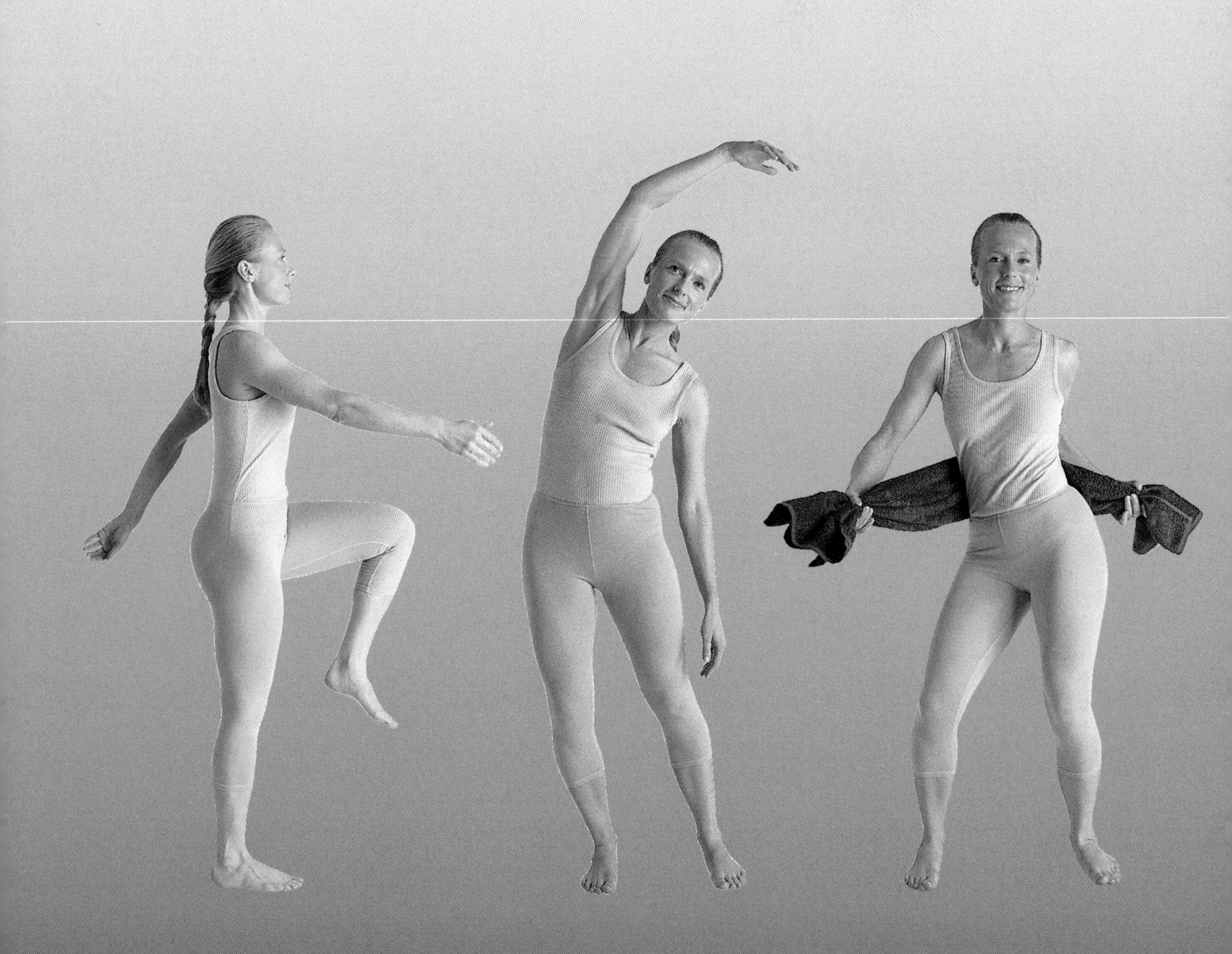

Prevention is better than cure is something of a cliché, but many clichés encapsulate a truth – and this is one of them. Unless muscles are put through their paces regularly they start to seize up, rather like a car engine; and tendons and joints lose their flexibility unless they are put through their complete range of movements regularly. And that makes them vulnerable to injury when they are expected to cope with physical activity, be it a game of tennis or a hard afternoon in the garden.

So, in a sense, you need to exercise in order to exercise, or to undertake any physical activity, for that matter. This irritating fact becomes even more important as you grow older, because muscles and joints inevitably lose some of their flexibility. The only consolation is that you can substantially slow down the rate at which you lose flexibility by doing maintenance exercises regularly.

This section of the book shows you how to maintain flexibility, reduce the risk of injury and work on any areas of your body that are relatively weak or prone to damage. First, I will show you how to warm up and warm down. This is a vital part of any physical activity but it is often neglected – and that is why so many muscles are pulled and joints strained in the home. A full warm-up might not be necessary before you start decorating a room, but warming up before digging the garden, say, might well save you from days of back pain.

Then there is a selection of exercises for specific muscle groups and areas of the body: choose from them according to your requirements. Finally, there is a ten-minute, once-a-day maintenance programme designed to fit into a busy lifestyle. Incorporate exercises from other sections of this chapter to suit your needs – and make it part of your daily routine.

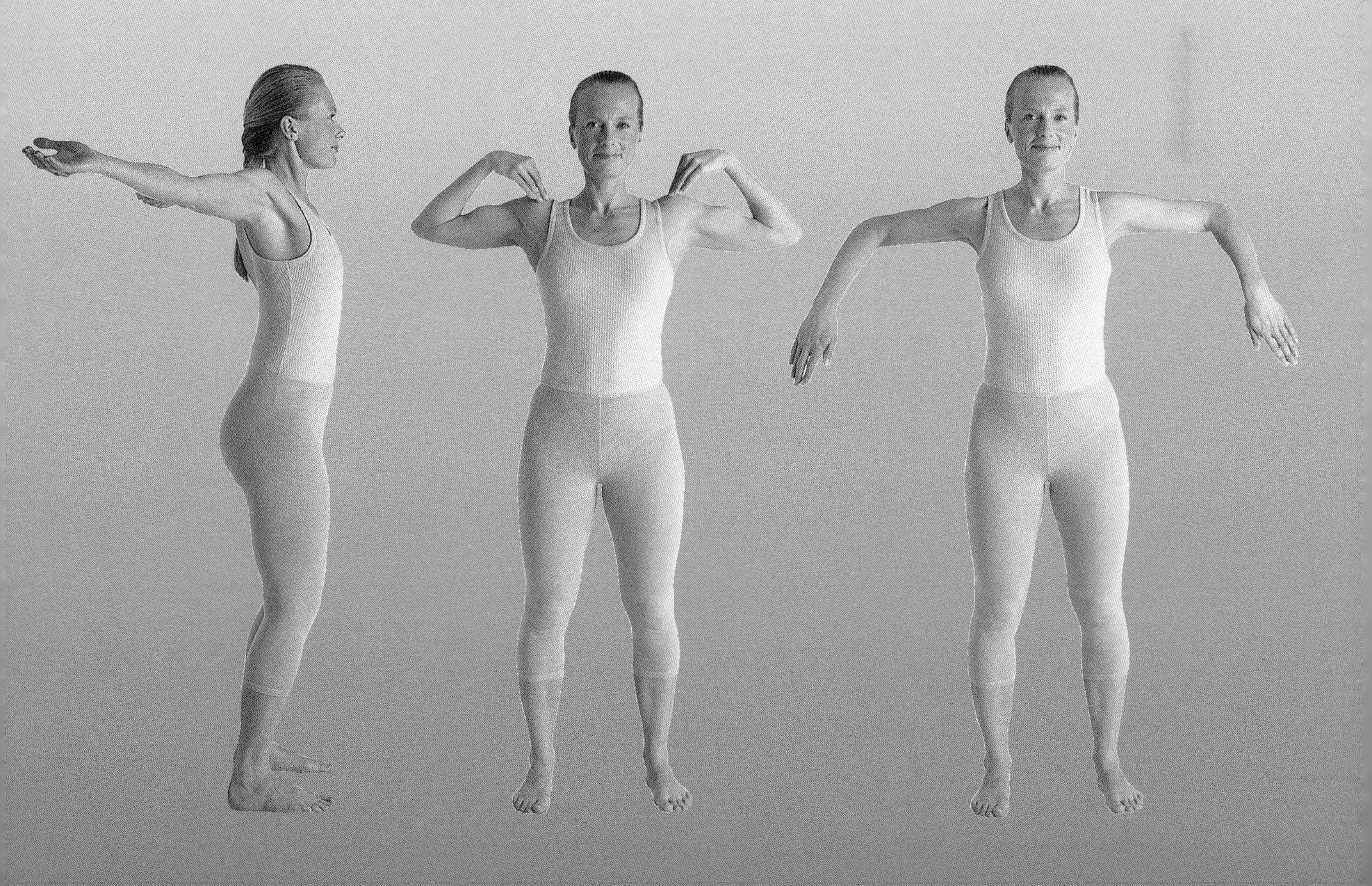

Warming up

MOBILISING EXERCISES

These exercises are designed to increase the activity of the heart gradually and so to steadily raise the amount of blood supplied to the muscles. This warms them, increasing their flexibility and their ability to contract, and reducing the likelihood of injury.

1 Stand in the middle of your exercise area and check your posture (see pages 20–23). Make sure that your shoulders are relaxed and back, your bottom is tucked under, your stomach is held in and that your knees are not braced back.

2 ◀ Walk on the spot, swinging your arms gently. Gradually increase the pace until you are marching on the spot and lift your knees up as far as is comfortable. Continue for two minutes. This exercise gradually increases blood flow and warms up the muscles.

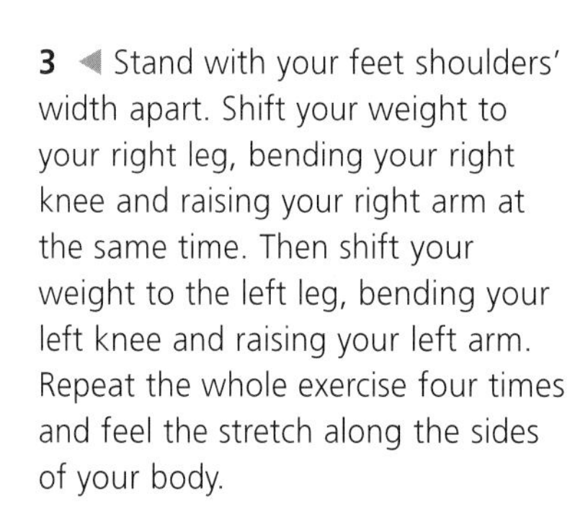

3 ◀ Stand with your feet shoulders' width apart. Shift your weight to your right leg, bending your right knee and raising your right arm at the same time. Then shift your weight to the left leg, bending your left knee and raising your left arm. Repeat the whole exercise four times and feel the stretch along the sides of your body.

4 ▶ Then repeat four times, but this time stretch your arm out in front of your body at right angles.

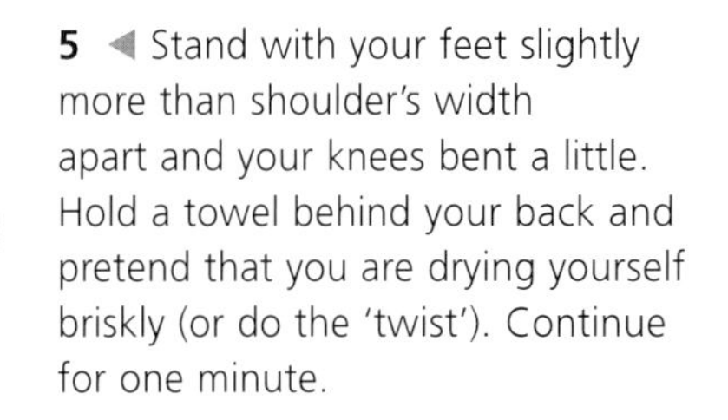

5 ◀ Stand with your feet slightly more than shoulder's width apart and your knees bent a little. Hold a towel behind your back and pretend that you are drying yourself briskly (or do the 'twist'). Continue for one minute.

6 ▶ Step to the side with your left leg, bring your right leg to it and transfer your weight from left to right and back again – it's a hopping, dancing motion. Then repeat the sequence, starting with your right leg, transferring weight to your left leg, and so on. You should be bouncing from side to side, doing a double leg movement (like a fast waltz: '**1**, 2, 3, **1**, 2, 3'). Repeat the sequence eight times.

7 ▶ Stand with your feet shoulders' width apart and knees slightly bent. Stretch your arms behind you, then swing them up and over your head, taking in a deep breath. Pause for a count of three, then swing your arms down, with your trunk curved forwards and down. Breathe out as you go and bend your knees until your arms point towards the floor (the classic downhill-skier's position). Pause, breathe in, then breathe out as you reverse the swing. Be careful to straighten your spine from the bottom up in a gradual, controlled, slow movement. Repeat four times.

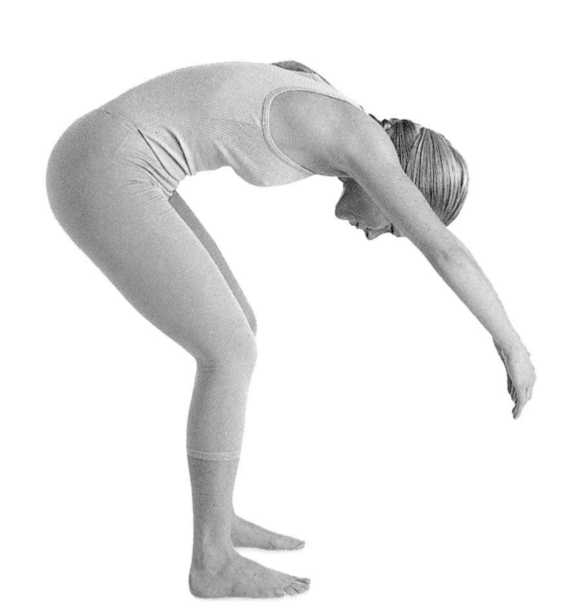

▲ **Safety watchpoint** If you feel faint at any stage of exercise 7, sit and rest with your head between your knees before trying again. If you still feel faint, stop completely.

STRETCHING EXERCISES

Once mobilising exercises have increased the flow of blood to the muscles and warmed them up, it is time to carry out a routine that emphasises flexibility and mobility of the joints in order to complete the preparation of the body for the exercises – or everyday activities – that have been chosen.

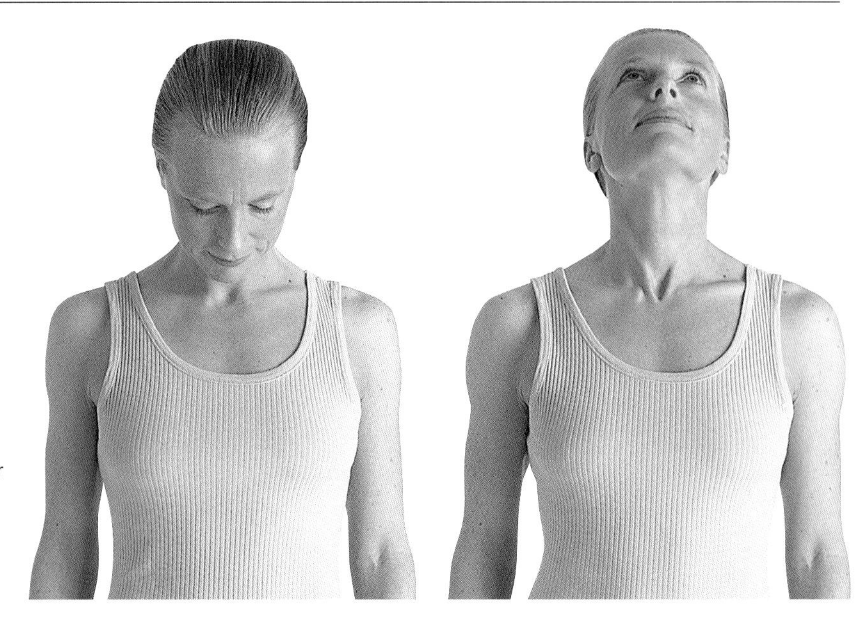

1 ▶ Stand straight with your shoulders down and relaxed. Tilt your head forwards onto your chest, then look up at the ceiling. Be careful not to arch your neck too far back. Repeat four times.

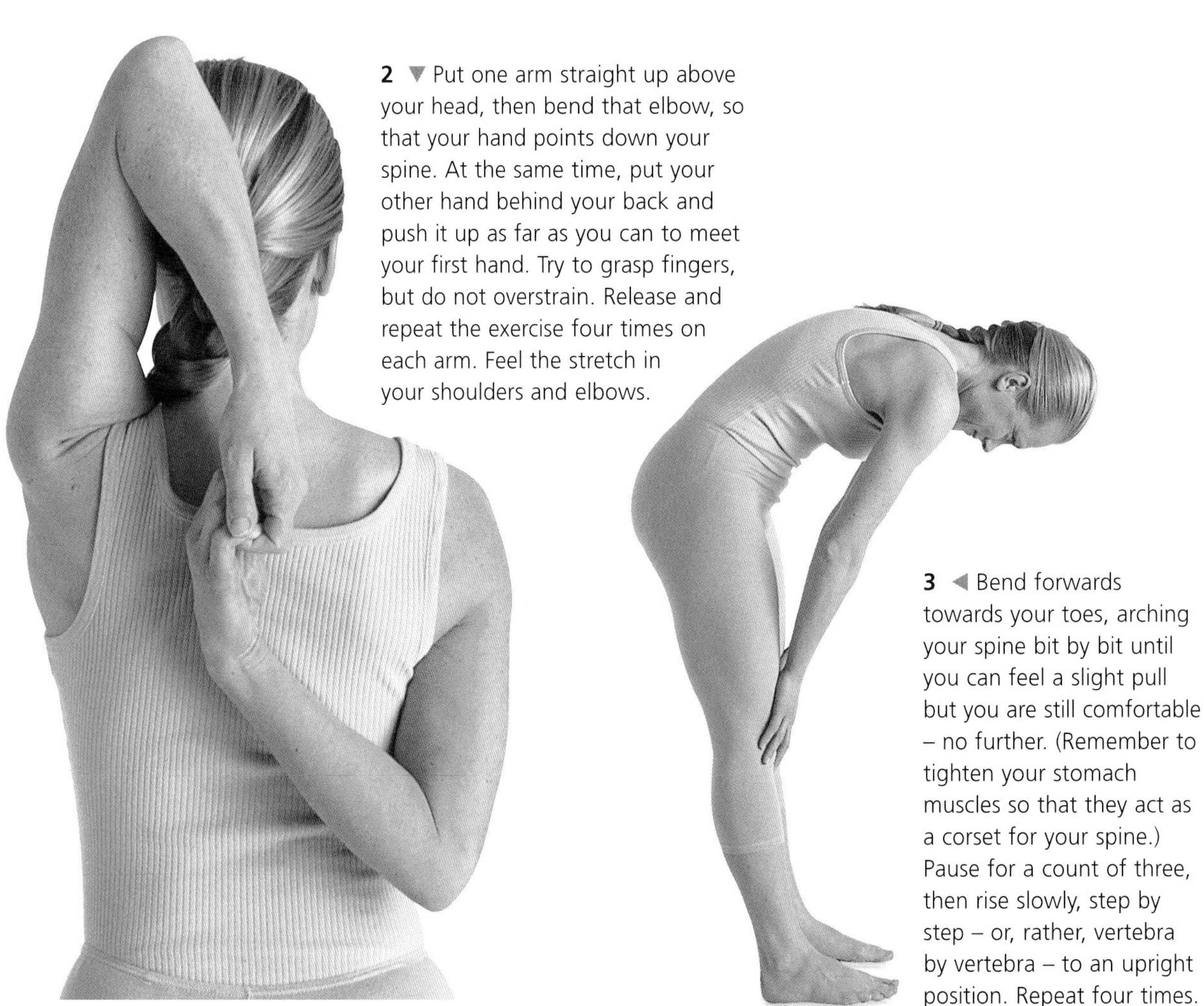

2 ▼ Put one arm straight up above your head, then bend that elbow, so that your hand points down your spine. At the same time, put your other hand behind your back and push it up as far as you can to meet your first hand. Try to grasp fingers, but do not overstrain. Release and repeat the exercise four times on each arm. Feel the stretch in your shoulders and elbows.

3 ◀ Bend forwards towards your toes, arching your spine bit by bit until you can feel a slight pull but you are still comfortable – no further. (Remember to tighten your stomach muscles so that they act as a corset for your spine.) Pause for a count of three, then rise slowly, step by step – or, rather, vertebra by vertebra – to an upright position. Repeat four times.

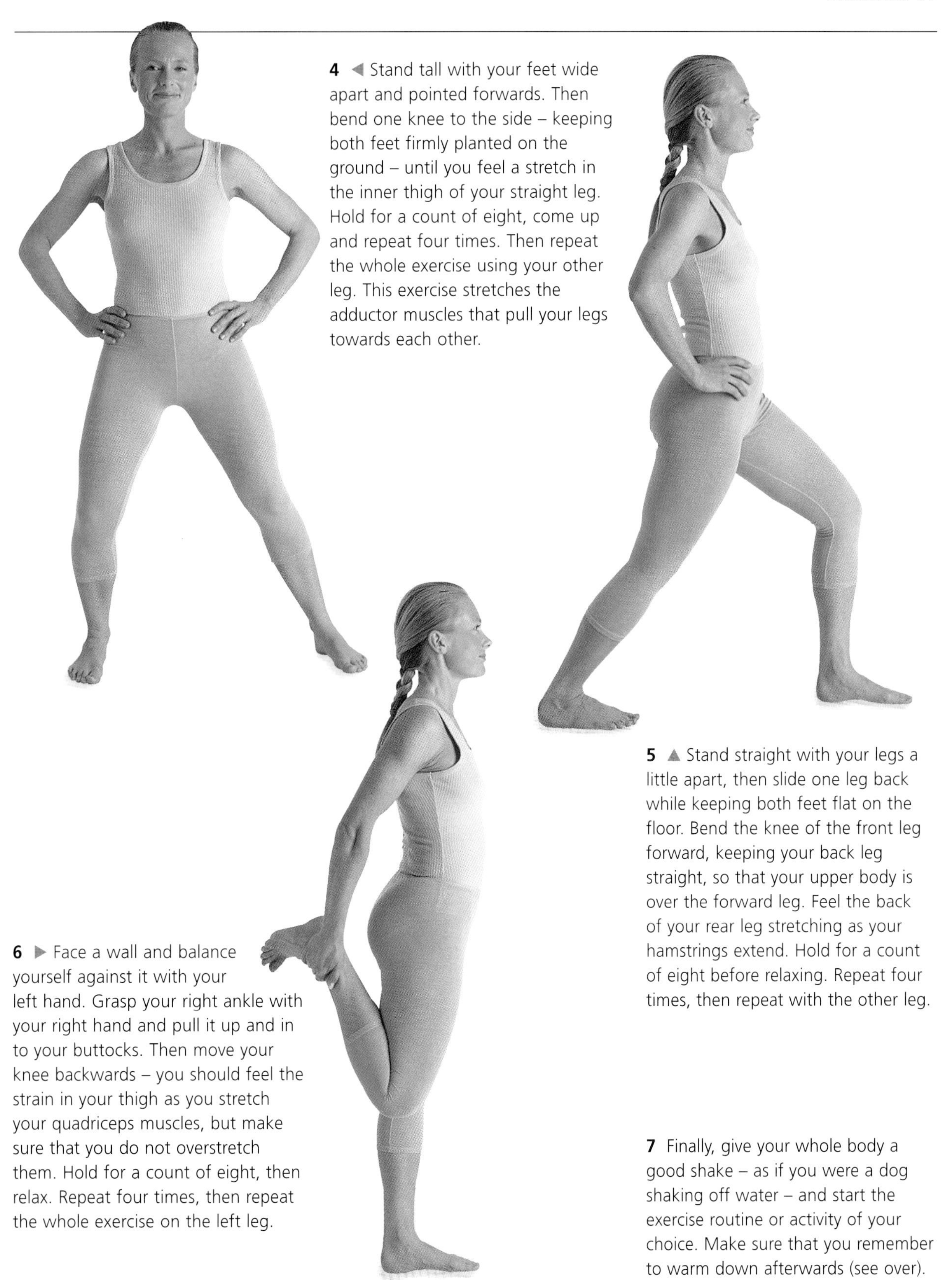

4 ◀ Stand tall with your feet wide apart and pointed forwards. Then bend one knee to the side – keeping both feet firmly planted on the ground – until you feel a stretch in the inner thigh of your straight leg. Hold for a count of eight, come up and repeat four times. Then repeat the whole exercise using your other leg. This exercise stretches the adductor muscles that pull your legs towards each other.

5 ▲ Stand straight with your legs a little apart, then slide one leg back while keeping both feet flat on the floor. Bend the knee of the front leg forward, keeping your back leg straight, so that your upper body is over the forward leg. Feel the back of your rear leg stretching as your hamstrings extend. Hold for a count of eight before relaxing. Repeat four times, then repeat with the other leg.

6 ▶ Face a wall and balance yourself against it with your left hand. Grasp your right ankle with your right hand and pull it up and in to your buttocks. Then move your knee backwards – you should feel the strain in your thigh as you stretch your quadriceps muscles, but make sure that you do not overstretch them. Hold for a count of eight, then relax. Repeat four times, then repeat the whole exercise on the left leg.

7 Finally, give your whole body a good shake – as if you were a dog shaking off water – and start the exercise routine or activity of your choice. Make sure that you remember to warm down afterwards (see over).

Warming down

A proper warm-down routine is just as important as a warm-up. Body tissues react much better to gradual change, rather than sudden stops and starts, so easing off bit by bit helps prevent damage. But warming down has other benefits, too. First, tapering off muscle activity means that extra blood is pumped around the body for longer, flushing out the toxins, such as lactic acid, that cause stiffness and pain. Second, the blood circulation in the legs is helped by the action of the muscles (this is known as the 'muscle pump'), and if the muscles stop working suddenly blood will pool in the veins of the legs, which have been widened by exercise. The result can be faintness and dizziness.

1 Jog on the spot and breathe deeply, making sure that you empty the lungs with each exhalation.

2 ▶ Still jogging, swing your arms in circles, starting them at your side and swinging up and back to open your chest. Repeat three times, then put your arms at shoulder height and swing across your chest and back. Repeat three times.

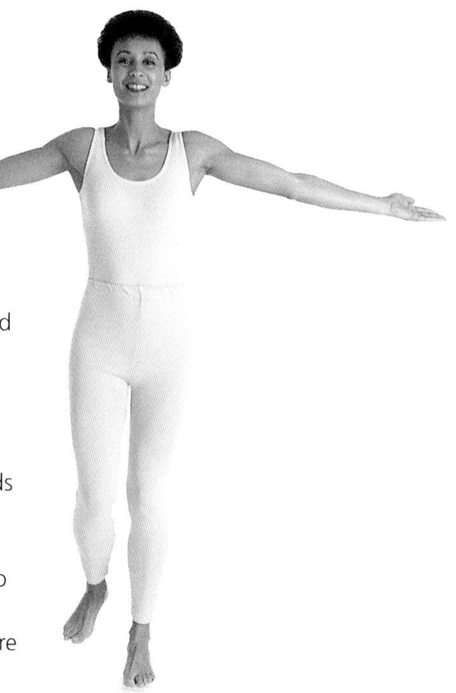

3 Skip three times on each leg, bringing the other knee high towards the chest.

4 Move from jogging on the spot to walking on the spot for one minute, reducing the pace slowly until you are at a standstill.

5 Stand with your feet shoulders' width apart and work your neck in a circle, rolling your head slowly. Alternate the direction after each circle, moving three times each way.

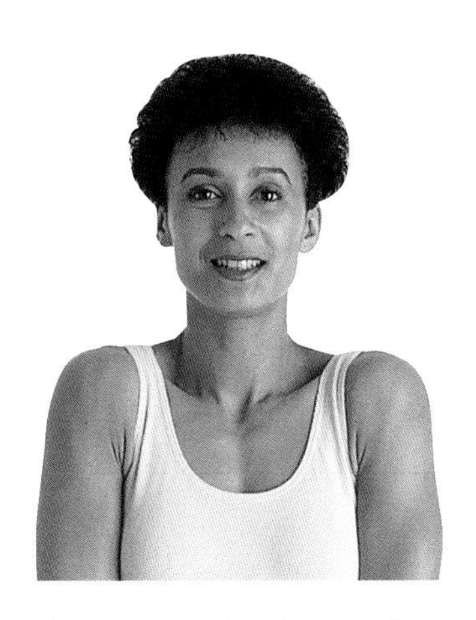

6 ▲ Hunch your shoulders and move them in a vertical circle. Alternate the direction of the circles, moving three times each way.

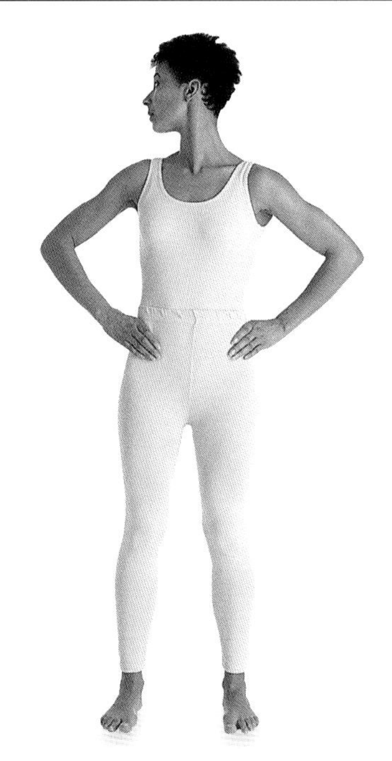

7 ▲ With hands on hips, twist your trunk from side to side three times to look over your shoulder. Then rotate your hips (as with a hula hoop).

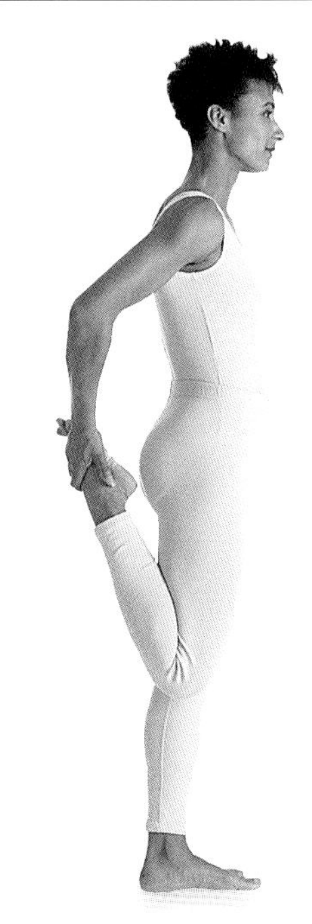

8 ▲ Put your hands behind your back and grasp each ankle in turn, stretching your quadriceps muscles. Repeat three times.

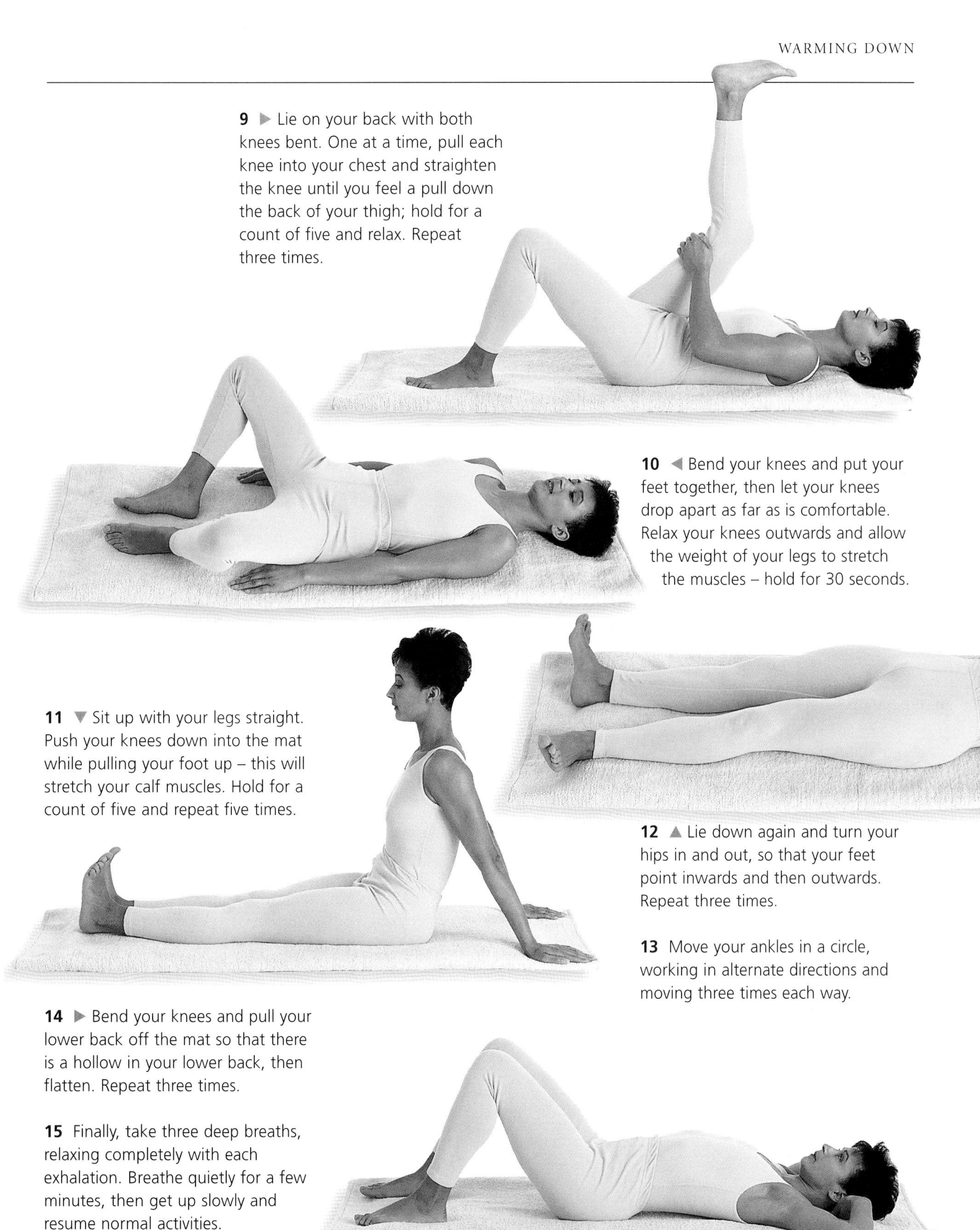

9 ▶ Lie on your back with both knees bent. One at a time, pull each knee into your chest and straighten the knee until you feel a pull down the back of your thigh; hold for a count of five and relax. Repeat three times.

10 ◀ Bend your knees and put your feet together, then let your knees drop apart as far as is comfortable. Relax your knees outwards and allow the weight of your legs to stretch the muscles – hold for 30 seconds.

11 ▼ Sit up with your legs straight. Push your knees down into the mat while pulling your foot up – this will stretch your calf muscles. Hold for a count of five and repeat five times.

12 ▲ Lie down again and turn your hips in and out, so that your feet point inwards and then outwards. Repeat three times.

13 Move your ankles in a circle, working in alternate directions and moving three times each way.

14 ▶ Bend your knees and pull your lower back off the mat so that there is a hollow in your lower back, then flatten. Repeat three times.

15 Finally, take three deep breaths, relaxing completely with each exhalation. Breathe quietly for a few minutes, then get up slowly and resume normal activities.

Upper-chest and shoulder maintenance

These maintenance exercises help to open the chest to aid breathing, align the ribs to the spine, and so encourage good posture, and keep the joints – the shoulder joints, in particular – loose. Try them three times a week if you have had an upper-chest problem or suspect you might develop one.

1 ▶ Place one hand on your hip and raise the other high over your head. Stretch your hand up, feeling the pull down that side of your body, then relax before repeating the exercise with your other arm. Repeat four times for each arm.

2 ▶ Imagine that you are swimming using a crawl stroke (but with your elbows straight) and swing your arms like a windmill. Then swing in the opposite direction – as if doing backstroke. Repeat four times in each direction.

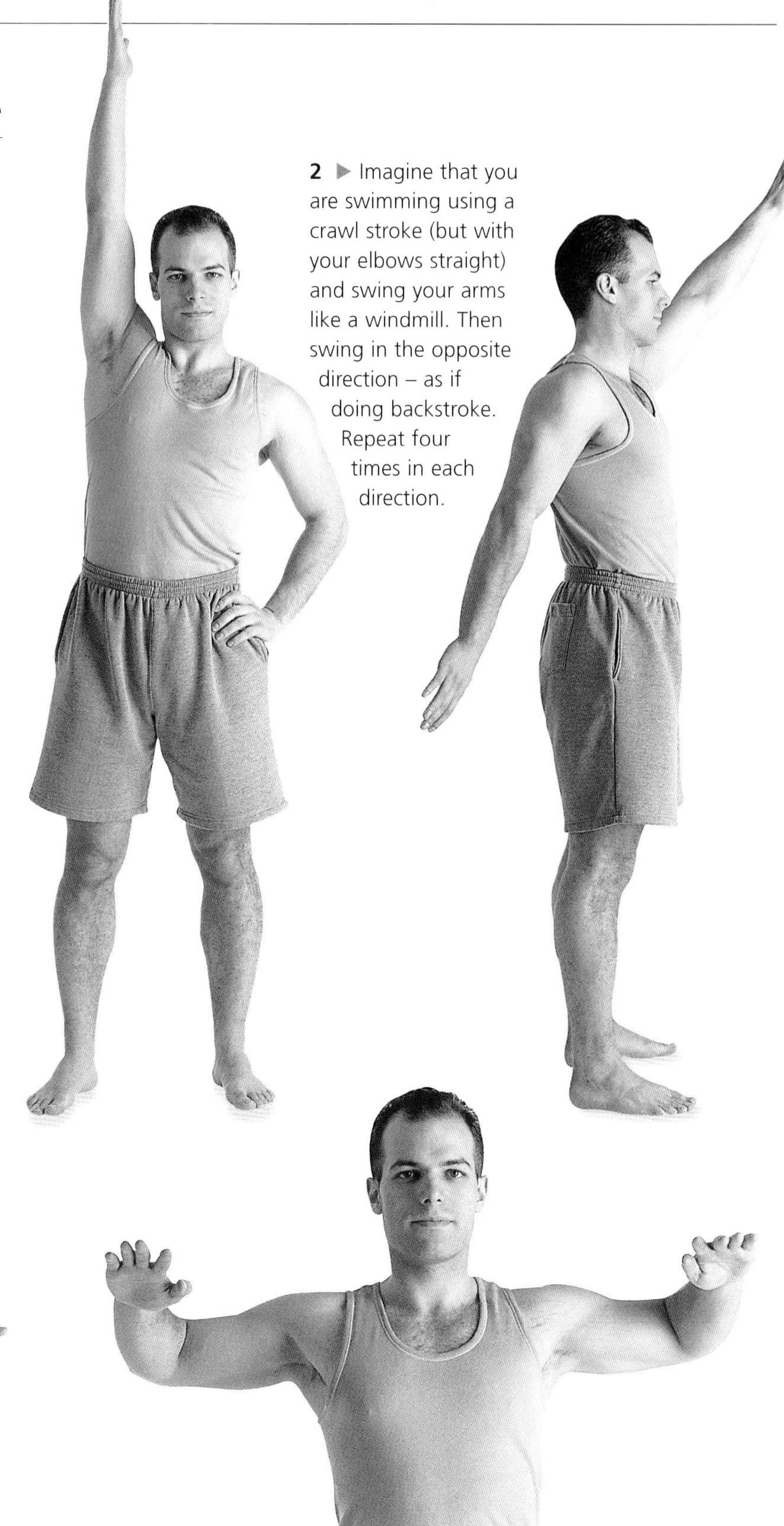

3 ▼ Raise your elbows to the level of your shoulders and cross your forearms. Keeping your elbows high, swing your upper arms back to pull your shoulder blades together. Feel the stretch across the front of your chest and the front part of your *deltoid* muscles. Repeat four times.

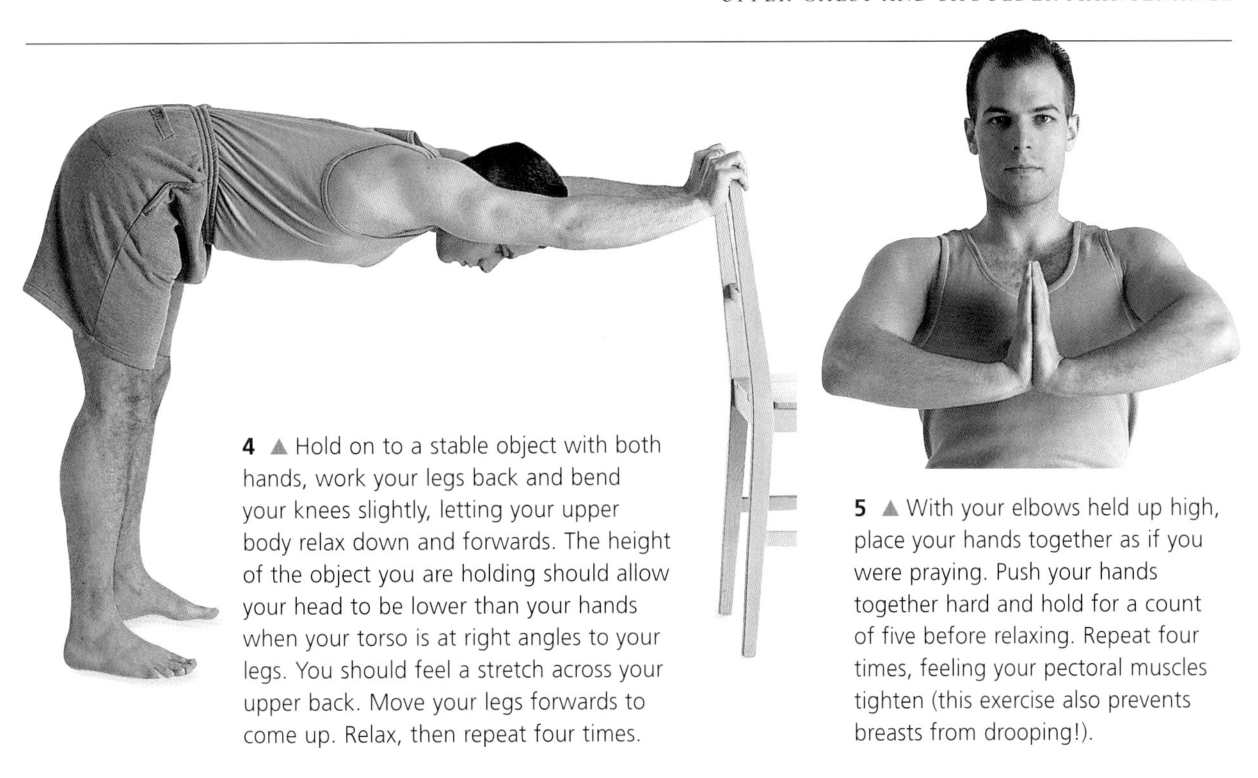

4 ▲ Hold on to a stable object with both hands, work your legs back and bend your knees slightly, letting your upper body relax down and forwards. The height of the object you are holding should allow your head to be lower than your hands when your torso is at right angles to your legs. You should feel a stretch across your upper back. Move your legs forwards to come up. Relax, then repeat four times.

5 ▲ With your elbows held up high, place your hands together as if you were praying. Push your hands together hard and hold for a count of five before relaxing. Repeat four times, feeling your pectoral muscles tighten (this exercise also prevents breasts from drooping!).

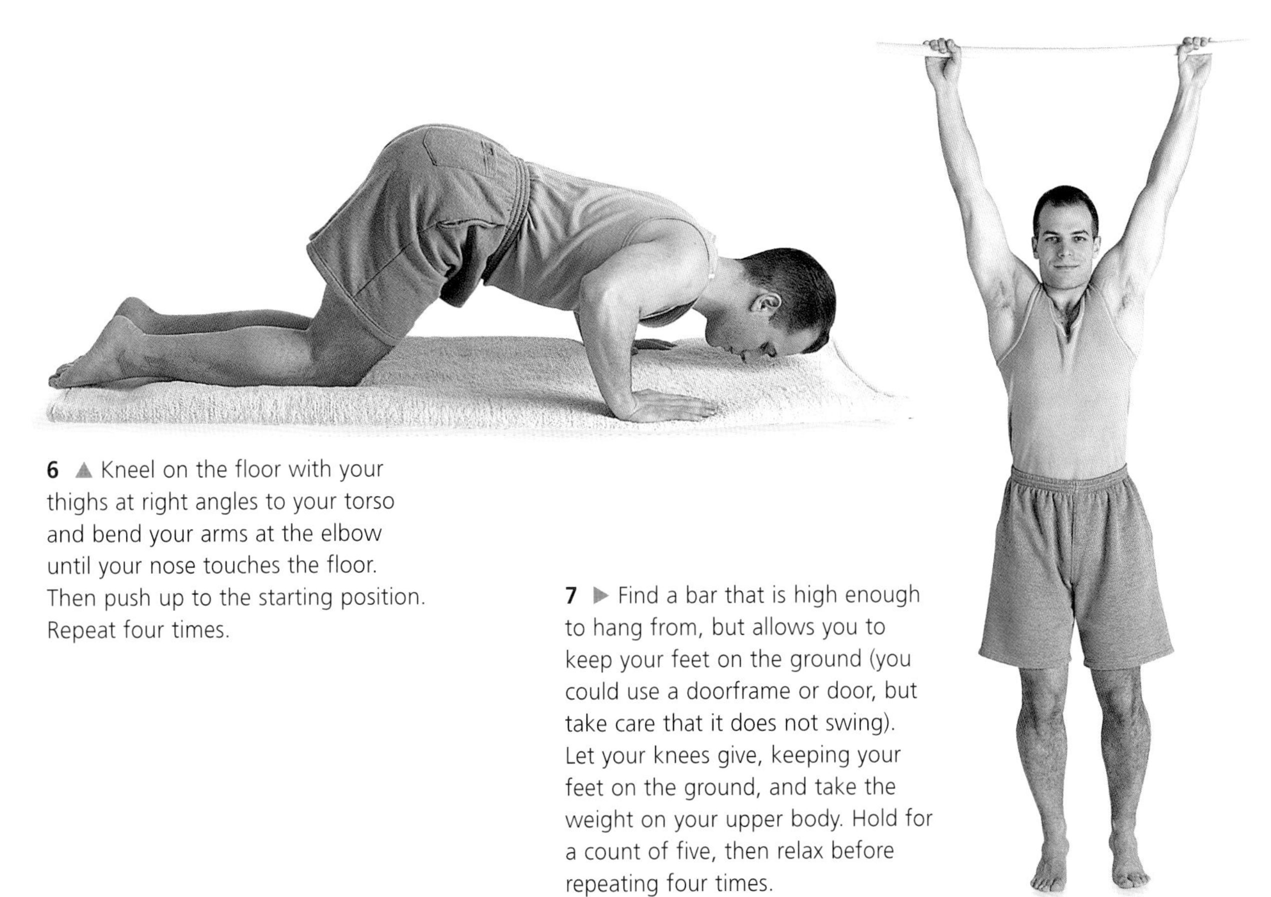

6 ▲ Kneel on the floor with your thighs at right angles to your torso and bend your arms at the elbow until your nose touches the floor. Then push up to the starting position. Repeat four times.

7 ▶ Find a bar that is high enough to hang from, but allows you to keep your feet on the ground (you could use a doorframe or door, but take care that it does not swing). Let your knees give, keeping your feet on the ground, and take the weight on your upper body. Hold for a count of five, then relax before repeating four times.

Shoulder and arm maintenance

For most of us, heavy manual labour, or even chopping wood for the fire, is a thing of the past. And our sedentary lives make us particularly susceptible to problems of the hands, wrists, arms and shoulders. Try this maintenance programme three times a week – especially if you do repetitive work involving computers.

1 ▼ Making sure that your shoulders are in the neutral position, stand with your arms out at right angles to your body. Bend your elbows until your fingers touch your shoulders with your palms down, then reach up high to the ceiling. Lower your hands back to your shoulders – still with your palms down – and repeat four times. You will feel a stretch along the sides of your torso, in the front of your chest and along the length of your arms.

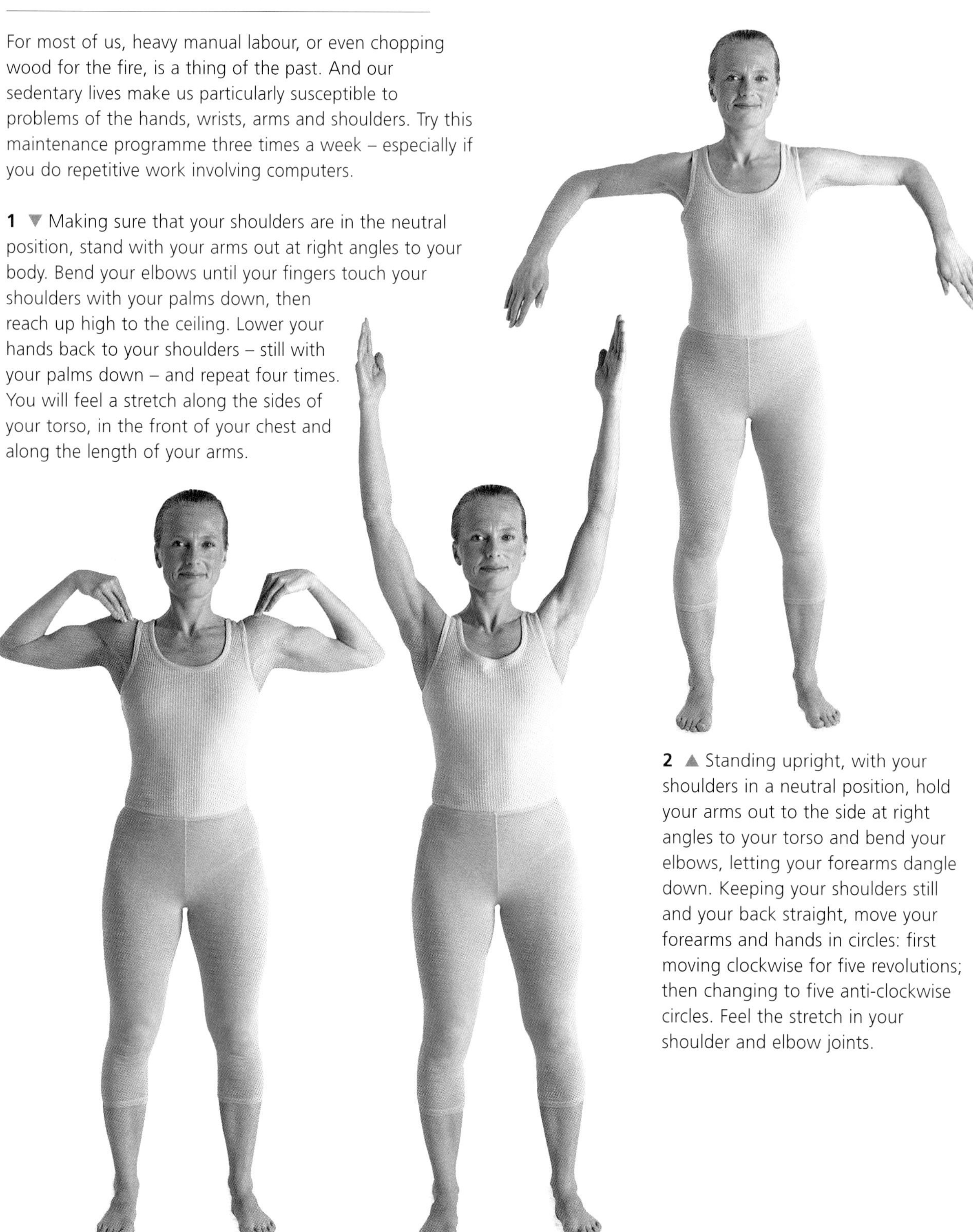

2 ▲ Standing upright, with your shoulders in a neutral position, hold your arms out to the side at right angles to your torso and bend your elbows, letting your forearms dangle down. Keeping your shoulders still and your back straight, move your forearms and hands in circles: first moving clockwise for five revolutions; then changing to five anti-clockwise circles. Feel the stretch in your shoulder and elbow joints.

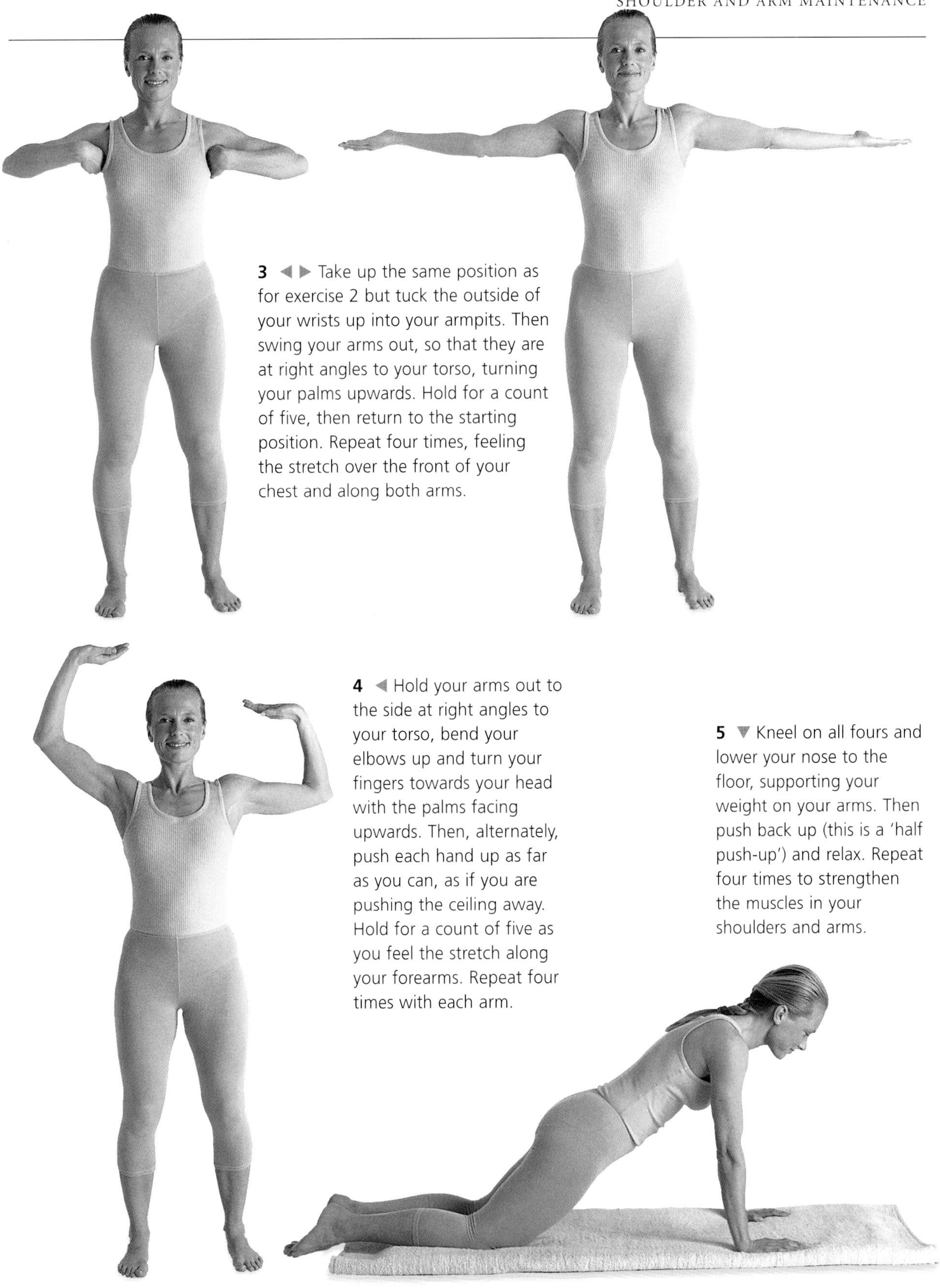

3 ◀ ▶ Take up the same position as for exercise 2 but tuck the outside of your wrists up into your armpits. Then swing your arms out, so that they are at right angles to your torso, turning your palms upwards. Hold for a count of five, then return to the starting position. Repeat four times, feeling the stretch over the front of your chest and along both arms.

4 ◀ Hold your arms out to the side at right angles to your torso, bend your elbows up and turn your fingers towards your head with the palms facing upwards. Then, alternately, push each hand up as far as you can, as if you are pushing the ceiling away. Hold for a count of five as you feel the stretch along your forearms. Repeat four times with each arm.

5 ▼ Kneel on all fours and lower your nose to the floor, supporting your weight on your arms. Then push back up (this is a 'half push-up') and relax. Repeat four times to strengthen the muscles in your shoulders and arms.

Wrist and hand maintenance

If you have once had a forearm, wrist or hand problem there is a danger that it will recur, so it is sensible to follow this simple maintenance routine two or three times a week. It is also useful if your lifestyle puts you at particular risk – if you use a keyboard a lot, for example, or if you play squash, tennis or the piano, or simply knit.

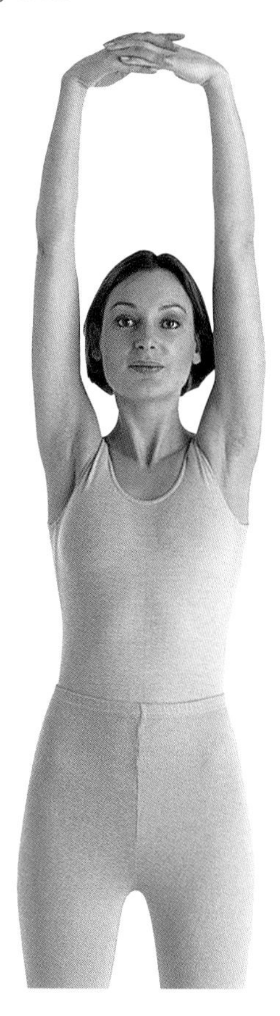

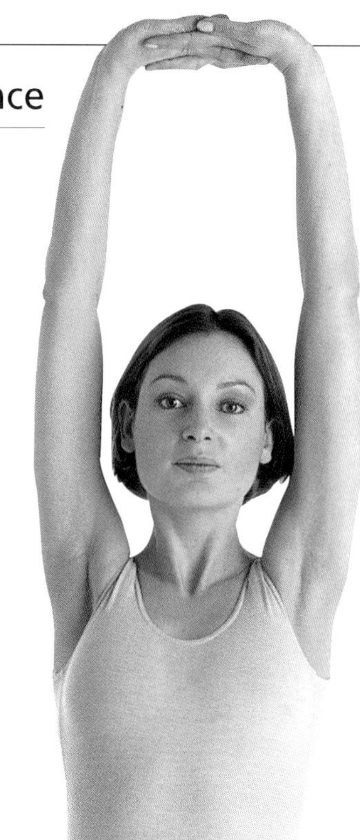

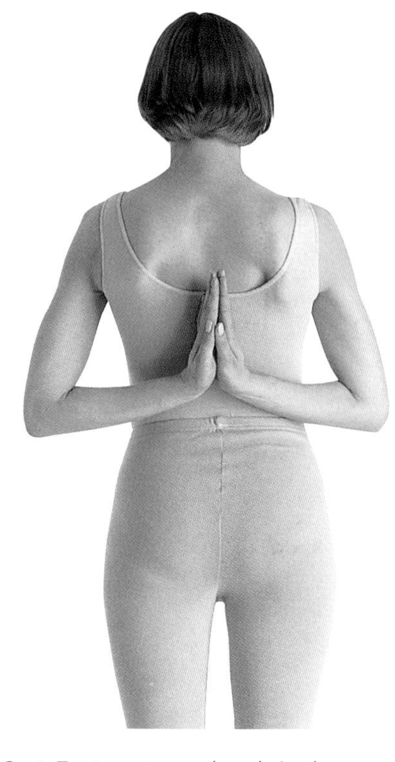

1 ◄ ▲ Lace your fingers together and raise your hands up above your head. Then turn your hands in and out three times, so that your palms are up and down alternately. Feel the stretch inside your wrists and across your palms.

2 ▲ Try to put your hands in the prayer position behind your back. Do not push yourself too far if this is difficult: it will become easier with practice. Hold for a count of five, then relax. Repeat three times.

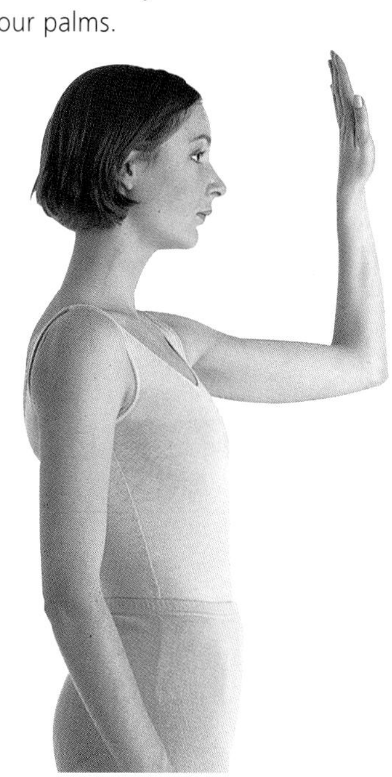

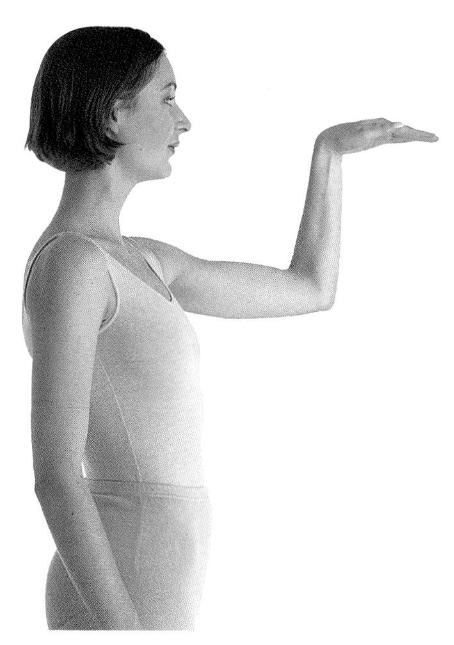

3 ► Put one arm out with your forearm bent up at right angles and your hand raised as if to signal 'stop'. Then push your hand down – do not just let your wrist go limp. Repeat six times with each arm, feeling the stretch in the ligaments over the back of your wrists.

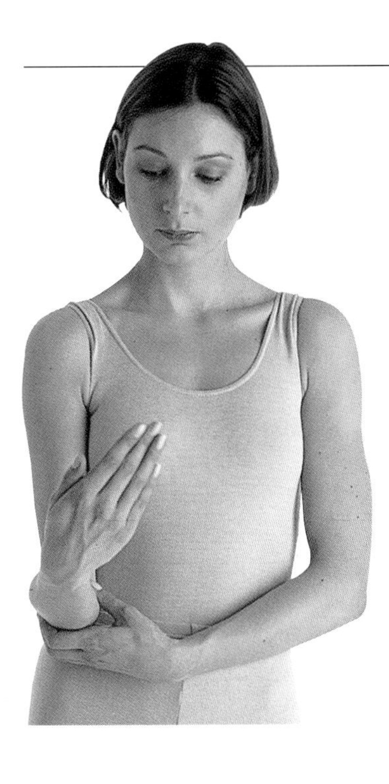

4 ◀ Rotate each wrist in a circle three times, then rotate it three times in the opposite direction. This movement keeps the small joints well-lubricated.

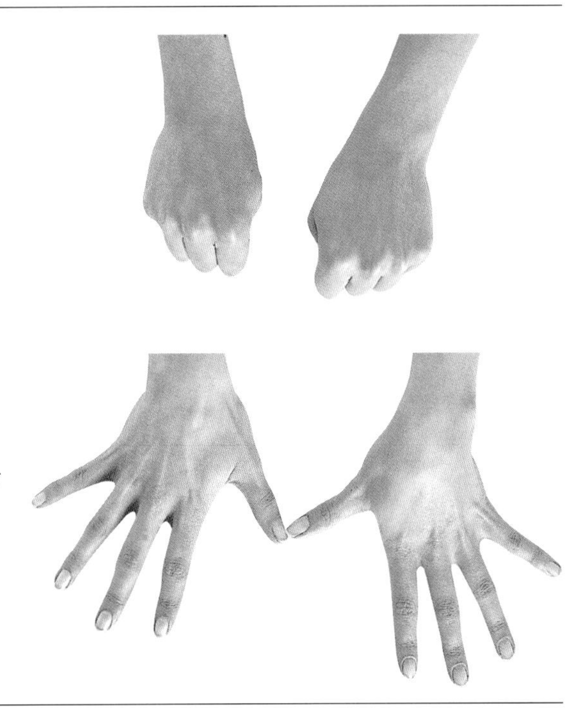

5 ▶ Hold both hands out straight and make a fist with them, then stretch your fingers as wide apart as you can. Hold for a count of five, then repeat the exercise: first with your wrists raised to the ceiling; then with them dropped towards the ground – the exercise is more difficult in this position.

6 ▶ Pick up something heavy between your fingers and thumb and turn your wrist out and back in again six times – as if you were turning a key in a lock. This helps with pronation and supination.

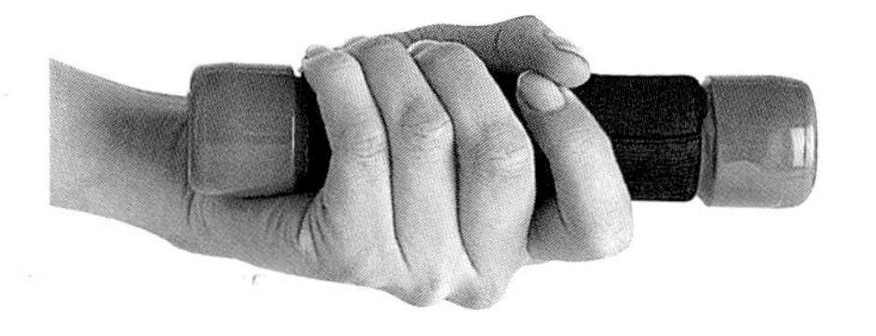

7 ▶ Pretend that the weight is a jug of water and pour the water out six times.

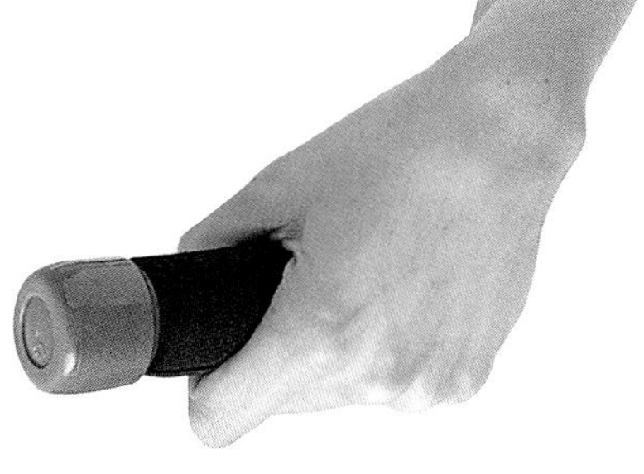

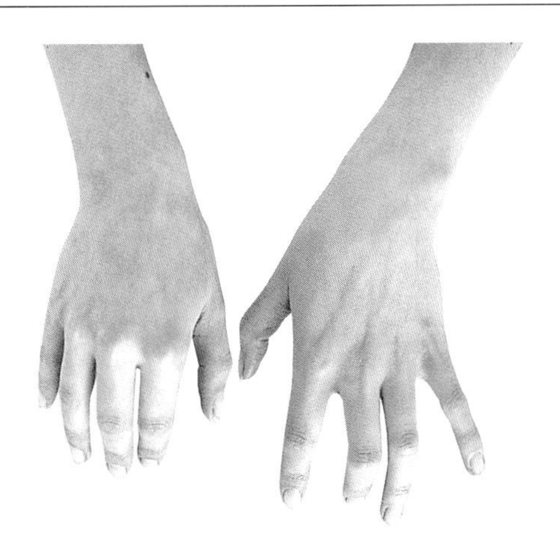

8 ▲ Pretend to play scales on an imaginary piano, making sure that you use each finger individually. Continue for 30 seconds, then reverse the direction and 'play' for another 30 seconds. This exercise loosens extensor muscle tendons.

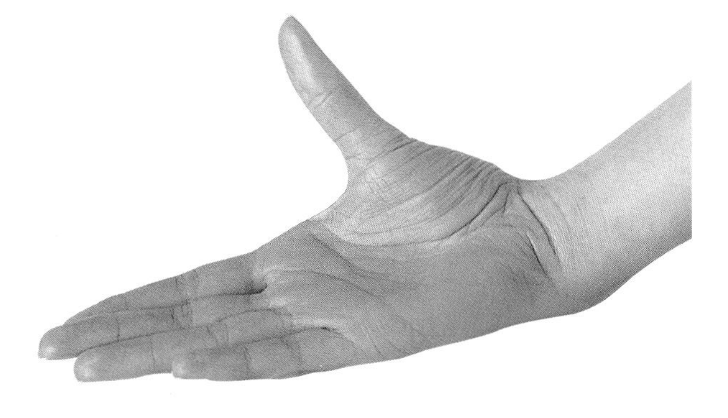

9 ▲ Rotate your thumb six times, describing as wide an arc as you can, then repeat in the opposite direction.

10 To finish off the sequence, loosen and relax your wrist and fingers by shaking your hands six times – as if you were trying to dry them.

Back and stomach maintenance

People often underestimate the importance of the part played by strong stomach muscles in the prevention of back problems. Together, strong stomach and back muscles act as a protective corset for the spine – which is why exercises for both are combined in the maintenance routine. Follow this programme three times a week.

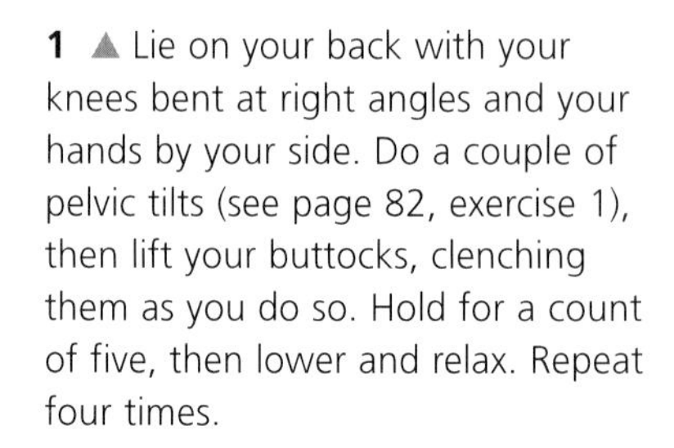

1 ▲ Lie on your back with your knees bent at right angles and your hands by your side. Do a couple of pelvic tilts (see page 82, exercise 1), then lift your buttocks, clenching them as you do so. Hold for a count of five, then lower and relax. Repeat four times.

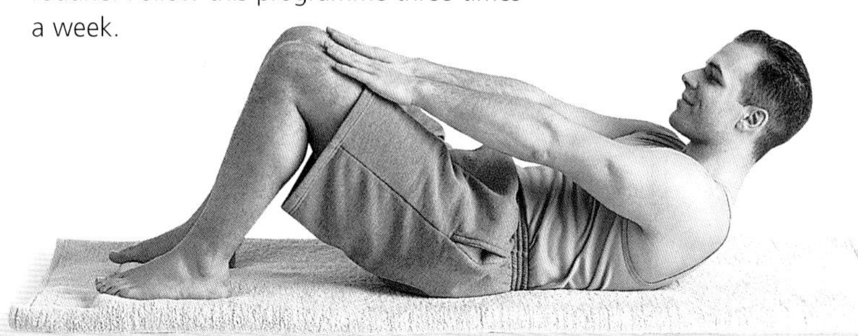

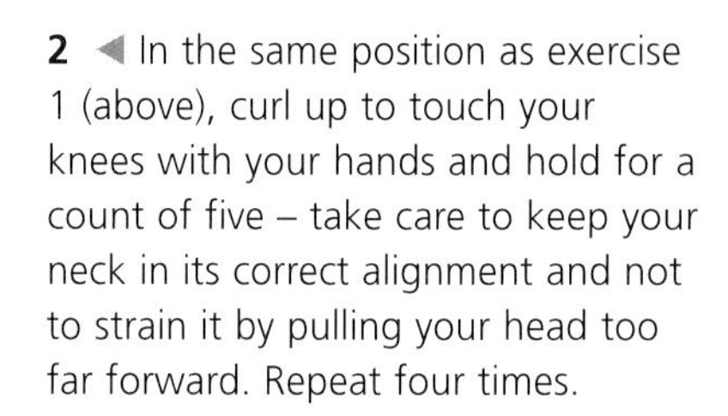

2 ◀ In the same position as exercise 1 (above), curl up to touch your knees with your hands and hold for a count of five – take care to keep your neck in its correct alignment and not to strain it by pulling your head too far forward. Repeat four times.

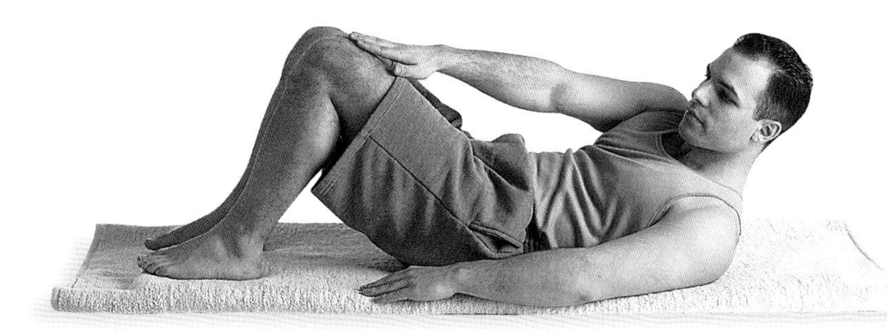

3 ◀ Repeat exercise 2, but this time stretch your right hand to your left knee, then your left hand to your right knee. Repeat four times.

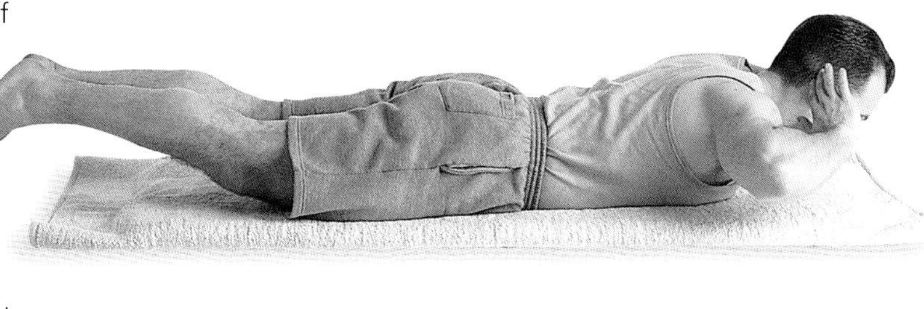

4 ▶ Lie on your stomach and raise your head, shoulders and feet just off the floor. Hold for a count of five, lower and relax. Repeat four times, feeling the small of your back tightening and your buttocks clenching.

5 ▶ In the same position as exercise 4, stretch one arm out in front of you and raise your opposite leg off the floor a little. Hold for a count of five, then lower. Relax and repeat with the opposite hand and leg. Repeat the whole exercise four times and feel the tension in your buttocks and the stretch down both sides of your body.

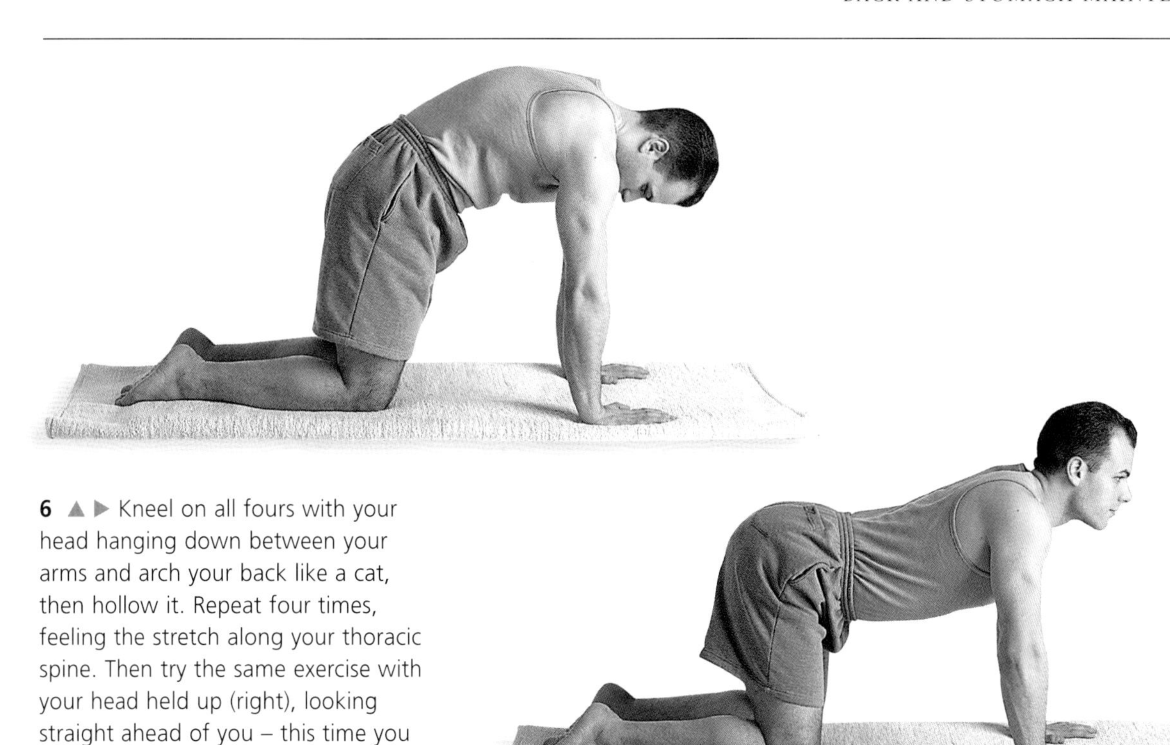

6 ▲ ▶ Kneel on all fours with your head hanging down between your arms and arch your back like a cat, then hollow it. Repeat four times, feeling the stretch along your thoracic spine. Then try the same exercise with your head held up (right), looking straight ahead of you – this time you will feel the tension between your shoulder blades.

7 ◀ Remaining on all fours (but with your head and neck straight ahead of you, parallel to the floor) raise one arm and its opposite leg until they are level with your trunk. You may find balancing difficult at first, but you will improve with practice. Stretch out, hold for a count of five, then lower your limbs and relax before repeating with the other arm and leg. Repeat the whole exercise four times.

8 ▶ With your knees on the mat and your hands out in front of you, curl up so that your head is as close to your knees as possible. Then swing your body forwards, straightening it, but also making sure that you keep your hands and knees still and your stomach muscles tightened. Swing back, then repeat the exercise four more times.

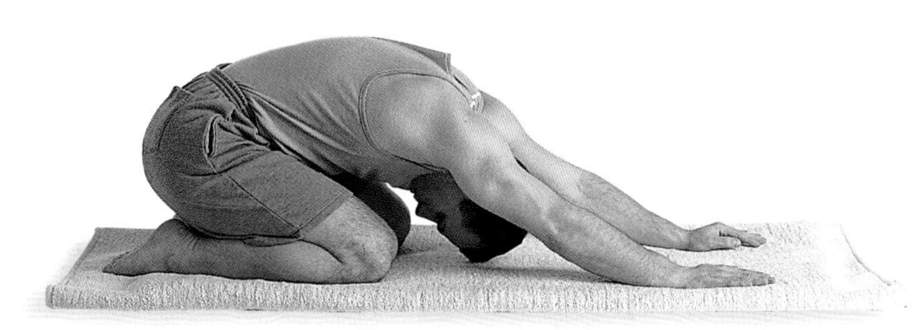

Hip and thigh maintenance

Osteoarthritis of the hip is a fairly common problem in the West but is seen far less often in the East. This is because Westerners tend only to extend and flex the hip joint when walking, while people in the East often sit cross-legged, which moves the joint far more. Help remedy the problem, and strengthen your thighs, by following this simple maintenance programme three times a week.

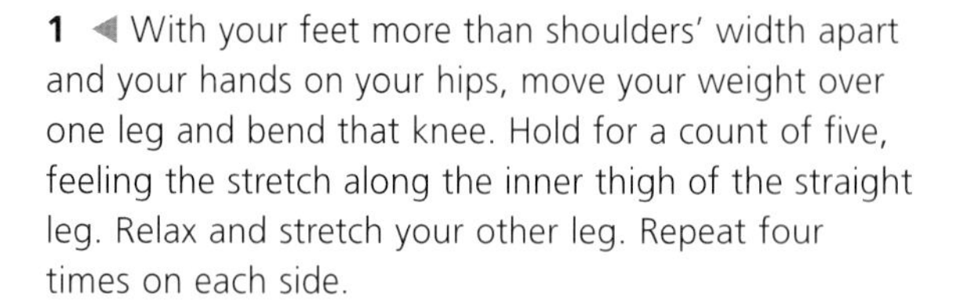

1 ◄ With your feet more than shoulders' width apart and your hands on your hips, move your weight over one leg and bend that knee. Hold for a count of five, feeling the stretch along the inner thigh of the straight leg. Relax and stretch your other leg. Repeat four times on each side.

2 Move your feet to shoulders' width apart and shift your weight onto one leg, then jut that hip out as far as you can, keeping both knees straight. Hold for a count of five, then relax before repeating with the other leg and hip. Repeat the whole exercise four times.

3 ▲ Kneeling up on a mat, bend one leg forward. Put your weight over your front leg and hold for a count of five, feeling the stretch in the front of your back leg. Do the same with the other leg and repeat the whole exercise four times.

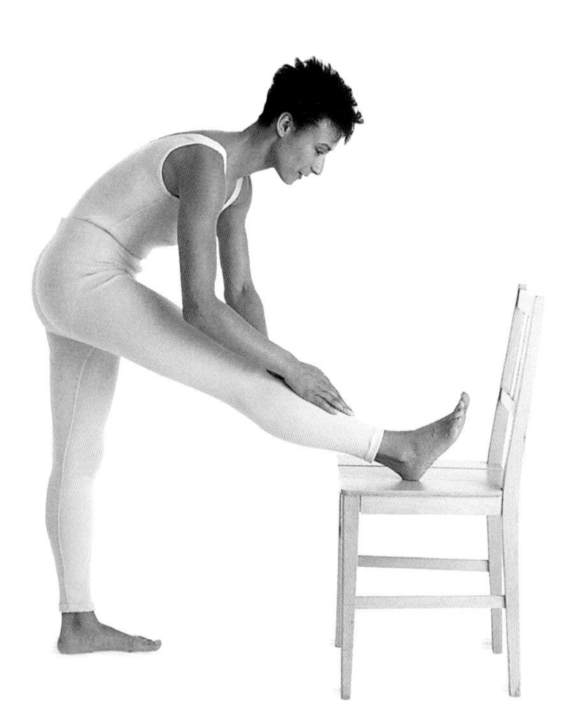

4 ▲ Place one foot on a stool or a chair and bend over from the hip towards it, keeping both knees straight. Hold for a count of five, then repeat with the other leg, feeling the stretch in your hamstrings. Repeat four times.

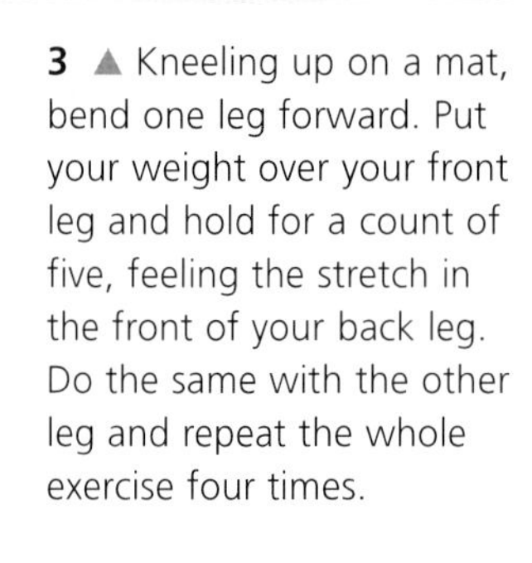

5 ◄ Standing up straight, pull one leg back as far behind you as you can, keeping your knees straight – you may need to hold on to the back of a chair for support. Hold the position for a count of five, then return the leg slowly, maintaining the tension. Do the same thing with the other leg, then repeat the whole exercise four times.

6 ▶ Lie on your back with your knees bent, then cross one leg over the other so that the ankle is resting on the opposite thigh. Using one hand, pull your lower thigh towards you until you feel a stretch on the outer thigh. Hold for a count of five, then repeat with the other leg crossed over. Repeat the exercise four times.

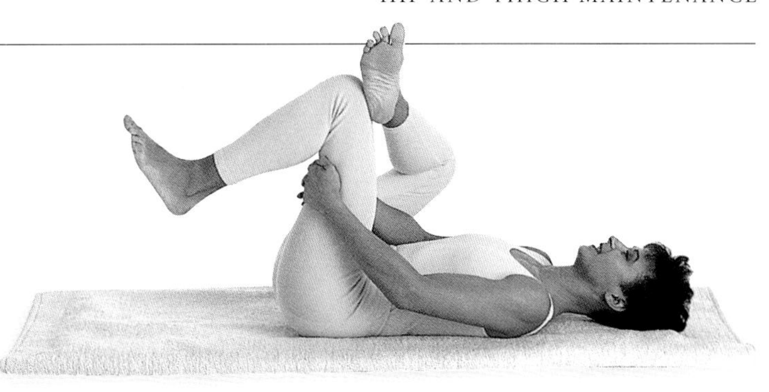

7 ▶ Lie on your back with your knees bent and raise one leg up, keeping the foot pulled up. Hold for a count of five, then lower back slowly, maintaining the tension. Relax, then do the same thing with the other leg. Repeat the whole exercise four times to strengthen your quadriceps muscles.

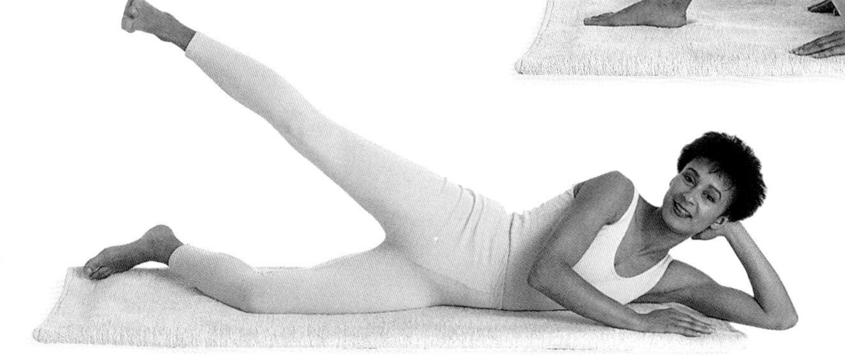

8 ▲ Lie on your side with your bottom leg bent. Raise your top leg, without twisting, and hold for five. Lower slowly, turn over and repeat with the other leg. Repeat the whole exercise four times to strengthen abductor muscles.

9 ▼ Lie on your back and squash a ball or cushion as hard as you can between your bent knees. Hold for a count of five, relax, then repeat four times. This works the little-used adductor muscles. Reduce the risk of cramp by following it with exercise 10.

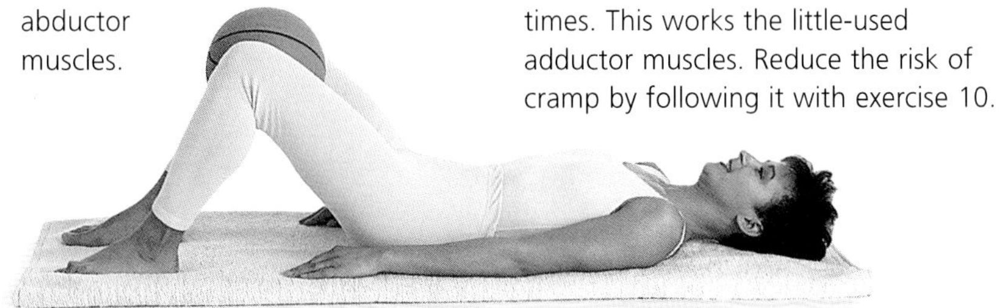

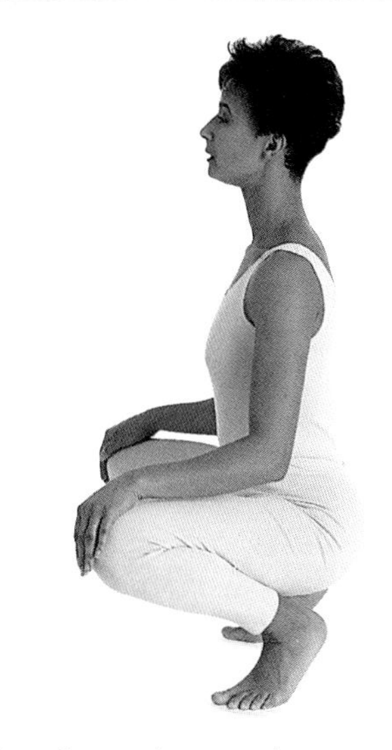

10 ▲ Squat down and use your hands to push your knees as far apart as you can without straining. This increases external rotation of the hip and strengthens abductor muscles. Hold for a count of five before relaxing. Repeat four times.

11 Stand up and swing one leg (with the foot flexed) forwards, backwards and sideways. Then describe circles: five clockwise, then five anticlockwise. Do the same with the other leg, then repeat with your feet pointed.

12 Finish off by shaking each leg vigorously a few times to release any tension and loosen up the muscles, ligaments and joints.

Lower-leg and foot maintenance

When it comes to the lower leg, ankle and foot, prevention is definitely better than cure. This is because the ankle joint is generally only moved in one plane, when walking, leaving ligaments that support other movements weak – thus strains in this area often recur. Follow this programme three times a week to help prevent problems.

1 ◀ Place one foot directly in front of the other, as if walking. Then – keeping the heel of your back foot on the ground – bend the knee of your front leg and move the weight of your body over it. Hold for a count of five, feeling the stretch in your calf muscles, then relax. Repeat with the other foot in front, then repeat the whole exercise four times. To increase the stretch, lift up the front of the back foot.

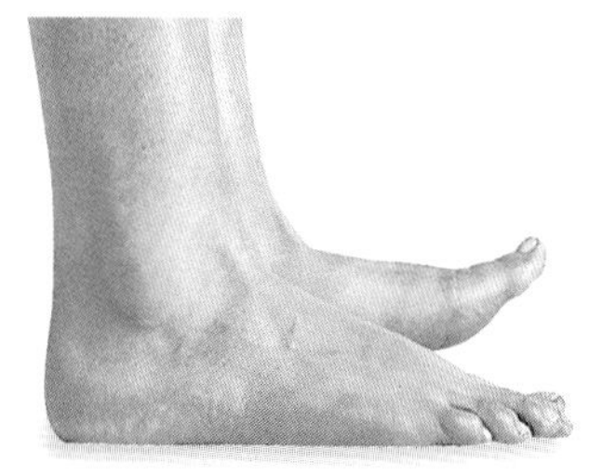

2 ▲ Pivoting on your heel, pull the front of one foot as far up as you can without overstraining. Hold for a count of five, feeling the stretch in your lower leg muscles. Relax, then do the same with your other foot. Repeat four times.

3 ▼ Raise one foot on tiptoe, pushing the front of your instep as far forward as possible; hold for a count of five and relax. Do the same with the other foot, then repeat four times.

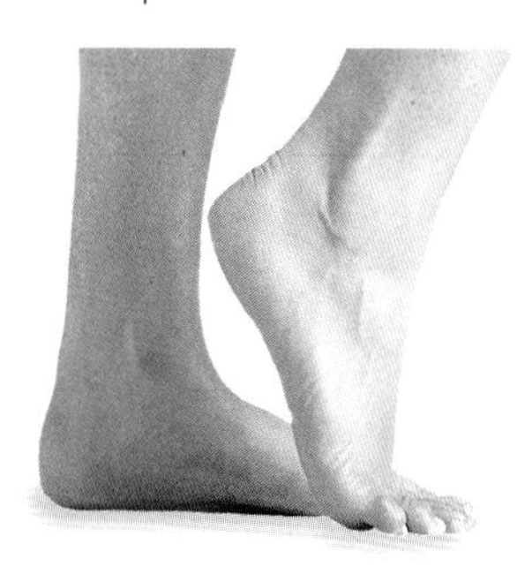

4 ◀ Lean against a wall with your arms and knees straight. Move your feet back, then raise the toes of both feet off the ground while keeping your heels in place. Hold for a count of five, then relax. Repeat four times, feeling the stretch in your calf muscles.

5 ▶ Stand with your feet apart. Keeping your outer toes on the ground, raise your inside toes and the inside part of your soles up as far as you can. Hold for a count of five, then try to flatten the same area into the ground; hold for a count of five. Relax, then repeat four times. Feel the pull along the inside of your ankle as you pull up then flatten the long medial arches.

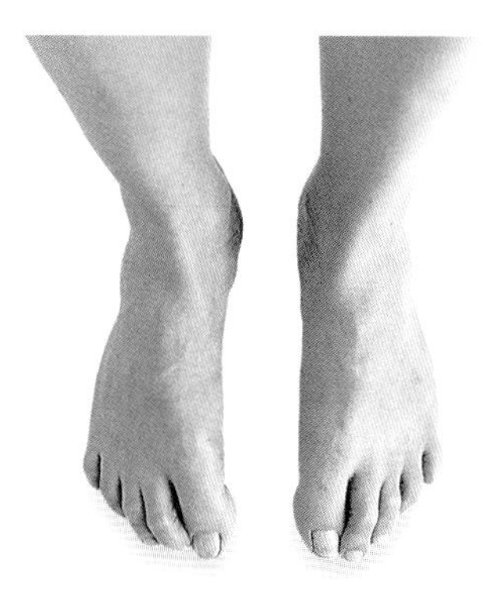

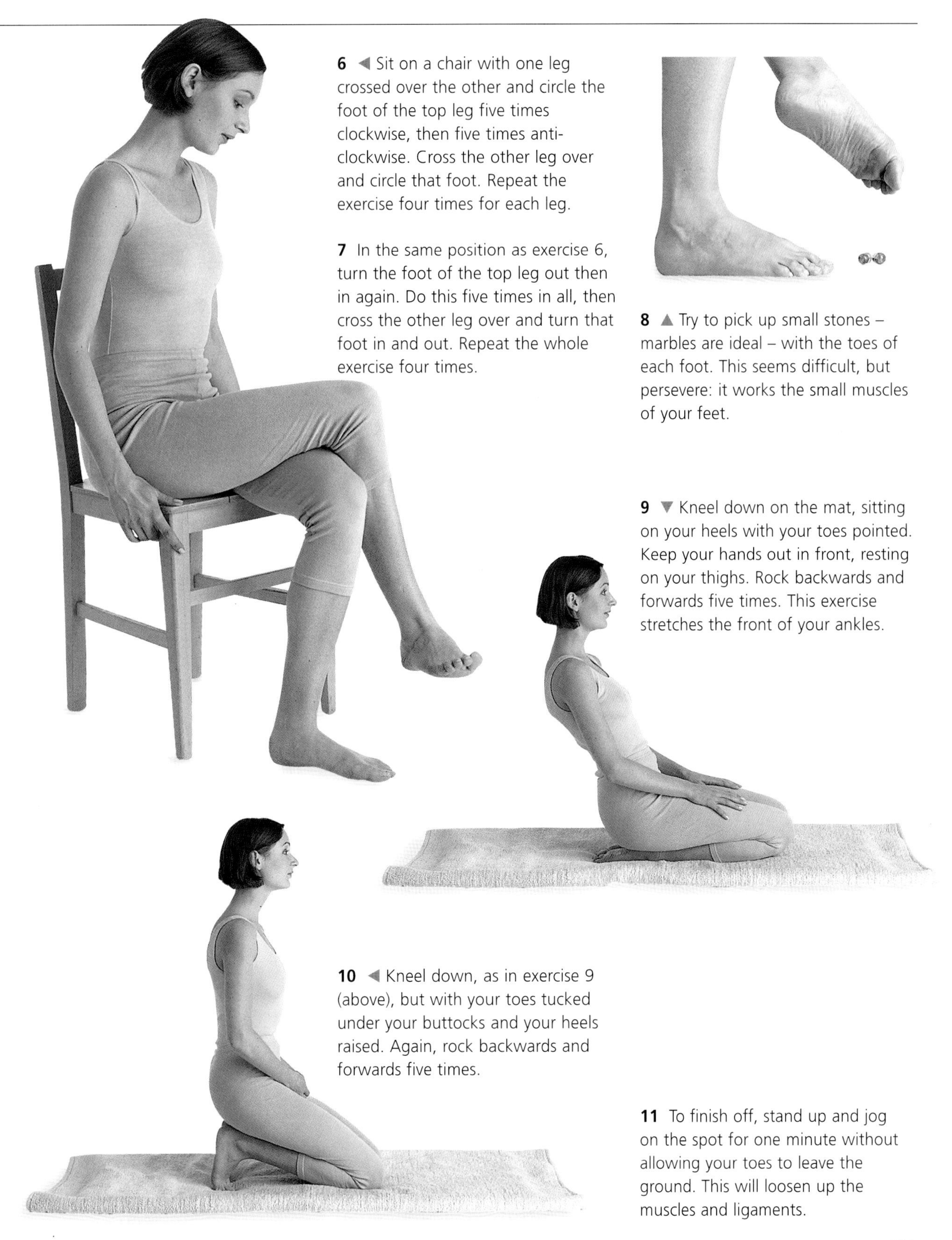

6 ◀ Sit on a chair with one leg crossed over the other and circle the foot of the top leg five times clockwise, then five times anti-clockwise. Cross the other leg over and circle that foot. Repeat the exercise four times for each leg.

7 In the same position as exercise 6, turn the foot of the top leg out then in again. Do this five times in all, then cross the other leg over and turn that foot in and out. Repeat the whole exercise four times.

8 ▲ Try to pick up small stones – marbles are ideal – with the toes of each foot. This seems difficult, but persevere: it works the small muscles of your feet.

9 ▼ Kneel down on the mat, sitting on your heels with your toes pointed. Keep your hands out in front, resting on your thighs. Rock backwards and forwards five times. This exercise stretches the front of your ankles.

10 ◀ Kneel down, as in exercise 9 (above), but with your toes tucked under your buttocks and your heels raised. Again, rock backwards and forwards five times.

11 To finish off, stand up and jog on the spot for one minute without allowing your toes to leave the ground. This will loosen up the muscles and ligaments.

Ten-minute daily workout

If your lifestyle allows it, do this routine first thing in the morning for maximum benefit, as it will prepare your body to work efficiently during the day ahead. It boosts the circulation, makes muscles more pliable, ligaments more resilient and joints more flexible. But if the mornings are impossible for you, make sure to find ten minutes at some time during the day. The routine is designed to minimise joint stress, but – especially if you are elderly or unfit – you should build up the number of repetitions gradually until you feel comfortable with those given below. If you have a specific problem, add at least four exercises from the appropriate self-help section (see pages 78–111) after the first standing and lying exercises. If some of these are already part of this workout, choose different ones, making sure that the joint involved is put through its full range of possible movements.

1 Stand upright and breathe in and out deeply and slowly three times. This increases the level of oxygen in the blood and so available to the muscles.

2 ▶ Jog on the spot for one minute. Start slowly, then speed up to make your heart pump more blood. Gradually lift your heels further off the floor and bring your knees up higher.

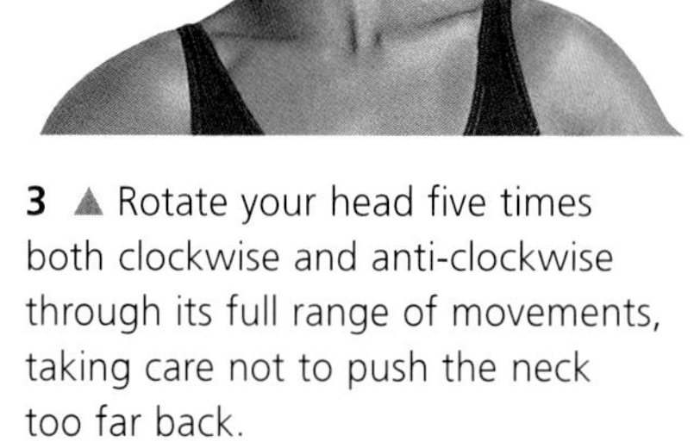

3 ▲ Rotate your head five times both clockwise and anti-clockwise through its full range of movements, taking care not to push the neck too far back.

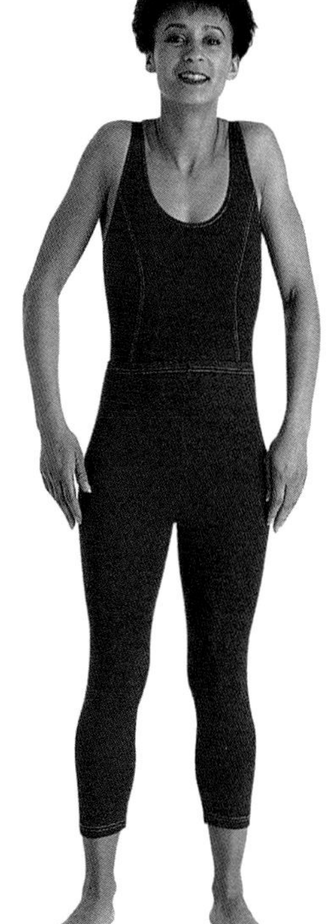

4 ◀ Hunch up your shoulders and rotate them in one direction and then the other. Repeat the whole exercise four times to open up your rib cage, but make sure to finish with an upwards rotation.

5 ◀ Hold your arms out to your sides, level with your shoulders, and swing them in large circles, first backwards, then forwards. Repeat four times to loosen up your shoulder joints.

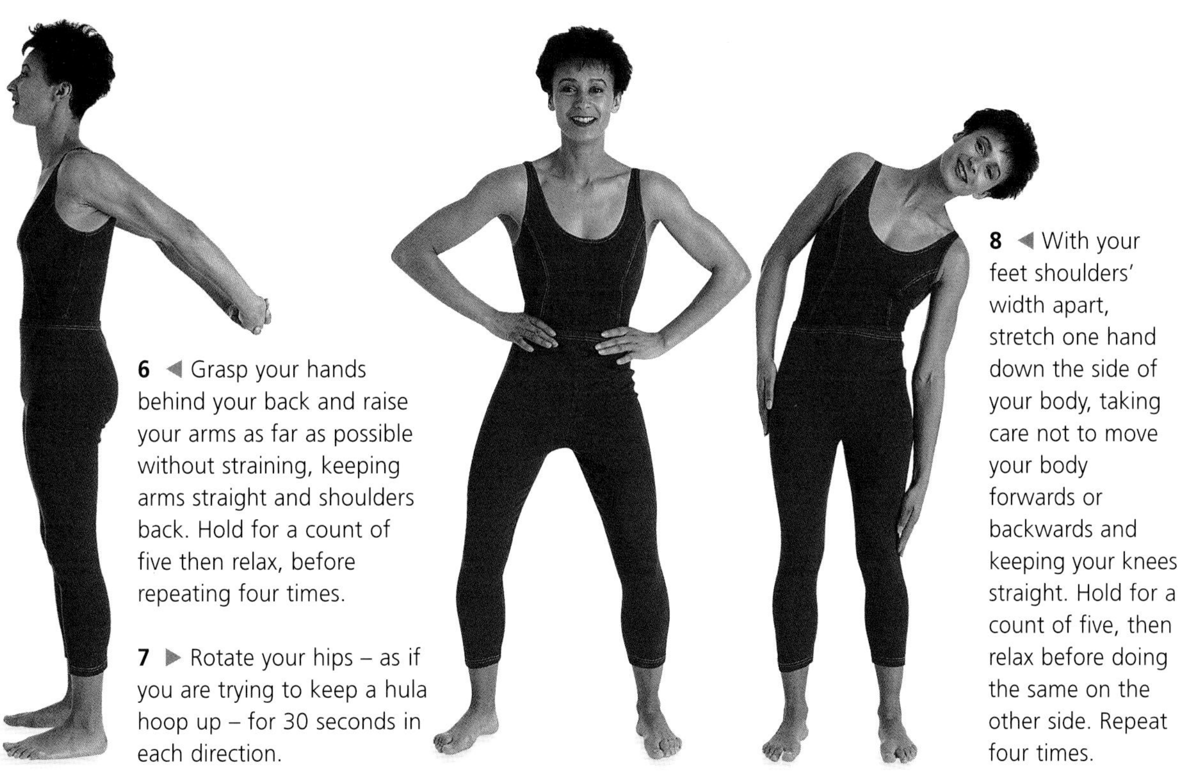

6 ◀ Grasp your hands behind your back and raise your arms as far as possible without straining, keeping arms straight and shoulders back. Hold for a count of five then relax, before repeating four times.

7 ▶ Rotate your hips – as if you are trying to keep a hula hoop up – for 30 seconds in each direction.

8 ◀ With your feet shoulders' width apart, stretch one hand down the side of your body, taking care not to move your body forwards or backwards and keeping your knees straight. Hold for a count of five, then relax before doing the same on the other side. Repeat four times.

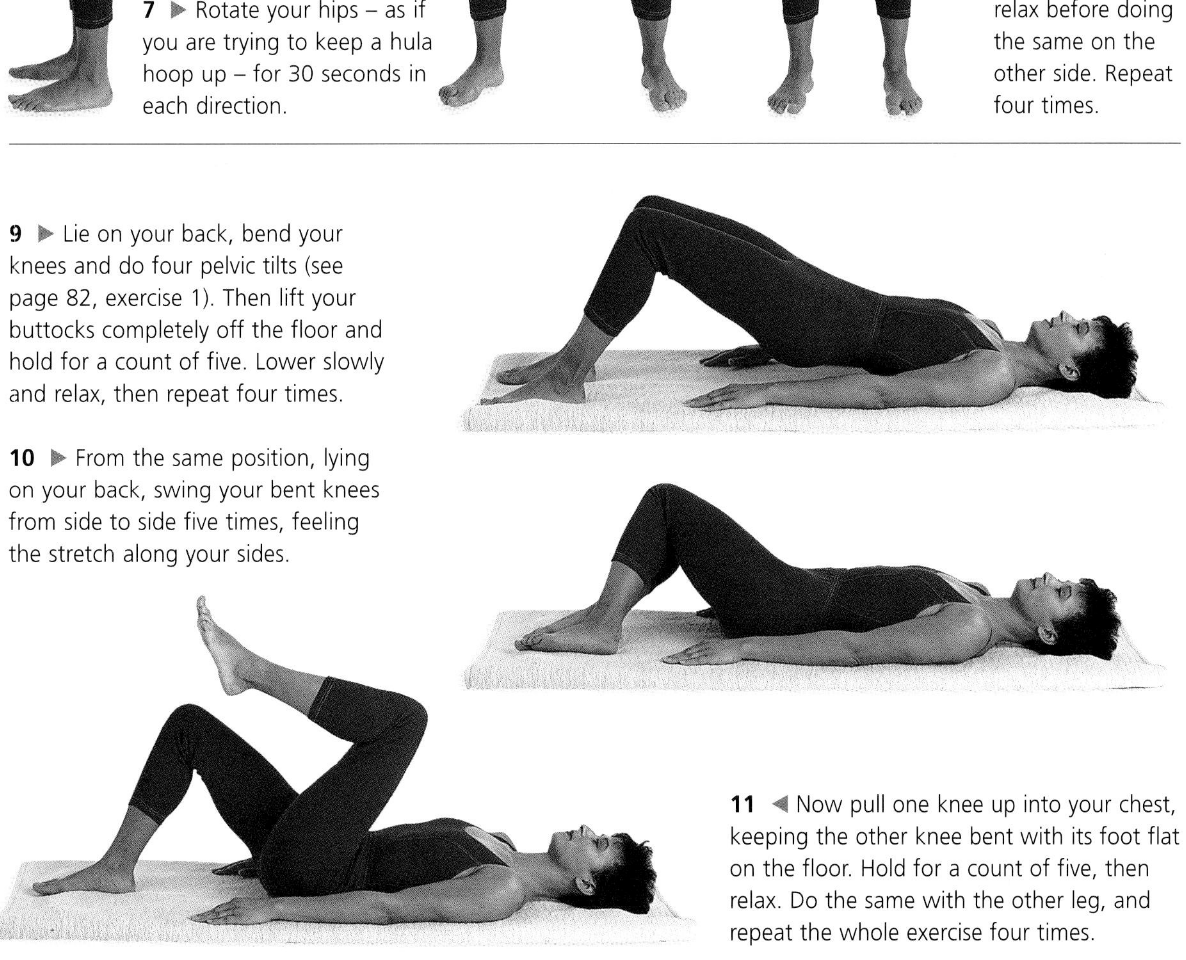

9 ▶ Lie on your back, bend your knees and do four pelvic tilts (see page 82, exercise 1). Then lift your buttocks completely off the floor and hold for a count of five. Lower slowly and relax, then repeat four times.

10 ▶ From the same position, lying on your back, swing your bent knees from side to side five times, feeling the stretch along your sides.

11 ◀ Now pull one knee up into your chest, keeping the other knee bent with its foot flat on the floor. Hold for a count of five, then relax. Do the same with the other leg, and repeat the whole exercise four times.

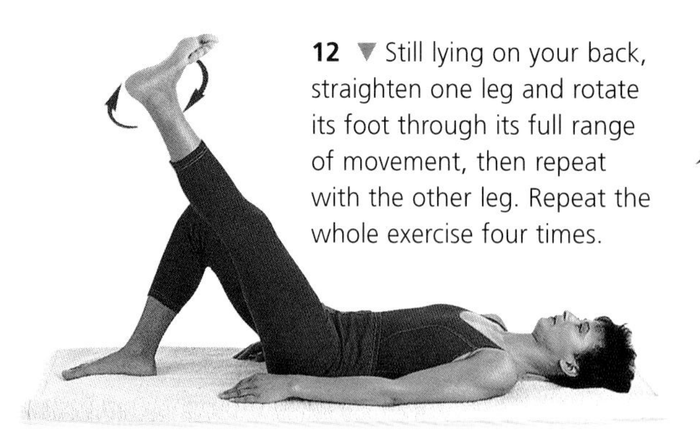

12 ▼ Still lying on your back, straighten one leg and rotate its foot through its full range of movement, then repeat with the other leg. Repeat the whole exercise four times.

13 ▼ In the same position, raise one leg and turn the sole of your foot out and then in as far as possible. Do the same with the other leg and repeat the whole exercise four times.

14 ▼ In the same position, raise first one leg, holding for a count of five, then the other. Repeat the whole exercise four times to strengthen quadriceps and stomach muscles.

15 ▼ Do five 'curl-ups': raise your head off the ground and touch your knees with your hands. Hold for five, lower and relax between each one.

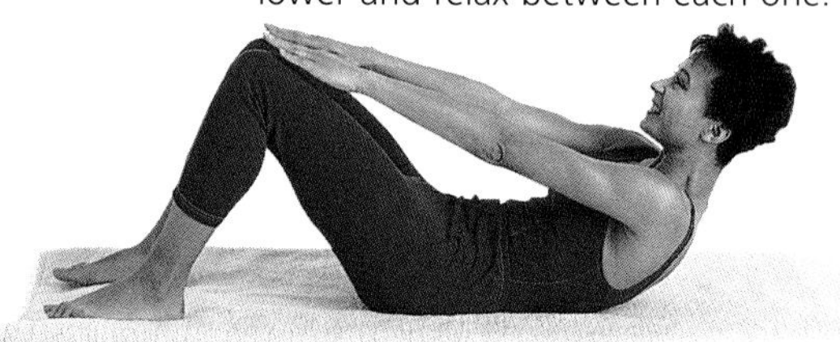

16 ▶ Turn to lie on your side with your lower knee bent back behind you. Raise your top leg, hold for a count of five, then lower slowly and relax before repeating four times. Turn over and do the same thing with your other leg.

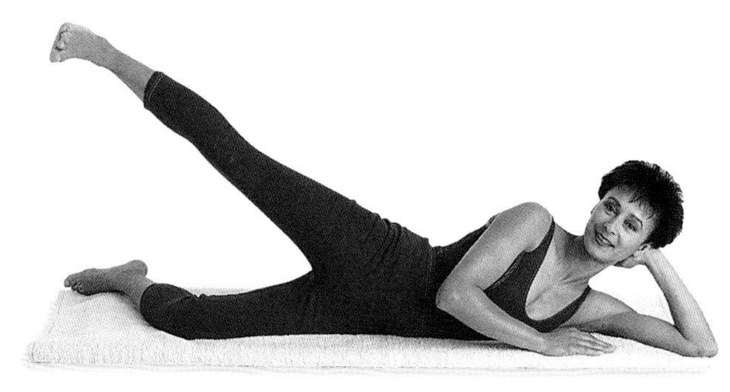

17 ▶ Again, lie on your side, but this time bend the top leg over in front of your body. Raise your bottom leg – this is only a small movement – hold for a count of five, then lower and relax before repeating four times. Turn over and repeat with the other leg.

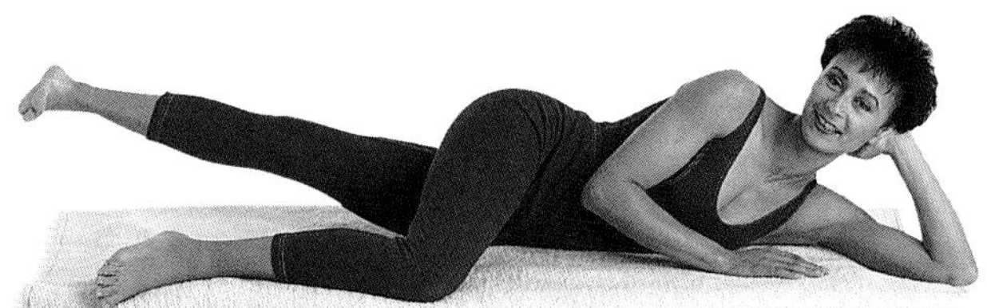

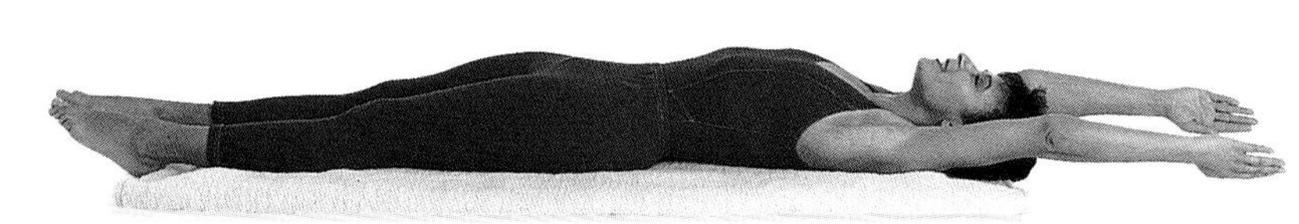

18 ◀ Lie flat on your back with your legs straight and your arms by your sides. Then point your toes and stretch your arms out and back over your head, elongating your body as much as possible. Hold for a count of five then relax to the starting position, before repeating four times.

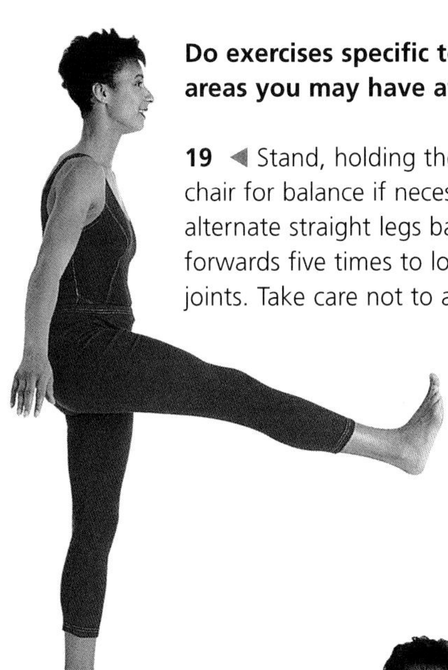

Do exercises specific to any problem areas you may have at this point.

19 ◀ Stand, holding the back of a chair for balance if necessary, and swing alternate straight legs backwards and forwards five times to loosen your hip joints. Take care not to arch your spine.

20 ▶ Again, holding a chair if necessary, swing your legs alternately in a diagonal across your body five times, keeping your knees straight.

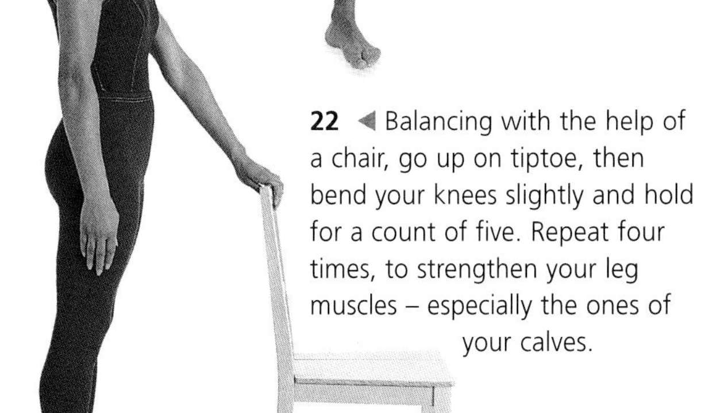

21 ▶ Put your hands on your hips and turn your feet out, then bend at your knees – a plié in ballet. Hold for a count of five and then come back up slowly. Repeat four times.

22 ◀ Balancing with the help of a chair, go up on tiptoe, then bend your knees slightly and hold for a count of five. Repeat four times, to strengthen your leg muscles – especially the ones of your calves.

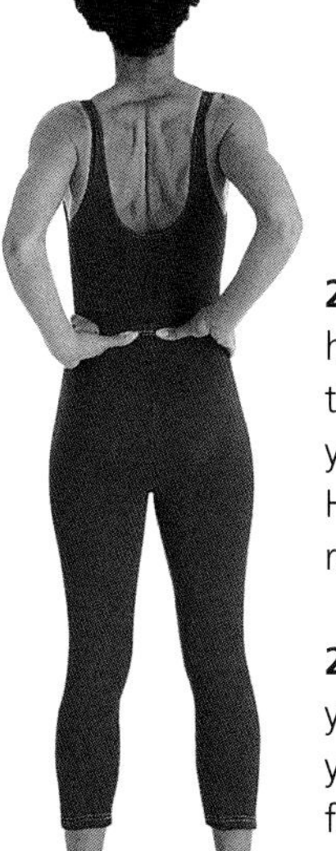

23 ◀ Put your hands over your hips and the small of your back, then arch backwards, pulling your shoulder blades together. Hold for a count of five, then relax. Repeat four times.

24 ▶ Bend over slowly, sliding your hands down the front of your legs. Hold for a count of five, then relax and come back up slowly. Repeat four times.

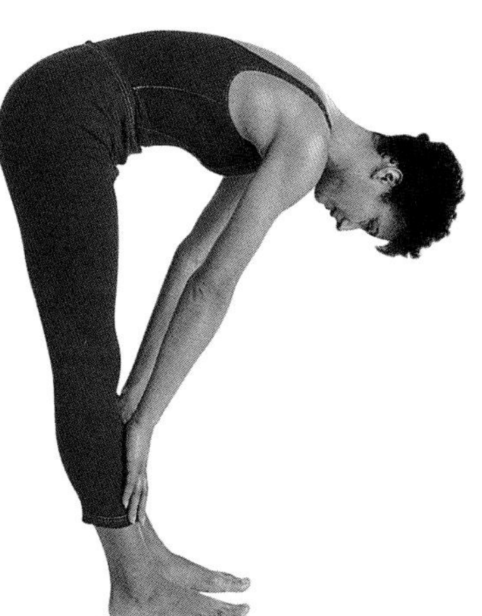

25 To finish off, shake yourself all over like a dog, to release any tension. Next jog gently on the spot for two minutes. Finally, take three slow, deep breaths to increase the level of oxygen in your blood and help speed the breakdown of the waste products of exercise.

APPENDIX: getting professional help

However scrupulously you follow the maintenance exercises in this book, and however carefully you carry out the self-help treatments that I have suggested, there will always be occasions when you have to seek professional help. And – as I have advised throughout this book – you should always take medical advice when you are in any doubt about your condition, both to rule out any underlying disorder and to ensure that you receive appropriate treatment.

The first port of call should be your family practitioner. He or she will take your medical history, conduct an examination and make a preliminary diagnosis, and then, if necessary, suggest who else it might be appropriate to see. Practices vary from country to country, but your doctor might suggest that you see a consultant – either an orthopaedic surgeon or a rheumatologist, if your condition involves tissue damage – a physiotherapist, an osteopath, a chiropractor or a teacher of the Alexander Technique.

It is sensible to ask your family practitioner for a referral, or for advice about which practitioner to choose. However, if you decide to consult any such practitioner directly, it is important that you make sure that he or she is properly qualified, and, preferably, has professional indemnity insurance cover, because any physical manipulation involves some degree of risk. The contacts listed here will be able to put you in touch with a practitioner in your area, or with your local registering body.

MEDICAL CONSULTANTS

If your family doctor suspects that you may be suffering from a problem that might require an operation, you will probably be asked to see an orthopaedic surgeon; if a degenerative disorder is thought to be at the root of your problem, you may be advised to see a rheumatologist. In both cases, you will see a hospital consultant who has qualified as a doctor and then received extra, specialist training. The consultant is likely to suggest a course of treatment that may include drug treatment, surgery, in some cases, and treatment by a physiotherapist (see below).

PHYSIOTHERAPY

Physiotherapy has been accepted as a branch of mainstream medical treatment for longer than any other form of manipulative therapy. Physiotherapists are found on the staff of nearly all hospitals, are state-registered in most countries, have their own professional indemnity insurance and cannot practise unless they have qualified at the end of a demanding course of study.

Physiotherapy treatment varies according to the condition being treated, but may involve manipulation and mobilisation, heat or cold treatments, ultrasound treatment, traction, hydrotherapy and a structured programme of exercises. Do not be surprised if your physiotherapist is blind: the extra sensitivity of touch that blind people have makes them particularly suited to the profession.

UNITED KINGDOM

The Chartered Society of Physiotherapy
14 Bedford Row
London WC1R 4ED
Tel. 0171 306 6633
Fax. 0171 306 6611

CANADA

Canadian Physiotherapy Association
2345 Yonge Street, Suite 410
Toronto, Ontario M4P 2E5
Tel. 416 932 1888
Fax. 416 932 9708
Email: information@physiotherapy.ca
Website: www.physiotherapy.ca

AUSTRALIA

Australian Physiotherapy Association
PO Box 6465, Melbourne
Victoria 3004
Tel. (03) 9534 9400
Fax. (03) 9534 9199

NEW ZEALAND

New Zealand Association of Physiotherapists
PO Box 27386, Wellington
Tel. (04) 801 6500
Fax. (04) 801 5571
Email: nzsp@mail.netlink.co.nz

OSTEOPATHY

Twenty years ago, osteopaths were on the fringes of mainstream medicine. Since then, however, osteopathy has become accepted as a valid and useful therapy, whose efficacy has been proved. Indeed, it will soon become illegal in most countries to practise as an osteopath without being registered with the appropriate association – which registration will only be possible on demonstration of adequate training and skills.

Osteopathy is based on the premise that many ailments are the result of a misalignment in the bones, muscles and ligaments. As part of treatment, osteopaths use deep, kneading massage, 'trigger-point' massage, localised massage, passive stretching of muscles and joints and manipulation.

UNITED KINGDOM
General Osteopathic Council
Premier House
10 Greycoat Place
London SW1P 1SB
Tel. 0171 799 2442

CANADA
Canadian Osteopathic Society
575 Waterloo Street
London, Ontario N6B 2R2
Tel. 519 439 5521
Fax. 519 439 2616

AUSTRALIA
Australian Osteopathic Association
PO Box 699, Turramurra
NSW 2074
Tel. (02) 9449 4799
Fax. (02) 9449 6587
Email: aoa@tpgi.com.au
Website: www.osteopathic.com.au

NEW ZEALAND
New Zealand Osteopathic Association
PO Box 14697, Wellington
Tel/Fax. (04) 387 3454
Email: marykind@clare.net.nz

CHIROPRACTIC

Chiropractic is believed to be the most widely practised complimentary therapy in the western world. Like osteopaths, in many countries chiropractors will soon only be able to practise if they can satisfy the requirements of the relevant associations.

Chiropractors believe that misalignment of the spine, with its extensive nervous and musculo-skeletal system, is responsible for many disorders – even those in parts of the body distanced from the back. They use more than 100 different manipulations, involving 'lever pulls' that twist the whole body, localised thrusts and ice treatments, to realign the spine and reduce pain. Research has shown that chiropractic benefits many patients, when undertaken by a qualified practitioner.

UNITED KINGDOM
British Chiropractic Association
Blagrave House, 17 Blagrave Street
Reading , Berkshire RG1 1QB
Tel. 0118 950 5950
Fax. 0118 958 8946

CANADA
Canadian Chiropractic Association
1396 Eglinton Avenue West
Toronto, Ontario M6C 2E4
Tel. 416 781 5656
Fax. 416 781 7344

AUSTRALIA
Chiropractor's Association of Australia
PO Box 241, Springwood
NSW 2777
Tel. (02) 4751 5644
Fax. (02) 4751 5856
Email: caa_nat@pnc.com.au
Website: www.caa.com.au

NEW ZEALAND
New Zealand Chiropractors Association
PO Box 2858, Wellington
Tel/Fax. (04) 9426 4529

THE ALEXANDER TECHNIQUE

Devised by F. M. Alexander, an Australian actor who found that retraining his posture helped cure a voice problem, the Alexander Technique has a proven record in correcting postural problems and eliminating unnecessary – and potentially damaging – stress on the musculo-skeletal system.

The Alexander Technique must be taught, and qualified teachers must complete a three-year course before they can be registered by the Society of Teachers of the Alexander Technique. Teachers first look at a student's whole body, both stationary and in motion, and make him or her aware of any 'poor use' movements. Then the student is shown how to stop using any bad postural habits and taught the balanced and correct way to sit, stand, walk and change position.

UNITED KINGDOM
The Society of Teachers of the Alexander Technique
20 London House, 266 Fulham Road
London SW10 9EL

CANADA
The Canadian Society of Teachers of the Alexander Technique
PO Box 47025, Apt. 12
555 West 12th Avenue
Vancouver V5Z 3X0

AUSTRALIA
Australian Society of Teachers of the Alexander Technique
16 Princess Street, Kew
Victoria 3101
Tel. 1800 399 571

Alexander Technique International Inc.
11 Stanley Street, East Sydney
NSW 2010
Tel. (02) 9331 7563

NEW ZEALAND
Alexander Technique Association
29 Brandon Street, Wellington
Tel. (04) 473 5543

Glossary

Abductor a muscle that acts to move a bone away from the midline of the body.

Acute pain a sharp, intense stabbing sensation that is felt immediately, but dies away to be replaced by chronic pain.

Adductor a muscle that acts to move a bone towards the midline of the body.

Aerobic exercise, such as a brisk walk, that is fuelled by oxygen and the nutrients you eat.

Agonist a muscle that contracts to cause movement while an opposing muscle – an antagonist – relaxes.

Anaerobic exercise, such as playing squash, that is fuelled by the body's stores of food.

Antagonist a muscle that relaxes to allow an opposing agonist to contract and cause movement.

Anterior situated at the front of the body.

Articulate connect by a joint.

Brachial relating to the arm.

Bursa a hollow area in fibrous tissue, containing synovial fluid, that reduces friction between tendons and bones.

Carpal relating to the bones of the wrist.

Cartilage a substance that is hard yet flexible and, with bone, forms part of the skeleton. Cartilage lines the ends of long bones, and also forms the disc in each vertebral joint.

Chronic pain a dull, throbbing, nagging sensation that follows acute pain.

Clavicle collar bone.

Condyle rounded projection on a bone.

Dermatome an area that is supplied by a single spinal nerve.

Endorphin naturally occurring painkillers released in the brain.

Extensor a muscle that acts to increase the angle between the surfaces of the bones (straighten the joint).

Facet a flat area on a bone, forming an articular surface.

Fibrocartilage a mixture of fibrous tissue and cartilage that forms the intervertebral disc.

Fixators short muscles that hold the fulcrum of a joint still in order to allow a lever (a bone) to move.

Flexor a muscle that acts to decrease the angle between the surfaces of the bones (bending the joint).

Isometric describes a muscle contraction that does not result in movement of the body.

Isotonic describes muscle contraction or relaxation that results in movement of the body.

Lateral situated at the side of the body.

Ligament a strong band of fibrous tissue that links and binds together bones at a joint.

Medial situated at the middle of the body.

Meniscus a crescent-shaped piece of fibrocartilage, as found, for example, in the knee joint.

Metabolism the physical and chemical changes in the body that produce energy and repair and replace damaged tissues.

Metacarpal bones of the hand, connecting the wrist to the fingers.

Metatarsal bones of the foot, connecting the ankle to the toes.

Myofilaments the smallest constituent of a muscle fibre, which slide over each other as the muscle contracts and relaxes.

Glossary

Orthopaedic describes anything to do with skeletal and structural aspects of the body.

Osteophytes bony projections that develop inside a joint as a result of wear and tear, causing osteoarthritis.

Patella kneecap.

Periosteum the membrane surrounding a bone that contains blood vessels and nerves.

Phalanges bones of the fingers and toes.

Phasic muscles muscles that are used to perform specific actions, rather than just hold the body in position.

Posterior situated at the back of the body.

Postural muscles muscles that maintain posture against the force of gravity.

Sprain injury caused by overstretching a ligament.

Strain injury caused by overworking or overstretching a muscle or tendon.

Synergist a muscle that works with an agonist to improve the precision and accuracy of a movement.

Synovial joint an articulation between bones that is lubricated by synovial fluid within a joint capsule.

Tarsal relating to bones of the ankle.

Tendon a bundle of fibrous tissue that attaches the end of a muscle to a bone and is generally surrounded by a synovial sheath.

Trauma physical damage to the tissues.

Further reading

Brennan, Richard, *The Alexander Technique Manual.* London: Little, Brown and Company, 1996. Boston: Journey Editions, 1996. Sydney: Simon and Schuster, 1996.

Harrold, Fiona, *The Massage Manual.* London: Connections, 1997. New York: Sterling Publishing, 1992. Sydney: Simon and Schuster, 1992.

Hazeldine, R, *Fitness for Sport.* London: The Crowood Press, 1993.

Key, Sarah, *Body in Action.* London: Penguin Books and BBC Books, 1992. Sydney: Transworld, 1993.

Milroy, Patrick, *Sports Injuries.* London: Ward Lock, 1994.

Needham, Alix, *The Stress Management Kit.* London: Virgin, 1996. Boston: Journey Editions, 1996. Sydney: Simon and Schuster, 1996.

Rosser, Mo, *Body Fitness.* London: Hodder Headline, 1995.

Sutcliffe, Jenny, *Solving Back Problems.* London: Marshall Publishing, 1999.

Index

Page numbers in *italics* refer to illustrations

Acknowledgments

I would like to thank Nigel Perryman for his ruthless criticism of my grammar and urgings to 'get on with it'; Rupert Eckersley for his constructive assistance and advice on all medical matters, though I should make it clear that any errors are my responsibility rather than his; Robert MacDonald for his ability to be politely rude; and Sarah Bloxham, another member of The Red-headed League. Lastly my thanks to my five children and stepson, who all acted as guinea pigs for the exercises in this book and who nearly prevented the book being finished by being on holiday.

My thanks to Sophie Bevan, my editor, for her limitless patience and enduring cheerfulness even through the sticky patches when she must have been tearing her hair out with an author who moved house and has far too many children to make any book production a smooth process.

EDDISON • SADD EDITIONS
Project editors Zoë Hughes and Liz Wheeler
Editor Sophie Bevan
Indexer Dorothy Frame
Proofreader Slaney Begley
Art Director Elaine Partington
Designer Phil Kay
Illustrator Aziz Khan
Photographer Laura Wickenden
Models Sue Atu, Sarah King, Alan Orr and Emily Outred
Make-up Caterina Liasis
Production Karyn Claridge and Charles James

Eddison Sadd Editions would like to thank Stephen Marwood for the photographs on pages 9, 24 and 29, and BACK 2 of 28 Wigmore Street, London W1H 9DF, for the loan of equipment used on pages 25 and 71–73.